The Family Doctor

The Family Doctor

his life and history

SIR RONALD GIBSON
CBE, MA, DM, LLD, FRCS, FRCGP

Published in association with **Pulse**

London
GEORGE ALLEN & UNWIN
Boston   Sydney

First published in 1981

© Sir Ronald Gibson, 1981.
This book is copyright under the Berne Convention. No reproduction
without permission. All rights reserved.

**George Allen & Unwin (Publishers) Ltd,
40 Museum Street, London WC1A 1LU, UK**

George Allen & Unwin (Publishers) Ltd,
Park Lane, Hemel Hempstead, Herts HP2 4TE, UK

Allen & Unwin Inc.,
9 Winchester Terrace, Winchester, Mass 01890, USA

George Allen & Unwin Australia Pty Ltd,
8 Napier Street, North Sydney, NSW 2060, Australia

British Library Cataloguing in Publication Data

Gibson, *Sir* Ronald
 The family doctor: his life and history.
1. Family medicine – Great Britain – History
I. Title
 362.1'0425   R729.5.G4

ISBN 0–04–610017–2

Set in 11 on 12½ point Bembo by Alan Sutton Ltd., Gloucester
and printed in Great Britain
by Mackays of Chatham

*Dedicated to
my wife, Betty, and
daughters, Janet and Sally*

Foreword

It would give me pleasure to write a foreword for this book, even if I had not read it; such is my respect for its writer. As it turns out, the typescript has been hard to put down. There is in it a mixture of directness, warmth, variety and fresh enthusiasm which reminds me of 'satchels and shining morning faces'. Yet Ronald Gibson is a grandfather, with four decades of experience in clinical medicine and of involvement in the discussions and conflicts which have guided the development of medical care in this country.

I see this book as an autobiography of a life in two professions. It will appeal first to general practitioners who had shared one experience and watched the other with intimate concern. It offers an important source for future historians of medical institutions after the start of the National Health Service. Younger doctors training for general practice will find that the author had them especially in mind and that the book aims above all to protect and promote certain permanent values. They will find very useful the short account of how general practice developed historically within medicine.

The whole text is imbued with Ronald Gibson's unshakeable belief in the absolute necessity of family doctoring.

DR JOHN HORDER, CBE
President of the Royal College
of General Practitioners

Contents

List of Illustrations

Preface

I have written this book for various reasons: because I was a family doctor for forty years and thoroughly enjoyed the contented and fulfilling life it gave me; because I thought it would be a good idea to build a history of the last three turbulent decades on the foundation of general practice as it has evolved over the centuries; and because I would particularly like young students and newly qualified doctors to know all about the discipline they are contemplating as a career.

Many excellent books and articles have been written about the history of medicine. I have drawn gratefully on these for my own history, which is not intended to be comprehensive but sufficient to trace the development of the family doctor from his very early days to his entry into the 1948 National Health Service, throughout the years of which I have been able to follow him because of my own particular involvement in primary care. The references are as complete as I feel is necessary, but not so exhaustive as to distract the reader from the main narrative.

In the post-war chapters I have concentrated on developing evidence for my concept of a health service in the 1980s and a description of today's family doctor. I am conscious that this has meant a recapitulation of some of this evidence in chapter XII and the epilogue, but my story would have been incomplete and my conclusions invalid without it.

I have tried hard not to be biased. Most, if not all, of the opinions I express have developed from my own experience over the years and my confirmed and unshakeable belief in the existence of family doctoring as an absolute necessity in any health service, delivered by a fully comprehensive and integrated primary health care team with the total care of the whole patient as its objective. Anything less than this is, in my view, not tolerable.

I am deeply indebted to so many people that I am at risk

The Family Doctor

in failing to remember them all: to Mr Bernard Naylor, Librarian of the University of Southampton; Mr F. M. Sutherland, Librarian of the BMA's Nuffield Library; Miss Margaret Hammond, Librarian of the Royal College of General Practitioners and Mrs C. Dobson, Librarian of the Post-graduate Library of the Royal Hampshire County Hospital, Winchester; Miss Linda Beecham (staff editor) and Mrs Ann Shannon (indexer) of the British Medical Journal, for searching out material and references for me and for their tolerance with my persistent inquiries. My thanks are also due to Mr I. A. P. Dillow, press and public relations officer of Wessex Regional Health Authority, for his great help with the illustrations.

To Dr Douglas Whittet, CBE for making so many of his historical works available to me, for the support he has been to me in my writing, in searching for references, and for his sound advice; likewise Major Charles O'Leary, Clerk to the Worshipful Society of Apothecaries of London and Mr Tony Thistlewaite, chief press officer of the British Medical Association. All three have been tremendously helpful in providing me with illustrations.

To the Editors of *The Lancet* (Dr Ian Munro) and the *British Medical Journal* (Dr Stephen Lock), and the Honorary Editors of the *Proceedings of the Royal Society of Medicine* for generously giving me their permission to quote extensively from my articles on 'Introducing the Family Doctor' (1955), 'The Impact of Malignant Disease on the General Practitioner' (1964) and 'The Origin and Progress of Organised Medicine in Britain' (Anglo-American Conference, 1971).

Mr John Stevenson, past Group Editor of *Pulse* and *The Practitioner*, deserves and has my special thanks for having spurred me into writing the book which I had thought about and put off for so long, for distilling my ideas for me, reading the draft and final manuscript and assisting in bringing the book to the attention of the most important element of my audience – the medical profession itself.

It was in 1956 that Mr Phillip Unwin wrote to me about the possibility of a book on general practice. I started on this but failed to complete it for lack of time. I am doubly grate-

ful to Messrs Allen & Unwin for accepting this present book
a quarter of a century later, at the end of my career, and in
particular to Mr Peter Leek for the encouragement he has
given me throughout and to Janet Clayton for her editing.

I am indebted beyond words to my wife and daughters,
to Mrs Nancy Wansbrough and Mr Cuthbert Roberts,
FRCS for their generous help in reading and criticising the
book in its various drafts. Without their constructive
suggestions it would never have reached the publishers.

It is impossible for me to thank personally the many
general practitioners I have spoken to during the course of
my writing, and for several years before that. As always,
this band of individualists has produced many different
opinions. I have found this very useful for they have opened
up for me the wide panorama of family doctoring. Adding
them all together, they have given me a central core of
opinion which has underlined my own views on the nature
of family doctoring and how it should develop in the future.

Like many other people, I have been worried about
present day general practice and I have found the writing of
this book helpful, even soothing, in setting out over the
years the reasons why the family doctor of 1981 seems so
different from his predecessor in 1950 and how government,
doctors and patients should accept the new type of primary
physician and, working together, mould him successfully
into the pattern most of us want to see as our own personal
and family doctor.

Lastly, I must record my very sincere thanks and lasting
debt to my secretary, Mrs Mary Offord, whose patience,
sympathy and understanding would make her the perfect
family doctor, and to Dr John Horder for his kindness in
writing a Foreword to the book and also for allowing me to
reproduce his painting of the Royal College of General
Practitioners.

Prologue

The family doctor, 1950

Traditionally in Britain the doctor first consulted in an illness is known 'as a general practitioner. Occasionally he is called a primary physician or a doctor of the first instance.

The doctor responds to patients' calls either by treatment in the surgery or by visiting the home. He may be the only doctor involved in an illness or he may have to arrange for admission to hospital, taking over care again when the patient is back home.

It is likely that a GP will be a doctor to all the members of a family and will look after them throughout his practising years, being involved in many important events in their lives, including births, marriages and deaths. He becomes used to being asked for and giving advice with very little relation to health in the strict sense and is regarded as a counsellor and friend as well as a doctor. So he is known as a family doctor and, particularly in rural areas, is an ex officio member of the family.

This was and is the ideal. There has always been a place for such a person within society and never so much as now. Yet I would not pretend that such a desirable doctor-patient relationship exists throughout the country as a whole.

Indeed, one of the difficulties of writing about the family doctor is that he has to adapt his method of practice to suit the area in which he lives. This was brought home to me whenever I travelled round the country (as Chairman of the Council of the British Medical Association) talking to

1

doctors, seeing their places of work and chatting with patients.

Yet a family doctor's role is basically the same wherever he is. He may practise from a village hall or a sophisticated health centre, alone or in partnership with others. He may work in an intensely overpopulated city centre, being responsible for some 4,000 patients within walking distance of his practice; or he could have a very small list scattered over a wide area, involving daily journeys of a hundred miles or more.

In some parts of the country a GP can be treated by his patients as merely a one-off doctor for a single illness, a certificate, or a repeat prescription. His services as a family doctor are little used or ignored, whilst a mile or two away, at the other extreme, a colleague is being called on for crises only marginally medical, with his willingness to practise as a family oracle being over-used.

Between these extremes are the vast majority of GPs going about their daily round and enjoying undiluted family doctoring. At the outset, therefore, I should make it clear that I am aware of all these variants. In nearly all that I say I shall be talking of family doctoring in general, particularising only when I must.

If, in doing this, I seem to concentrate on the 'middle classes', this will only be because, after all, they are in the middle and in the majority. For my aim is to draw a picture of an average family doctor, practising the well-tried type of general practice built up by his forefathers, a type both recognisable to the majority of his patients and satisfying to himself.

I shall also try to show whether this particular kind of doctor has changed over the past decades, as his environment and his patients have changed, and whether he has been able to adapt to the awe-inspiring scientific and technological advances of the twentieth century without losing those qualities which make him a family doctor – qualities which have given him a place second to none in the affection and respect of his patients and, indeed, of society as a whole.

The family doctor, 1950

First I shall consider the family doctor as he appeared in the 1950s; then, in the epilogue, will look at him again in the 1980s, over a quarter of a century later, for it is important to know the man whose history we are relating. His or her image is, of course, coloured for each of us by our own experience, either as the patient of a particular GP or as a member of the patient's family. People tend to be kind to their doctor, perhaps on occasions too kind, and are much more likely to overlook his faults than to advertise them; patients are quick to extol his virtues and do not quickly forget them.

General practitioners become inured to being the centre of conversation. Medicine, indeed, is a sure-fire winner at any party when it comes to starting off a conversation and guaranteed to keep it going. Round and round the stories go, gathering ghastly and intimate details on their journey, yet building up to the $64,000 question: 'What did the doctor say?' It is of no great significance whether what he said was accurate or even relevant for, after all, medicine is an inexact science. The whole episode is enhanced medically, socially and environmentally if it be of sufficient importance to attract the attention of the family doctor.

Medicine is a highly emotive subject. So is the doctor, who is such an essential part of it. Once he qualifies he can never be a completely private person again. Whether at work or at play, he will be just that little bit different from other mortals – more so than practically any other member of society and even more so as a general practitioner than as a specialist. For the family doctor is expected to be part physician, part priest and part social worker, dealing with humanity when it is at its most sensitive and most fragile. This is equally true of the family doctor of 1950 or 1980 – indeed, of any age.

How can we describe the family doctor and characterise his work? I remember a film which (for me, at least) had a particularly dramatic beginning. It was early morning in a small American township, and the whole scene conveyed the peace and quiet of early spring morning in England. The paperboy was cycling along the pavement, throwing

3

the morning papers down the garden paths to end up against the front doors. There was no one else about to break the silence until a car came down the main street, the camera following it until a close-up revealed the identity of the occupant – the local doctor.

This short scene filled me with tremendous nostalgia. I felt a oneness with this celluloid doctor, recollecting the satisfaction of driving back in the early dawn after a night call; a comfortable sense of achievement entirely transcending the original upsurge of annoyance which had greeted the importunate telephone message an hour or two earlier.

I wondered what he had been up to – a complicated maternity case, a heart failure, even an appendix? Since calls in the night are usually about genuine emergencies, the odds are that it was one of those. His return home in the early morning in such a relaxed and contented mood suggested that his efforts had been successful. He and the milkman, the postman and the newspaper boy were members of that early morning fraternity who, for the moment, had the world to themselves and shared a somewhat exaggerated sense of superiority over their fellows still asleep.

I was sure he had left his house with that rather uncertain feeling which is always present on an urgent call. Was the emergency bag in the car? Was it fully equipped? When was the patient last seen, what was the condition then, will a transfusion or an anaesthetic be required? So many thoughts crisscross his mind as he drives that he is probably unaware of any detail of the journey.

On arrival at the scene he can expect, as often as not, a thankful greeting from the waiting family. It indicates confidence in his ability to deal with the crisis, but also warns that every detail of his performance will be keenly watched, criticised, and discussed for months to come.

From the first, he takes on the role of leading actor in the drama. No matter how worried he may be, or uncertain, he takes care that no sense of strain is allowed to reach the patient or family. Automatically the most sensible-looking person present is picked out to help him, and all the others are given jobs to occupy their minds and their hands while the crisis is on. Soon everyone is well–disciplined and under control, there is a feeling of confidence in the air, a cup of tea downstairs, and the doctor's car outside ready to proceed homewards.

On the other hand, of course, the GP can be regarded merely as the man a sick person consults first and whose job is to act as a sieve separating those who need referring to a hospital specialist from those who can be given an aspirin for a common cold, a soothing tonic for their nerves or a sleeping tablet for their insomnia.

Indeed, in 1950 this was the young house doctor's view of the GP, for he received from his teachers a constant indoc-trination against general practice and those who dabbled in it – a view that patently ignored the fact that general practice is a most stimulating, exciting and worthwhile occupation for any man or woman with a keen sense of dedication and a flair for hard work.

After qualification the new doctor, it is said, must immediately forget most of what he has learned about medicine, and start again. Although over 50 per cent of their pupils eventually go into general practice, medical schools, today as yesterday, still tend to concentrate on the diagnosis and treatment of obscure illnesses which a GP will be very lucky (or unlucky) to encounter in the course of a long career. Why this is so I have always failed to understand, and so have 99.9 per cent of my medical contemporaries.

One must not, however, make too much of this point, but the hospital and medical school environment as a whole is too refined and unrealistic to be of constant use to the potential GP. Once the hospital doors close behind him he has to start again as he moves from the academic to the practical.

In those days the young doctor could be said to have left medical school knowing nothing about general practice, unless he had a doctor in his immediate family. He carried with him an exalted sense of his own importance after having been a house doctor in hospital, surrounded by his senior and assistant physicians, the registrar, sister and nurses, pathologists, radiologists and pharmacists; and after

5

having been taught to deal peremptorily with phone calls from desperate GPs begging for a bed for a patient in need.

In the 1950s, the young doctor suddenly found himself in another unexpectedly specialised world as a tyro and, in consequence, often displayed an ignorance that would have brought a blush to the cheek of a schoolboy. In those days (as now) a student after qualification might first become the junior member of a specialised hospital team, a sort of professional closed shop, which operated on a stage with a heavy curtain between it and the medical world outside.

Yet the day was bound to come when this part-of-a-doctor was cast into outer light – alone for the first time. If he was methodical-minded he would have brought a book of 'favourite prescriptions' with him, which was as well because up until then it is doubtful whether he would have been taught how to write a prescription. With any luck, he would also be equipped with some knowledge of human nature gleaned from six years of undergraduate existence.

In no time at all he would be cut down to size. The difficulty was that the cutting down had to take place without his patients knowing, for in their eyes he was already a doctor, already overwise for his age and already capable of dealing with any of their difficulties – from advising them about their unmarried sister's prognosticated, though unwelcome, pregnancy to rescuing them from the very jaws of death itself. Thousands of individuals entrusted themselves to such a man each day. During our travels through history we shall see what unremitting and unrelenting efforts have been made to improve their chances of survival and his fitness for such responsibility.

As for the patient, he was usually less apprehensive than the new doctor, for he would probably have gleaned some knowledge of his illness and its possible treatment from the young man's predecessor and could tactfully pass this on with some hope of achieving continuity. He might, of course, have to combat the new boy's traditional reaction of mistrusting anyone's diagnosis but his own, and of automatically cancelling treatment of proven value because he had not first thought of it himself.

However, it was surprising how little the book of favourite prescriptions in the top drawer of his desk came to matter. He soon learned that he himself was the prescription his patient most enjoyed taking and from which both could achieve the greatest benefit. Nor was it long before he had forgotten the confined hospital stage and was enjoying the vast and fascinating vista of family doctoring.

In short, in the 1950s it took very little time to convert a newly qualified and inexperienced doctor into a comparatively knowledgeable and efficient family physician, wise beyond his years. He soon became capable of dealing with any type of patient, any emergency and any unpredictable situation, yet deep down the uncertainty and the excitement never left him. Each day brought a new adventure, each patient a new problem, each birth a new triumph and each patient lost a new heartbreak. He had to be a self-taught GP, learning his job by trial and error and trying to do as little damage as possible in the meantime.

It is no wonder that this particular type of doctor, as he existed then, is difficult to describe. I remember, in the summer of 1954 when on holiday, standing on a ferry waiting for the cars to embark. One middle-aged man drove on in a rather dated, open two-seater. There was a BMA badge perched on the front of the car and a half-closed blood pressure machine thrown on the back seat, but I did not need either to tell me that he was a family doctor. (He was to become a good friend of mine, the late Dr R.M.S. McConaghey, first honorary editor of the *Journal of the Royal College of General Practitioners*. He was everything I thought he was when, then unknown to me, I saw him in his car on the ferry.)

He looked very comfortable and placid, sitting there smoking his pipe; I decided that I would have no hesitation in trusting my life to him, even though I did not know his name. Most people seemed to know him and to offer him some sort of greeting. One old lady even leaned on the car and started chatting; I reckoned I could have repeated the conversation word for word. I doubt if there had been any crisis in her family for three generations which he had not

7

shared. From the way she spoke to him you could see that he was not just her doctor, he was her *family* doctor, an old friend and an honorary and ex officio member of her family.

By the time we reached the other side of the river I had decided that he was a very good doctor, and I did not care which end of the stethoscope he put into his ears. He stood out on that ferry for the very reason that he was a family doctor; his BMA badge and his blood pressure machine were as nothing, they need not have been there.

When we come to 1980, we shall see what the years have done to this doctor, We must hope that time will have done nothing to change the innate, basic qualities we can discern from our so-far incomplete picture of him. Already we have seen that the man who goes into family doctoring confident that he is going to make a success of it just because he knows a textbook of medicine off by heart – how to give a blood transfusion or deal with a complicated maternity case – is going to flop from his first day in general practice. This was so in 1950 and should still be so today.

The attributes which go to make a family doctor do not appear in any textbook. In 1950 these were rarely if ever included in the undergraduate's medical curriculum and barely relevant to a book of favourite prescriptions. Preferably they were inborn but they could be acquired through long experience. In either case they were reflected in the face of the man sitting in his car on a sultry summer's afternoon when his luckier colleagues were on holiday. It will be unfortunate if history is found to have changed this man as we have so far described him. For he was such a man long before 1950 and, for his patients' sake, should remain so for as long as general practice is recognisable as a separate and highly specialised branch of medicine.

It is fair to ask why hospitals for so long failed to impress students with the fundamental attributes required by the man or woman proposing to enter general practice, and why most medical textbooks ignored the special training required for this branch of the profession, because there were those who chose to spend a lifetime working in it and there were, above all, some 55 million people who expected to have their own family doctor. So, in theory we should expect some good news by the time we reach 1981 both in the development of teaching in general practice and in the type of material produced to form the up-to-date model of a family doctor. Whether or not this expectation has been fulfilled is one of the more important questions which I shall attempt to answer.

There was some excuse for the lack of preparation of students and young doctors for general practice while at medical school. Unless teachers and authors had themselves experienced general practice, they would be unaware of the need to talk or write about the fundamental qualities required by the potential GP. Equally, they would be ignorant of the fact that a man responsible for primary care in the community required at least as much education as the specialist in his more limited field. They were right in assuming that basic education was necessary for both GP and specialist. They were desperately and dangerously wrong in taking the line that the GP could safely be left to learn the rest of his job on his own.

The three great qualities of a GP of any century are compassion, sympathy and understanding: the ability to feel at one with a patient in an illness and to show him that, once having consulted his GP, he is no longer alone in his struggle. And the patient has not only to know this but to feel happy and more secure as a result. These properties form the foundation upon which *all* treatment, or care, in general practice is built.

As the years go by a GP encounters more and more human problems. His tolerance grows and his compassion is intensified. Unspoken words, conveyed by a worried look, can tell an eloquent story. They tell, for instance, of the nagging mother-in-law living on the premises or an inability to cope with the housekeeping; of the fences to hide poverty or unhappiness from neighbours; or of the deaths and separations in the family, mixed up with happy things, such as births and weddings and achievements of the younger generation. All of these appear in the GP's consulting room sooner or later, wrapped in some obscure disguise or another.

9

The other all-important qualities needed are faith, hope and affection. Let me offer an example: patients generally expect to leave the GP's consulting room with a prescription or at least some positive advice. If this does not happen the consultation can be regarded as highly unsatisfactory. Yet this is not enough in itself, for it is vitally necessary that the patient should be told why a certain medicine has been pre-scribed and what symptoms it is intended to cure. Without such information a patient may well return to the doctor with the wrong symptoms cured. This is embarrassing for the doctor, unless he realises that the faith and hope he has instilled into his patient are of such a degree that he is actually being complimented! The patient is on the doctor's side and wants the treatment to succeed, he knows that it ought to succeed and so, hopefully, faithfully and affection-ately he presents the wrong success to the doctor next time they meet. Such is life in its reality, unsuitable for the pigeonhole or the perfectionist.

Again, the consultant in hospital relies much on the build-up the GP gives him. 'You'll find him a bit abrupt, Mrs Jones, but don't mind him. He's incredibly clever, knows your sort of case inside out and I would certainly go to him myself.' Mrs Jones carries with her the GP's sympathy and understanding and passes on her faith and hope to the con-sultant. She is delighted to share the GP's confidence in this particular specialist and would positively hate him not to be abrupt. His very abruptness becomes part of the treatment she expects from him. The hospital doctor has to recognise, too, that in the absence of the GP with his knowledge of the patient, the patient might never have appeared at the hos-pital at all.

I hope I have said enough to show why it is difficult to teach general practice, and why in the past virtually no attempt was made at vocational training.

Since my retirement, from time to time frustrated former patients have regretfully complained to me that they cannot get on with their new doctor: 'He doesn't seem to under-stand me.' The answer is simple, and acceptable: 'I have known you for thirty years, he has known you for a few months. For heaven's sake, give him a chance.' But what does 'knowing you' matter unless it is a part of the whole spectrum of family medicine? For this reason alone general practice has, in fact, always been a specialty.

A preliminary skirmish with disease at home had enormous advantages in the short and long term. In the short term it gave both patient and doctor time to get to know each other, for preliminary investigations by the X-ray and pathology departments, and even for a visit to the home by a hospital specialist. The patient thus had a chance to get used to the idea of going into hospital. In the long term, a successful battle fought at home by doctor and patient against disease could bind both together for the rest of recorded time, while an unhappy outcome created a special relationship between family and doctor.

In the past doctors perhaps had more time to sit and talk and examine, although in those days there was a tendency to regard this as more necessary for the upper and middle classes. Yet if a GP has so little time for each patient that even the preliminary physical examination has to be curtailed or omitted, then the population is being badly served.

Lastly, I have already mentioned that medicine is an all-consuming profession. I can illustrate this best by a GP's walk along the platform of his local station. This can resemble a surgery. Do the waiting people tackle their solicitor, butcher or greengrocer about their daily problems and needs? Watch what happens to the GP. It can take him fifteen minutes to reach the end of the platform from the ticket office – and he must make for the end of the platform, or risk being mobbed.

Smiles of pleased recognition greet him yard by yard. He is approached to be told how successful, or unsuccessful, his last treatment was. He is given a list of symptoms and asked whether they merit a more official consultation. He is required to take a note of some 'more of the same' and to remember to ring the chemist with a prescription on his return to the surgery. He is expected to recognise a face and put a label to it even though he has not seen it for five years or more, to remember the names of children and the date of

11

arrival of the last grandchild, and he must be ready with relevant questions and satisfying answers to suit all occasions and all comers.

Even when the train arrives and he sinks into his seat he must watch out in case he sits next to an avid patient who has the whole length of the journey in which to concentrate attention on his ailments and would regard it as wasted time if he let the subject drop before the train reached its destination.

The same applies to the cocktail, lunch or dinner party. Host, hostess and guests alike will snatch some of the doctor's time to concentrate on their real or imaginary symptoms. Indeed, the reason for inviting him may not be for the pleasure of his company but the need for his out-of-hours advice. The interval between the acts in a theatre is God's gift to the professional GP lapel-clinger, and a GP soon learns not to go shopping in his native environment, for even buying a toothbrush can turn into a very lengthy expedition.

Yet should anything be done about it? It all adds up to an acknowledgement that the GP is a rather special person who needs a vast fund of patience and dedication. He would, in fact, have every reason to worry if he were not always being pestered when off duty. Hospital doctors are comparatively unknown outside their place of work and are regarded with especial reverence and awe, so are much less approachable in a social environment. They are, in short, protected by the GP.

I have tried in this prologue to give a picture of the GP as he was in the middle of the twentieth century, inevitably including some characteristics which he shares with his counterpart a quarter of a century later.

No one could expect the National Health Service to produce a perfect doctor, but with all the millions of pounds spent on health and welfare since those early days there is at least a right to expect a better service given by men and women of equal dedication who have been specifically trained as family doctors. Whether this comparison is to the benefit or shame of the National Health Service we shall see. Meanwhile, the intervening chapters will reveal exactly how the role of the GP has altered and the reasons for that change.

I

The early years

In the 1955 Linacre Lecture, delivered at St John's College, Cambridge, Sir Harold Himsworth said,

> Professions arise in response to the recognition of a social need, and their continued existence is dependent on their success in satisfying the expectations raised by the state of knowledge which they profess.[1]

This backs up a petition presented to the Parliament of King Henry V of England:

> A man hath three things to govern, that is to say, soul, body and worldly goods, the which ought and should be revealed by three sciences, which are divinity, physics and law.[2]

The doctor's role has, therefore, always been to care for man's body as part of a total social need.

There was no organisation to the beginning of the medical profession; it developed from a union of medicine, religion and superstition. In the days of ancient Britons medicine was practised by Druids, being largely tinctured with theology, astrology, magic and divination.

In Anglo-Saxon times the equivalent of what we would call medical practice was in the hands of leeches, who performed the functions of physicians, surgeons and apothe-

15

caries; wise women and the purveyors of magical incantations. Leech was an Anglo-Saxon term for healer and leeches were outstanding for their skill in the healing art. Such knowledge as they had was handed down by word of mouth for it was not until the early seventh century that the Anglo-Saxons took to keeping written records.

There were too few leeches for all needs and King Magnus the Good, after a victory in battle, 'Went to such men as seemed good to him, and felt their hands, then named he twelve men who had the softest hands, and told them to bind up the wounds of men, and yet none of them had bound up a wound before, but all these became the greatest of leeches.'[3] Most remedies were herbal mixtures but there is evidence of rudimentary surgery, such as removing arrowheads and splinting fractures.

Then came a period of monastic medicine during which there grew a cult of faith healing, an implicit trust in the miraculous powers of saints and holy relics. Men of piety, through their innate goodness, gave a sense of well-being to all with whom they came in contact. The church attributed diseases to devils, whereas common people thought them due to elves. The church met this difficulty by christianising pagan prescriptions through the simple expedient of adding a few words of church Latin to them.[4]

Throughout the Middle Ages monasteries provided a refuge for the sick and infirm. The monk who treated the poor in his infirmary is recognisable as a general practitioner and a very important person, for his duties were based on instructions from St Benedict who, in the early sixth century, required that the care of the sick – and notice the word 'care' and not just treatment – should be placed before and above every other duty as if Christ himself were being directly served by waiting upon them.

Cassiodorus (AD 490–585) reinforced St Benedict by instructing monks to 'learn the properties of herbs and the blending of drugs, but set all your hope upon the Lord, who preserves life without end.'[5] He also detailed particular rules for those caring for the sick. They were to be 'sad with others' suffering, sorrowful over others' dangers and

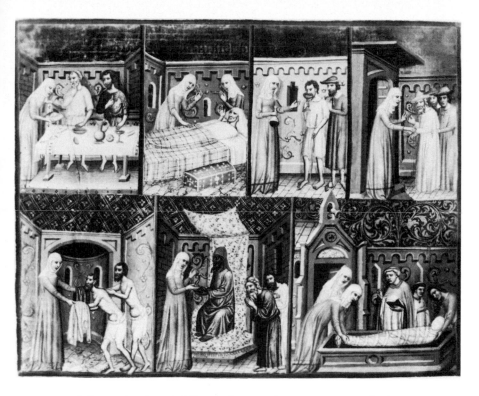

1 Scenes in a hospital from a fourteenth century manuscript in the Bibliothèque Nationale, Paris *(Mansell Collection)*

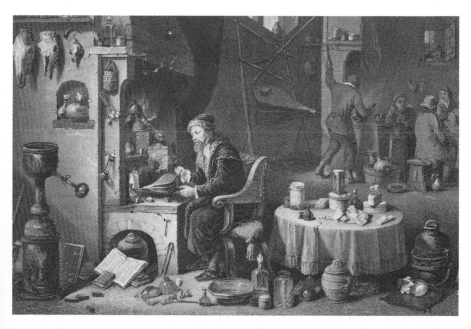

2 A medieval apothecary *(Society of Apothecaries)*

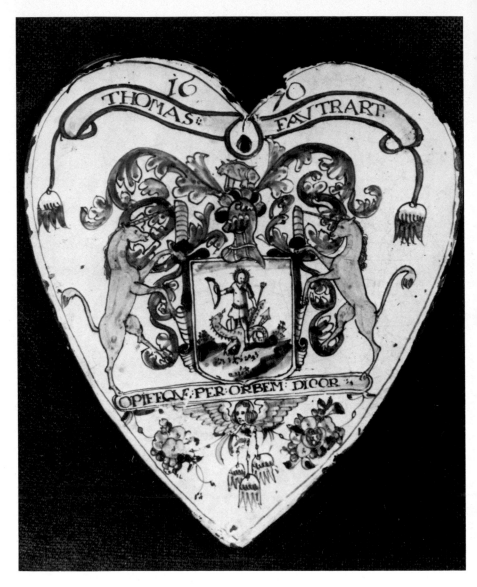

3 Blue delftware 'pill tile' bearing the arms of the Apothecaries'
Company and the name of Thomas Fautrart, believed to be an
apothecary of Huguenot descent, 1670 (*Pharmaceutical Society of
Great Britain*)

sympathetic to the griefs of those whom they care for and always zealously to help others' misfortunes.' This envisages the total care of the whole person, the role of the general practitioner.

Sir Arthur Bryant, in *The Mediaeval Foundation*, remarks that in the twelfth century the famous London hospitals, St Bartholomew's and St Thomas's, were established by Augustinian canons and that the Franciscans also made a cult of lazar houses, often establishing their friaries beside them. They were 'Enthusiastic practitioners of medicine – a science recently revived by contact with the Moorish and Jewish scholars of southern Spain – and administered it free to the poor among whom they worked.'[6]

Then came doubts: the seeking of fees to the detriment of other duties, the sight of many aspects of sickness which might offend modesty, and the possibility of being the cause of a patient's death, came to seem somewhat inconsistent with the original intention of holy orders. Monks were forbidden, by the Lateran Councils of 1139 and 1163, to practise usury in any form or to go out of their monasteries to study medicine or civil law, because such occupations might make them avaricious of worldly gain. Many new hospitals and asylums had been founded in addition to the monastic infirmaries, requiring the help of monks who had thus come to concentrate on medicine to the detriment of their other work.

So, with the enforcement of papal decrees and exhortations, notably those issued between 1131 and 1234 urging monks to leave outside interests alone, the practice of medicine and surgery was gradually transferred to the laity. It therefore became necessary to raise the status of the art of healing the sick, and this was done by improved medical legislation; by the foundation of the great medical universities, notably Salerno which was ecclesiastical; and by the foundation of gilds amongst the physicians themselves.

Medical ethics and etiquette were regulated in detail by stereotyped rules. The Salernitan treatises are interesting, even rather amusing. The physician is instructed to approach the bedside with the same 'humble mien and wall-eyed expression' which we find in so many paintings by the old masters. His remarks at table were to be 'punctuated by continued enquiries about the patient's condition, which he should always regard as grave, in order that a fatal or a favourable termination might redound to his credit as a wonder-making therapeutist or a shrewd prognostician.' Illusory treatment by harmless remedies was permissible (and, incidentally, still is today), since otherwise the patient's mind might be ruffled by not getting his money's worth, while a 'normal recovery by the healing powers of nature might injure the physician's therapeutic reputation.' (The prescription which marks the closure of today's consultation between doctor and patient obviously stems from earlier traditions.) A later authority suggested that if a convalescent showed signs of ingratitude in the matter of payment he might be 'temporarily sickened by some harmless drug'.

In England under the Normans the trade in drugs and spices was handled by mercers (merchants). In the latter part of the twelfth century the trade passed to the pepperers and spicers who were already an organised body known as a 'gild'. The pepperers were wholesalers and the spicers retailers, but the same person, for example Adam de Carlill in the reign of Edward III, could be called spicer, apothecary and grocer.

In 1338 the Gild of Pepperers went bankrupt. Later in 1345 they joined up with the Spicers and in 1373 the gild changed its name to the Grocers' Company of which the apothecaries formed a section, until they seceded in 1617.[7]

From about the time of Henry VIII (1507–47) there was a persistent struggle between physicians and apothecaries – the argument being basically whether apothecaries could prescribe for and treat patients as well as dispense medicine and drugs. At the other end of the scale apothecaries resented their association with grocers.[8]

During this reign, too, four major Acts were passed designed to regulate those who practised physic and surgery and to bring together the various types of practitioners. In 1512, in an attempt to eliminate 'ignorant persons', it was required that candidates should first be examined by a panel of expert physicians and surgeons and then licensed by the bishop of the diocese before being allowed to practise. By this Act, and for the first time, a number of practitioners who were neither university graduates nor members of a gild were brought within the legislative fold. This was to have a profound influence on the medical profession in Britain.

In 1518 an Act was passed confirming the foundation of a College of Physicians. This was a confusing and ill-considered Act. It seemed in conflict with its predecessor of 1512 for it said that no one could practise anywhere in the kingdom unless first examined by the president of the college and three of the elects. Clearly, these conditions could not be enforced and the licensing of practitioners in London and throughout the country continued to be carried out more by the church than the college.

There were by this time numbers of 'medical practitioners' scattered about the country in towns and villages. They were described as 'true students of human nature' and un-doubtedly some were unlicensed and practising with the knowledge of church, college and their patients in spite of possible legal action to prevent them.

Then came the Act of 1540, establishing the power of physicians over surgeons, the latter being considered as 'minding only their own lucre', and over apothecaries (who came from the lower orders).

Finally, in this busy reign, came an Act in 1542 which was, in effect, an amendment to the one of 1512, for it exempted from the penalties of unlicensed practice 'divers honest persons, as well men as women, whom God hath endowed with the knowledge of nature, kind and operation of certain herbs, roots and waters, and the using and ministering of them to such as has pain with customable disease'.[9] This could be said to let the quacks in again and no doubt it did but, in fact, it was accepting the existence of the good and much-loved 'true students of human nature'.

Midwifery was in the hands of midwives and local wise women. The bishop licensed the midwives who had to be of high moral character and skilled in their art. The destination of the infant's soul was more important than the preservation of the life and health of mother and child.[10]

The first major milestone in the history of the apothecaries came in 1614 when Gideon de Laune – apothecary to Anne of Denmark, queen of James I – obtained a charter separating the apothecaries from the grocers, and so was born the Worshipful Society of Apothecaries of London, which held its first meeting on 16 December 1617.[11] [12]

The apothecaries' proper occupation was the preparation and compounding of drugs according to the prescriptions of physicians and surgeons, but to these were soon to be added all the functions of the general practitioner. James I granted his charter 'to enable them to make up the physicians' prescriptions with greater nicety and accuracy'. What is more, he gave a sharp retort to the grocers when they protested! Apothecaries now had control of pharmacy in the City of London and within seven miles of the City, and thus it remained for two hundred years until an Apothecaries Act (1815) extended their powers to cover the whole of England and Wales.

The written word, by now, was playing an increasing part in teaching. One of the most helpful books for the general practitioner (i.e. the apothecary) was the *Boke of Chyldren*, published by Thomas Phayre in 1545.[13] It was the GP's guide to paediatrics and instructed in such troublesome conditions as 'terryble dreams, colyke and rumbling in the guttes, bedwetting, goggle eyes and of falling of the fundament'. Some of its advice is sound today.

The Society of Apothecaries gradually became pre-eminent in the training and licensing of apothecaries and it had completely displaced the barber-surgeons by the second half of the eighteenth century. Moreover, from the time of Paracelsus (1493–1541) their herbal remedies were augmented by various chemicals and their knowledge of these new and powerful remedies allowed them to depose the dispensers, who had to remain content with herbs.[14]

It was the Great Plague of London in 1665 which really set the apothecaries on their journey to becoming general practitioners. Physicians died, fled from the city, or were too overworked to cope with the number of patients; so apothecaries, by popular demand, left their shops to come to the patient's bedside. One apothecary, William Boghurst, wrote the best treatise on the plague at the time while another, Francis Barnard, remained at his post in St Bartholomew's Hospital when the physicians fled. He was eventually appointed a physician.[15]

Some idea of the growth of ill-feeling between apothecaries and physicians can be gained from a case that the physicians brought in 1703 against a London apothecary, William Rose, for treating a patient without supervision. Rose lost the case but subsequently obtained a reversal of the verdict from the House of Lords. From then on, apothecaries practised medicine and surgery quite openly.[16] [17]

The Rose case enabled them to come to the bedside and to give advice. They were, however, not allowed to charge fees for this advice; another century was to pass before this privilege was granted to them. So they gave free advice and charged for the medicine. On the other hand, physicians charged for their advice and then set up dispensaries to give medicine free to their poorer patients. In the latter part of the eighteenth century apothecaries were so taken up with practising medicine that chemists and druggists increasingly took over their pharmaceutical practice.

The apothecaries resisted this trend. They wanted the best of both worlds for, having vanquished the grocers, put the physicians in their place and encroached on the surgeons (numbers of them being licensed to practise surgery), they now turned on the pharmacists and formed a General Pharmaceutical Association of Great Britain.[18] Nothing came of its original terms of reference, however, so that by 1803 chemists and druggists had almost completely supplanted apothecaries as practitioners of pharmacy – although the latter continued to supply medicine direct to their patients (almost unique to this country). In those days too, and to some extent still existing up until the present time – which is as well from the point of view of easing the burden on the GP – patients consulted their pharmacists about their minor complaints.

It is interesting to follow the care of the poor over the centuries, because it was recognised only very slowly that the sick poor required treating. In the Middle Ages they depended to an extent on the religious foundations scattered throughout the country, usually either in or near the larger towns or in isolated places. Before the Reformation the lady of the manor (often skilled in compounding medicines), the village priest, parish clerk, poor wise women or wandering mountebanks and charlatans were their main sources of help.

In the fourteenth century barbers and barber-surgeons began to come into prominence in the boroughs and larger villages (and the emphasis on surgery is notable). In the larger towns they were formed into gilds. In the villages we know that the unqualified practitioners worked and continued to do so in spite of regulations in the sixteenth and seventeenth centuries designed to eliminate them.

In 1536 came an Act which encouraged local authorities to receive the poor 'most charitably' and to succour and help the sick poor. After this, some sort of medical and nursing care seems to have been provided, usually by handy or wise women. It was unusual for medical men to be employed by local authorities to treat paupers and as late as the turn of the eighteenth century the poor were not officially treated by recognised physicians. For example, there is no mention of the licensing of apothecaries in the diocese of Exeter until 1748 and there are only four entries for apothecary-surgeon and eight for apothecary-surgeon/man-midwife (Buckfastleigh and Plympton Morris). Although there is a record of a learned physician engaged by the mayor and corporation in 1629 'to be resident in the town of Barnstaple and give gratis to the poor at £20 per annum', it was not until the end of the eighteenth century that a parish doctor became a more usual feature of the parish economy.[19]

Physicians (often with degrees from Oxford or Cambridge) looked after the wealthier classes and were appointed to work in the hospitals, giving their services free to the poor. Doctors in olden times had two methods of getting about – walking or riding on horseback. There may have been carriage roads in some parts of the country but patients did not necessarily live on high roads and much time could be saved by riding across country. North country doctors could take a week to get round their patients, sleeping each night 'wherever darkness caught them'. Physicians would stay in the houses of their sick patients or put them up in their own houses.

In the eighteenth century, the age of the elegant physician, the physician came into his wards 'accompanied by the apothecary [equivalent to the hospital junior medical staff of today] and sat down in an armchair at the head of the table. The apothecary sat on one side and on the other side the sister of the ward. The patients who could sit up sat on benches on each side of the table, and moved to the physician's right, so that he saw each in turn and prescribed and the apothecary took down the prescriptions. The matron held a towel, and after seeing each patient the physician washed his mouth with water into a bucket and rubbed his hands with a towel.'

The duties of the hospital apothecary were many and varied. Indeed he was responsible for casualties, admissions and discharges, ensuring that the treatment ordered by the physicians and surgeons was carried out; doing morning and evening rounds of the wards to check that patients were properly attended to; never absenting himself from duty without arranging for a proper person to take his place; and doing all the dispensing. Since he was forbidden any private practice, he must have been quite a man. In Cambridge in 1767, for example, the only resident staff was the apothecary who had to be permanently on duty and was paid £25 a year, plus a £5 bonus.[20]

The only hospital in most towns was the infirmary adjoining the workhouses. Students were attached to practitioners in the town or to physicians and surgeons working in the infirmary.[21] Throughout the eighteenth century voluntary general hospitals were being established as charitable institutes for the sick poor, not for the middle classes. Home care for those who could afford it continued until the early twentieth century, by which time hospitals were becoming more and more 'hygienic' and thus available to and suitable for the middle classes. In the voluntary hospitals, physicians and surgeons gave their services free of charge. Yet still one could say that medical science in England concentrated on the disease rather than on the patient. As Rosemary Stevens says:

> The eighteenth-century physician . . . was able to collect his symptoms and analyse them from the conveniently increasing number of indigent patients found in hospital wards. Hospital beds thus rapidly became valuable vehicles for individual observation and for teaching apprentices, and access to beds by physicians and surgeons was at a premium. The social structure of the medical profession had already ensured a small élite of consultants attached to voluntary hospitals. The new medicine gave this élite a technological reason for limiting their number.[22]

Indeed by now medicine itself was making swift advances. To quote G. M. Trevelyan in his *English Social History:*

> An even greater check on the death rate was the advance in medicine. Throughout the eighteenth century the medical profession was moving out of the dark ages of sciolism and traditional superstition into the light of science. The physician, the surgeon, the apothecary and the unlicensed practitioner were all going forward apace in knowledge and in devoted service, especially to the poor, who had hitherto been horribly neglected. Science and philanthropy were the best part of the spirit of the 'age of enlightenment' and this spirit inspired the better medical training and practice of individuals.[23]

2

The nineteenth century

By 1800 the population of the British Isles had increased to about nine million, two million more than in the middle of the eighteenth century. The majority of the people lived in towns which were small by our reckoning. London, for example, had a population of only 800,000.

The coming of the Industrial Revolution, and factory owners' demands for labour on the spot, caught the authorities unawares. There was no town planning and London was the only city with any sanitary system at all. Lines of back-to-back houses and miserable tenements sprang up here, there and everywhere without restraint or design. Too many people were crammed into too small a space.

It is not surprising, therefore, that there were recurrent epidemics of enteric and typhoid fevers, joined by Asiatic cholera in 1832 and 1848. Malnutrition, scurvy, rickets, tuberculosis, smallpox, diphtheria, venereal disease and, no doubt, alcoholism were the doctors' main enemies. It is difficult to understand the comment that the increasing population was more likely to be due to improvements in hygiene and housing than to larger-sized families or advances in medical knowledge; even though those who came to the towns earned higher wages which led to higher standards of living and of education.[1]

25

One major influence on nineteenth-century medicine was the deep division between the doctors of the urban and rural areas and the differing standards of care available to them – a division accentuated by slow and poor communications. There were, therefore, contrasting outlooks and problems which resulted in the activities of national medical associations being more and more challenged by the provincial associations. E. S. Turner says that:

> In 1800, anyone could call himself a doctor, even if he had done little more than devil behind the apothecary's counter for a few months. Anybody could cut off anybody's leg without legal penalty. Within the British Isles were nearly a score of authorities, including the Archbishop of Canterbury, with powers to licence practitioners in physics and surgery, but any amateur was at liberty to thumb his nose at them and put up his own brass plate, red lamp or mortar and pestle. Many a surgeon-apothecary or general practitioner looked on diplomas as mere pedantry.[2]

The unlikely spark lighting the flame of reform turned out to be an exorbitant duty on glass imposed by the government in 1812. Two developments resulted: a surgeon-apothecary, William Pilkington, founded his own glassworks to ensure a reasonable supply of glass at reasonable cost, and a society called the Associated Apothecaries and Surgeon-Apothecaries of England and Wales was founded.[3] The glassworks still exists. The Association stimulated the government to approve the Apothecaries Act of 1815.

Until this time there had been little control over medical practice. Thanks to the narrow and short-sighted policy of the two Royal Colleges, a most important part of it had been left to a trading gild, the Society of Apothecaries. The colleges were bypassed and the universities ignored in favour of a society of shopkeepers.

Undoubtedly, therefore, the Apothecaries Act of 1815 is the most important landmark in the history of general practice. It created a 'body of qualified practitioners who were entirely independent of the Colleges of Physicians and Surgeons and were entitled to practice medicine not merely by sufferance, but by law.'[4] In other words, the Society of Apothecaries had *de jure* if not *de facto* control of general practice, at least where it was conducted by people calling themselves apothecaries.[5]

The Society, by this Act, was also enabled to undertake the examination and licensing of general practitioners and to appoint a court of examiners. No one was allowed to practise as an apothecary in England and Wales unless duly examined and in receipt of a certificate of examination. However, cutting out the Royal Colleges from a share in the control of education was a retrograde step.

After 1815, then, the standard of qualification became Member of the Royal College of Surgeons (MRCS), which was confirmed after an hour's examination in anatomy and surgery, and Licentiate of the Society of Apothecaries (LSA). Many practised on the strength of a single qualification, the LSA.

Candidates for an LSA had to serve an apprenticeship of not less than five years and to produce a certificate of attendance for at least six months in the medical practice of some public hospital or dispensary. They were examined in Latin, pharmaceutical chemistry, materia medica and in the theory and practice of medicine and surgery, but not of midwifery. In 1816 physiology and botany were added to the curriculum and in 1827 the Society demanded evidence of training in midwifery too.

In 1829 it was at last permitted that an apothecary might claim remuneration either for his medicine or his skills; but it was not until 1838 that the right to claim for both medicine and advice was confirmed by a judgement of Mr Justice Littledale.[6]

Before that case, in 1830, Mr James Handey, a surgeon-apothecary, brought an action against a patient for fees due in relation to medicine and attendance. He won his case. Thomas Wakley, that most renowned of medical editors, who later became an MP, said in *The Lancet*:

27

General Practitioners will no longer be regarded in families as plunderers, whose interested object is to convert the stomachs of their patients into drug shops, but will now be looked upon as men of experience and skill, and their ability to prescribe appropriate remedies for diseases will be valued rather more highly than the ability to mix those remedies in a bottle, or in a mortar.[7]

The *London Medical Gazette* of the same year summed it up by saying that general practitioners existed because the body of society had raised them up. The pure practitioners of surgery or of obstetrics, it said, could exist only in populous cities, and whilst the physician might earn his bread in the country, there was room for only one physician where there might be twenty general practitioners.[8]

Thus apothecaries, who had come to the bedside in that other momentous year in their history, 1665, progressed through the stages of being allowed to charge fees for medicine to fees for advice. They became known, after 1823, as general practitioners.

There remained an argument over the term 'general practitioner'. *The Lancet*, in particular, continued to have doubts about it. In the edition of 19 June 1830 a stinging editorial said,

If the regularly educated member of a College of Surgeons be equal, in point of learning and skill, to the man who has purchased an Aberdeen diploma for 15 or 20 pounds, why is the former to be stigmatised by the title of 'General Practitioner' while the latter is dignified by that of 'Doctor'?

This was followed on 17 July by a comment that it was a curious way of increasing respectability to descend from the title of surgeon to that of general practitioner. The reply was that 'man may degrade a title but the title cannot degrade a man', but this failed to quell the opposition and the next contribution was even more vitriolic: ' "Men of all work" would not be a bit more absurd or irrational. A more clumsy, a more vulgar, or a more inapplicable expression could not be found.'⁹

Personally I have always disliked the term 'general practitioner'. It does not seem to mean more than that one is a doctor who generally practises. 'Family doctor' has my vote.

An arrangement for medical care can now clearly be seen emerging, with apothecaries as the nearest to general practitioners, but they could also be pharmacists and might be surgeons. The surgeons might also be part general practitioners or work with apothecaries. So there was still some clearing up to be done.

However, a decision which was to have a profound effect on the origin of general practice as a discipline in its own right, with all that follows from this, was now made after much debate and many arguments. It is difficult to understand how such a misjudgement could have been made when, up until this point the main activity had been in creating a doctor who was to be called a 'general practitioner'. It all seems to have started in 1844. Sir James Graham, who was the Home Secretary, followed up three abortive Bills in 1840, 1841 and 1842 with one which was drafted 'for the Better Regulation of the Medical Profession throughout the United Kingdom'.

In that same year, on 7 December, the National Association of General Practitioners in Medicine, Surgery and Midwifery was instituted. A memorial was presented to Sir James, the last sentence of which said that it would prove to 'the best interests of the public generally and most conducive to the advancement of medical science and be also a measure most serviceable to the profession, if the general practitioners were incorporated by Charter into an independent College.'¹⁰ Between December 1844 and January 1845, support for incorporation came from all over the country.

On 14 March 1845, with 'about 1,200 present, including most of the respectable general practitioners in all parts of London', there was a harmonious issue of business at a general meeting of the National Association of General Practitioners in Medicine, Surgery and Midwifery and the concept of a college of their own was supported by an 'ardent, enthusiastic and unanimous meeting'.

Sir James Graham not having found favour with his 1844 Bill and presumably encouraged by the reports from doctors' meetings, produced an Amended Bill on 7 May 1845. This provided for the incorporation by charter of a college of general practitioners. So far, so good. It also included a board of six physicians and six surgeons appointed by their respective colleges to conduct a preliminary examination and then each of them, together with representatives of the college of general practitioners, was to conduct the final examination in their own particular field; and if provided for two GPs on the Council of Health. Objections were raised, on the grounds that in the preliminary examinations the college of GPs would be put in an inferior position to the two Royal Colleges.[11]

This was unfortunate because the Bill recognised, for the very first time, one portal of entry into the profession for all medical practitioners and it recognised general practice as a specialty in its own right. In retrospect, it would have been so much better if the Bill had been accepted in its entirety and the alleged 'inferior' implications haggled over later, even if this had entailed ten years of further argument. For the rejection of this Bill, and with it the concept of a college of GPs, took nearly a hundred years to make good.

Still trying to help and, like so many of his successors, desperately trying to get some sort of agreement out of a diversified and suspicious profession, Graham tried again in July 1845. What a year that must have been! This amended Bill switched round the order of things, which seemed to be what the GPs wanted. It stipulated that the first examination was to be conducted by the college of GPs and subsequent examinations, for those wishing to specialise, by the Colleges of Physicians and Surgeons.

This was one better even that his last Bill, for it ensured that all undergraduates would have a thorough knowledge of general practice before proceeding to their chosen speciality and what could be wrong with that? But, again, it was not to be. This time, the Royal Colleges were the dissenters. It is said that practitioners turned down Graham and his particular concept of a college in disgust. Doctors

seemed, too, to have lost confidence in their own representatives whom they described as making 'bigoted, irresponsible
and unforgivable blunders'.

In May 1851, after considerable bickering and toing-and-
froing, a deputation of the Associated Surgeons and of the
Provincial Medical Association (note the provinces moving
in here), led by Dr Charles Hastings, asked for the Colleges
of Physicians and Surgeons to be remodelled and said there
was no need for a college of general practitioners, which
would tend to lower the status and efficiency of the
surgeons engaged in general practice.

In 1852 the charter of the Royal College of Surgeons was
reformed and it was no longer thought necessary to demand
the incorporation of another college.[12] So, the opposite
opinion had prevailed; the idea that the College of Surgeons
should be the future home of all general practitioners. This
implied a reconciliation with the College of Surgeons at the
expense of the formation of an independent college of GPs.

What at first seems a crass mistake on the part of the
profession in 1851 is only explicable if we remember that
there was still no clear-cut division between one discipline
and the other, and that there was still doubt as to the necessity for the existence of this emerging type of doctor, the
general practitioner. So, in their hesitation and doubt the
profession clung on to the old nomenclature. 'Apothecaries'
or 'surgeon-apothecaries' were terms more understandable
to their patients.

They had not yet experienced general practice as a clear-
cut entity in itself with a very necessary role to fill in
society. They feared loss of status. Maybe, too, they
foresaw a loss of income. This must particularly have
applied to the provinces and it is significant that a major part
in the final outcome was played by a provincial medical
association, clearly at odds with the opinion of doctors in
the metropolis. But it was a seriously missed opportunity.

In 1858 the *sixteenth* Amended Bill was passed and by it
the General Council for Medical Education and Registration
was set up. This new Act regulated the profession as a
whole by establishing a body we now know as the General

Medical Council (GMC). It gave the right to legally qualified practitioners to practise throughout the realm and it created a register of practitioners which the public could recognise.[13]

As opposed to the Act of 1815, which had legalised an inferior grade of practitioner, the 1858 Act set up a standard of education below which a practising doctor could not fall. Its weakness was that it gave a man the right to register on a single qualification, through passing either of the incomplete examinations of the LSA or MRCS, but its strength was that it created one medical profession in the United Kingdom and isolated the unqualified. It thus made good the rejection of this part of the 1844 Bill.

In 1884 the GMC approved the conjoint diploma of the Colleges of Physicians and Surgeons, MRCS (Eng) and LRCP (Lond). This was the writing on the wall for the Society of Apothecaries which, up until now, must have been at the peak of its status and power. Two years later a new Medical Act made it obligatory for every practitioner to be qualified in medicine, surgery and midwifery and a committee of the Royal Colleges in the same year refused to admit the Society of Apothecaries to a Conjoint Examining Board in England. Physicians and surgeons, strange bedfellows, had been brought together by the growing importance of the Society of Apothecaries.

In spite of this rebuff and being, as it were, cast into outer darkness, the Society of Apothecaries remained an independent licensing body with powers to confer a 'triple' qualification. Nevertheless, from then on the Society, which had done so much to create the general practitioner and stood up so valiantly against the might of the two Royal Colleges, had to accept dwindling numbers of holders of its licence in favour of the London conjoint diploma.

As the Society's role in the life of the GP and its influence over the terms and conditions which governed them waned, that of the British Medical Association (BMA), formed in 1832, increased. General practitioners, therefore, were not left unprotected and indeed, particularly in the country districts, they were rising rapidly in public esteem and social

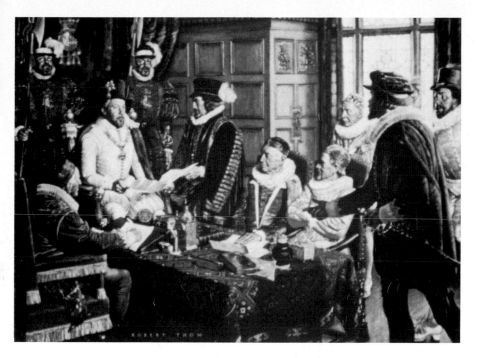

4 James I granting the Charter to the Society of Apothecaries of London, 1617 *(Parke-Davis)*

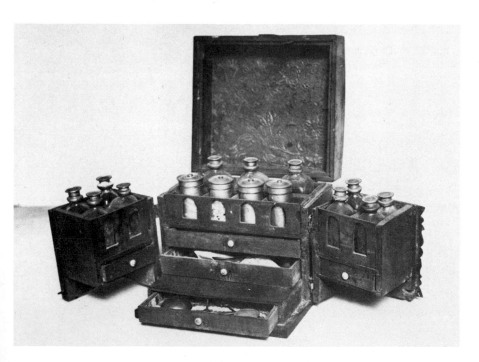

5 An apothecary's travelling case *(by courtesy of the Wellcome Trustees)*

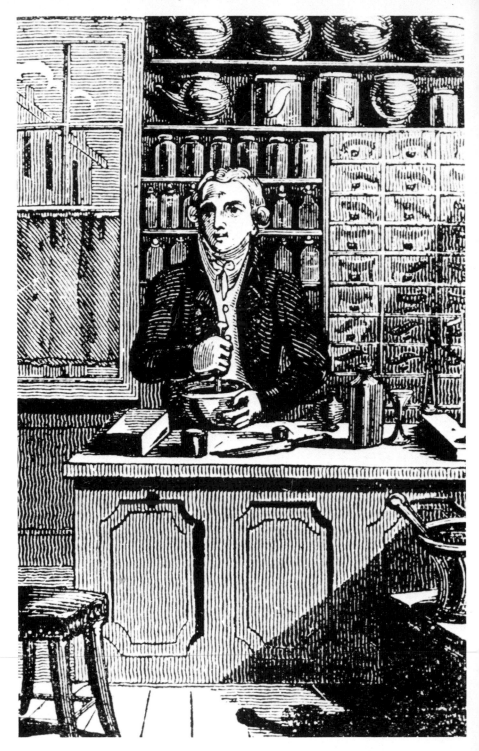

6 An apothecary's dispensary *(Society of Apothecaries)*

status. Incidentally, in 1876 an Act was passed allowing all licensing bodies to open their examinations to women 'at their discretion'. And how discreet they were!

In the first half of the nineteenth century, the apprenticeship system still existed in medical education and brought a welcome addition to the income of the surgeon or apothecary-teacher. Fees seem to have been moderate. In 1830, for example, Sir James Paget paid 100 guineas when bonded to his practitioner, the highest sum recorded being under £300. As well as teaching for five years with certification at the end, meat, drink, lodgings and even clothes were provided. Yet payment brought criticism, 'that a master had no inducement to correct any wrong view which a youth might have taken of the profession, nor to examine into his attainment, but has a direct interest in taking him merely for the money.'[14]

Paget gives an account of his duties: he had to be in the surgery from 9 a.m. to 1 p.m. and from 2 p.m. to 3 p.m. or 5 p.m. to 6 p.m., occupied in dispensing, seeing a few patients of the poorer classes, receiving messages and making appointments. Of the dispensing, he says 'the bottles [were] to be neatly corked and covered; the pills to be duly rolled and smoothly rounded; the leeches to be put in their boxes with scarcely struggling room; and all to look as neat as from any druggist's shop.'[15]

How much or how little a student learned during his five-year apprenticeship depended on him and his master. There seems to have been very little supervision. The apprentice, in case there is any risk of comparing him with today's student, was expected to sweep the surgery, wash the bottles and help to groom the horse.[16] He also was allowed to visit patients occasionally, dispense medicine and dress wounds. In return he was able to pick up scraps of medical knowledge. For example, he was advised to make himself acquainted with the dressing of ulcers, the treatment of accidents and the simpler operations in surgery. Through the post-mortems done by his master he learned the different parts of the body and he was recommended to acquire some knowledge of certain extra professional subjects.

There was no place in those days for the illiterate doctor.

There existed a diversity of opinion as to the value of apprenticeship. Apart from the worry about fees it proceeded, said the critics, on the supposition that everyone came to the profession 'with the mind cultivated alike, and therefore the same thing is required of all.' Again, compelling individuals to serve a certain time as apprentices could prevent some, who had the necessary talent but no taste for an apprenticeship, from joining the profession. This deprived the profession of many who might have been good doctors.

However, thanks to the Apothecaries Act, it soon became necessary for students to become more than servants or bottle-washers to busy doctors. They began to look for teaching in the large London hospitals and, later, in the provincial hospitals. Three 'seasons' for training in hospital were advocated, although it was sadly accepted that the student's stay would be influenced by his finances and by the degree of attention he might give his studies.

This programme may not have differed much over the years. The third season was to consist of 'a strict investigation of disease by clinical observation and pathological anatomy. The plan is to learn, as far as the patient or friends can give information, the history of the disease from its commencement to the time of observation; secondly, to examine carefully the present state of the patient and to retrace the examination of each organ that appeared to have any share in the malady.'

After this, it was considered that the student could present himself for the examination 'without any fear of the result'. The examination was in 'Latin, Pharmaceutical Chemistry, Materia Medica and in the theory and practise of medicine, but not in surgery nor midwifery.'[17]

By the middle of the nineteenth century five-sixths of the students at the London hospitals were studying for general practice as surgeon-apothecaries and Horner says that between 1815 and 1883 the LSA was issued to nearly 31,000 persons.[18] In addition, students destined for country practice and therefore obliged to become suppliers of drugs were 'almost forced to "pass the Hall" whether or not they arrived also at the diploma of the College of Surgeons.' But even by 1858 there were still five grades of the profession recognisable – from the 'pure' physician and the 'pure' surgeon to the dispensing and non-dispensing general practitioner, and from the surgeon-apothecary, with an open surgery but not a retail shop, to the surgeon-chemist, who added to his professional work that of a retail shop.

Rivington, in 1879, divides general practitioners into dispensing and non-dispensing orders. The first consisted of surgeon-chemists or the red-bottle and blue-bottle practitioners. These combined the work of medical men with the retail business of a chemist. They kept shops and sold such things as tooth and nail brushes, patent medicines, soaps and feeding bottles. They were retailers. The second was that of surgeon-apothecaries, with an open surgery and a red lamp. They did no retail trade but charged for advice and a bottle of medicine. Some of these men kept dispensaries and attended patients.

Gradually these groups of general practitioners 'shaded off one into the other' and the open shop, with its red and green bottles, was closed for good.[19]

Between 1858 and 1886 the better class of English general practitioner was described (by Sir Clifford Allbut in his 1920 Presidential Address to the BMA) as favouring Hippocrates or Paré rather than the modern graduate. 'His University . . . was nature: in his clinical experience he enriched the instructions, half empirical, half dogmatic, of his medical school by the shrewd, observant, self reliant, resourceful qualities of the naturalist. His science and his practice were of the naturalist, not of the biologist . . . his rules of thumb were not without their efficacy and his flair for the issues of disease marvellous.'[20]

Such men were skilled in their craft because they were partly born to it, largely self-taught and self-disciplined yet learning from experience day by day. The family doctor was learning his medicine by practising it, but with improved education came also better conditions of practice and progress in medical knowledge.

Auscultation, percussion and urine analysis were essential requirements for every practising doctor. Quacks were now becoming unacceptable and in 1890 the permanently unqualified assistant who acted as understudy to his master was banned by the GMC.

Diagnosis was a new science, arrived at by careful history-taking, searching for signs at the bedside and correlating these with the findings of autopsy. GPs could now bring into their practices the scientific learning and research they had watched develop in the hospital wards. Their work was becoming increasingly rewarding and satisfying. Their status was raised accordingly.[21]

In 1890, the instruments recommended for the GP's surgery included the microscope, laryngoscope, ophthalmoscope and urinary cabinet, and those to be taken on rounds were a clinical thermometer, female catheter, bistoury, small forceps, hypodermic syringe, probe and needles.[22]

How did the GP live in those days? Some patients still liked a medical man to be on a footing with the servants, but there is no doubt that a better class of student was being attracted to hospitals. A GP would worry lest he should gain the reputation of a doctor who 'looked after the servants' for he had to acquire most of his income from his richer patients, the remainder from his 'club' patients. The poor looked to the apothecary whom Dr Percival in his *Medical Ethics* described as 'the physician to the poor in all cases and of the rich when the distress or danger is not too great.'[23] Even in 1938, when I first went into practice, I was told that I had to climb 'over the heads of the poor into the pockets of the rich' and I obtained some private patients by first entering the house (by the front door) to see a servant.

In the mid 1880s there were bitter complaints of poverty amongst practitioners and taxation was a particularly sore point. They were, it was said (in 1840), unable to keep the wolf from the door when expected to pay £24 a year for taxes, increased by Sir Robert Peel from £12 a year. 'We live as frugally as possible indoors; but, unfortunately we have an expense without which we cannot lessen – I mean the purchase and keep of a horse.'[24]

The doctor's rounds were done with his horse and gig or pony and trap, which might be used alternately. The more prosperous had a small dogcart or brougham. A hansom cab might be hired or a patient could even be visited by train. With the coming of the motor car, or 'horseless carriage', in 1896, some doctors took to these, being thus able to speed up their mode of travel to about 25 m.p.h., although mechanical failures, and tyres which disliked the un-macadamed roads, were distinct disadvantages. Bicycles were popular with the young but distinctly disapproved of by the more mature GP as being undignified.

These new methods of transport were largely responsible for the gradual disappearance of the top hat, frock coat, tan breeches and shiny top boots. It must have been difficult to keep on a top hat in an open car and not easy to change a tyre in a frock coat!

A hundred years ago, then, the sufficiency of general practitioners in an area depended on the distribution of the minority of the population who could pay worthwhile fees. Patients were visited within the range of a horse and it was not always easy to obtain treatment. An Irish Member of Parliament said he would 'rather go through the heaviest fire of battle than submit to medical treatment in an English village!'[25]

Yet as the years passed a fundamentally important change was taking place. Physicians were gradually coming to accept surgeons as equals and were patronisingly accepting apothecaries. Some physicians and surgeons, Paget' and Brodie for example, started life as apothecaries and thus had first-hand knowledge of medical practice in the raw.

Another important development was the referral system whereby the patient could reach the specialist via the generalist. The value of this system to patients in this country over the years has been enormous and should be particularly appreciated when compared with alternatives as practised in some other countries. GPs, physicians and surgeons do not jockey for patients here. There is little undignified competition between the disciplines.

Sickness benefit clubs had their origins in the seventeenth

century and were well established by the middle of the nineteenth. Most doctors ran sickness clubs for their poorer patients and Dr Alfred Cox says that, in Gateshead, a subscription of 3d a week was collected at their homes by a collector who was paid a commission but was not supposed to canvass.[26] There were also a good many friendly society clubs in which members could get their doctor's services for 2s 6d or 3s 0d a year. Employers also ran their own clubs. It helped them to keep their workers active if their health was looked after.

In return for paying into a club, workers could receive a limited standard of medical care together with sickness or injury benefits and help with funeral expenses. Some pension was payable to members over sixty years of age if they continued their contributions.

By the 1850s the practice was fairly general of employing medical men as club doctors and it was no secret that some appointments were obtained by bribery and corruption. Appointments were almost auctioned to the lowest bidder. In the cities, the 6d doctor was a common phenomenon.[26] If the doctor gave offence he could be summarily dismissed and his place immediately filled by one of his neighbours, which does not say much for medical ethics in those days.

The club contract, as it covered both attendance and medicine, did not encourage any pretence at real prescribing. Medicine was usually supplied from one of six stock mixtures suitably diluted. A most popular remedy was described as a mixture of burnt sugar and ginger, which 'gripped, had a robust colour and was regarded as a specific for all diseases of the alimentary canal.'[27] These clubs were undoubtedly popular among some doctors. Similar clubs were being run by friendly societies, public houses, and doctors for National Health Insurance families until the 1939–45 war.

They were abused in two ways: patients were sometimes admitted who were quite able to pay fees, and Guardians of the new poor law, who founded 'clubs' to provide the medical relief for the independent labourer and the pauper, could add to the number of 'paupers' any name they might think proper, paying at the same rate as those originally included.

The underpaid medical profession complained about the 'gratuitous medical assistance that has at all times been afforded to the needy by all grades of the profession', and an investigating committee found four main evils: the system of letting the sick poor of parishes for an annual stipend to the lowest bidder, a system open to obvious abuses; some practitioners held a monopoly of parishes; ignorant and unqualified persons were often employed; and medical relief was extended improperly.[28]

As to the work of the GP at the end of the last century, Lucius Nicholls describes how his grandfather's working-class patients sat on wooden benches on either side of a passage leading to the dispensary, from 8 a.m. onwards.

> The clinical examination consisted of feeling the pulse, looking at the tongue and maybe turning down the eyelid . . . the stock questions were about abdominal pain and the state of the bowels. He used a wooden tubular stethoscope which, when going round his practice, he carried by fixing it across a space just above his head in a square felt hat, a little higher than the bowler hat of today. I do not remember him using a thermometer . . . he judged the amount of fever by placing his hands on the bare belly skin. Each patient received a bottle of medicine and/or pills . . . .
>
> Knowledge having no obvious application for the treatment of patients gave busy practitioners of the past no incentive to keep up to date. When there was little or nothing that could be done to cure infectious diseases the personal approach may have been more important than it is today. Charm, kindness and good manners were a necessity for high success and some of the practitioners of old had these in abundance.[29]

William Pickles described the life and thoughts of his predecessor Dr Alfred Baker, who began to practise in 1873.[30] Baker's assistants, 'ardent Listerians', boiled their instruments and stitches so that nasty gashes in arms and legs and scalp wounds healed in no time and without the intervention of laudable pus. He exclaimed at their stipulation for holidays. His recreations were at home (apart from the Grand National), a few hours down by the stream and days on the moors after driven grouse. His assistant actually had a surgeon who came by the last train to see a lad with inflammation of the bowels. 'These two,' he said, 'with only a paraffin lamp for a light and a table to operate on, removed the vermiform appendix.' They were now opening the bladder above the pubis and the age-old spectacular lateral lithotomy was a thing of the past. His 'young fellow' was actually intending to spend part of his holiday at his own hospital, keeping up to date.

And so, in 1903, died a typical country GP of the latter part of the nineteenth century.

3

1900 – 1938

Rosemary Stevens contrasts two medical archetypes at the end of the nineteenth century:

> The hospital consultant, a brilliant bluff empiricist, impressing his group of students at the bedside with a barbed, self-conscious wit; and the kindly omnicompetent general practitioner who knew and loved all his patients.[1]

By the opening of the twentieth century the practice of medicine was becoming more technical and, with the linking of the laboratory and the wards, the methods of diagnosis and treatment became more intricate. The GP found it increasingly difficult, therefore, to keep pace with the new knowledge and the demands of an educated public for new methods.[2] Doctors existed in those days more to prevent suffering than to save life and there is a well-known comment that they had 'no more control over disease than meteorologists today have over the weather'.

To give a picture of the medical scene in the first decade of this century I cannot do better than quote from Sir Robert Hutchison, the physician, and Mr Grey-Turner, the surgeon.

Sir Robert says that it was more exciting to find out things for oneself and to try to come to a conclusion on insufficient data than simply to collate the reports, often conflicting, of a number of technical experts. Diagnosis, he

41

says, was achieved with astonishing accuracy by the physicians of those days as a result of careful history-taking, thorough physical examination and the exercise of their clinical intuition.

He says, too, that disease seems to have been more varied, indeed florid, than it is now and modern treatment has made it impossible to follow the natural course of many diseases. In those days, physicians were supposed to be general physicians. Patients were not segregated according to their disease and every ward afforded a varied assortment of cases. He comments that disease has probably become less picturesque with each generation. 'Should medicine ever become an exact science,' he says, 'it would probably become so dull no one would want to practise it.'

At the beginning of the century, a great deal of therapeutic scepticism was prevalent. Bacteriology was proving disappointing and it was widely believed that drugs were at the end of their tether. A medical ward full of advanced cases of organic disease was rather depressing; 'one felt so helpless to do anything'.[3]

Mr Grey-Turner vividly describes conditions in the old Newcastle-upon-Tyne Royal Infirmary (the new one was built in 1906). In 1900 there was a complement of about 250 beds. Overcrowding was a very serious problem, especially on the surgical side. He remembers a double row of beds all up the middle of a female ward, with one or two patients lying on mattresses on the floor and two patients in one bed, an adult at one end and a child at the other. By the end of a firm's weekly duty (a 'firm' being a consultant's team of registrars and junior house doctors) the wards were often in an appalling state of congestion, with 'nurses distracted and house staff worn out'.

The surgical wards took more than half the admissions. Stomach surgery of the 'cold' type was just beginning; strangulated hernia was much more frequent than today, as were urethral strictures, many of the latter being complicated by periurethral abscess or extravasation of urine. Every year two or three cases of tetanus were admitted with appalling consequences to the sufferers, as anti-tetanus serum was not yet a 'practical proposition'. In one year twenty-six cases of thoracic aneurysm were admitted (many being quite obvious externally). There were fourteen cases of liver cirrhosis.

Gynaecology in those days was dealt with by the general surgeons. An X-ray department had just been started but only 157 cases were examined. Cystoscopy was still a 'curiosity' and catheterisation of the ureters was not employed. Bacteriology was in its infancy (and maybe that is why Sir Robert Hutchison found it 'disappointing'!) Antiseptic surgery was in full swing but not aseptic methods, so rubber gloves were not used and face masks were unknown[4].

Dr Charles Marsh graphically describes life in Bath at the same time. There was no pathological department except for post-mortems. If he wanted a sputum test for TB the patient had to pay for it. Blood counts were done privately and sedimentation rates had not yet come in. An ambulance service, as we know it, simply did not exist. Other writers comment on this and describe how patients were transported by train in guard's vans. There was a nominal ambulance but it was horse-drawn and so seldom used that the driver was full time on other work. The system of district nurses was being developed but there were very few qualified midwives.[5]

Dr Hime succeeded Dr Baker to the Yorkshire practice mentioned in chapter 2 (until Dr Pickles took over in 1913). He set about modernising the midwifery practice. He insisted on cleanliness and considered the prevailing practice of retaining the used nightdress or even day clothes to be a gypsy habit. He had been taught not to give ergot before the birth of the child. The night bell was often the first intimation that a birth was expected. If there was a specialist attending the wealthy, he would like to make the lady's acquaintance before the event, 'but seldom thought it necessary to do more'.[6]

Sir George Godber describes the range of effective drugs available at that time: the alkalies in urinary infection, salicylates in acute rheumatism, digitalis in some forms of heart disease and quinine in malaria. These, he says, were all within the compass of the well-trained generalist, providing an accurate diagnosis had been made. Only a few, such as the arsphenamines, were used almost entirely by specialists.[7] An electro-cardiogram was in use in 1902.

The advance of preventive medicine was robbing the field of some chronic specimens, of which typhoid fever, rickets, infantile scurvy and chlorosis are examples.

Perhaps one rather special example of effective surgical intervention is highlighted by the increasing rarity of advanced cases of pyloric stenosis with gastric fomentation in which the patient belched marsh gas so that 'sometimes when lighting his pipe the gas took fire and he seemed like a dragon breathing flame'.[8]

This detailed description of the work of physicians, surgeons and GPs in the early years of the century reveals the positively enormous advances that have been made in all directions over the past decades, something which tends to be forgotten as the years go by. Secondly, although doctors' professional lives were full of excitement and even adventure in those days, they too had their frustrations and felt helpless at times. In addition they had, in many ways, a more exhausting life than doctors have today.

Communications were growing easier, but motor cars were still rare. Surgeons would arrive at the hospital in a barouche and pair, physicians alight from a one-horse brougham, and the assistant staff travelled on foot, on a bus or occasionally by hansom.[9]

Income was still a source of worry, however. In spite of the fact that the sovereign was supreme and worth twenty shillings, living cheap and taxation light, some doctors did not travel by car because they could not afford one and William Pickles was distressed at being no longer able to employ regular labour. That picturesque figure, the 'doctor's man', began to disappear from practices. Yet at night the horse still had to be saddled or harnessed or the bicycle fetched out.

A week's salary of a locum in 1906 would just about pay for a suit of clothes. Juniors were exploited – housemen received no pay at all and registrars had to work very long hours for practically nothing. There were few recognised consultant posts outside London, except in the very large cities.

Soon the telephone, which was at first a source of irritation and an invasion of privacy, came to be accepted as a necessity, and electric light, taking over from the paraffin lamp or the candle, was undoubtedly a great boon.

In 1912 the government employed an independent firm to inquire into the income of GPs. Six towns were selected. The average income of all the doctors (225) whose books were examined, for every kind of service rendered, was £493 a year, or 4s 3d a head, including every section of the local population.[10]

Then in 1914 came a major crisis which doctors shared with the rest of the population. They not only had to qualify but also to face service in the First World War, in which 9 per cent of all men under forty-five were killed.

Undergraduate years took their toll health-wise, too, mainly through septicaemia or tuberculosis. Writing (in 1964) of his years in general practice, Dr H.H.A. Elder says that 'in the 70's and 80's the bogy was typhus. Nowadays, from what I read, the main danger to the undergraduate is psychoneurosis and suicide.'

He agrees with his nineteenth-century predecessors when he comments that the medical syllabus had changed very little over the years and students were turned out as doctors who had very little knowledge of paediatrics, dermatology and psychiatry. In other words, they were not trained as potential GPs. This he regarded as 'pure folly' and he adds that all doctors who intended to make their career in hospital work should have had some experience of general practice.[11]

The cottage hospital system was developing by now in many parts of the country. These hospitals were open to all local practitioners and added greatly to the fulfilment of their professional lives. Patients, too, liked the cottage hospital, particularly because they could be looked after by their own doctors close to home, relatives and friends.

Doctors of the 1920s tell hair-raising stories of their inadequacy on entering general practice. In midwifery, the majority of deliveries took place at home or in nursing homes. Up to 200 deliveries a year could be encountered, probably with only a 'handywoman' present. Only 'desperate' conditions like failed forceps deliveries and haemorrhage were sent to hospital. Adherent placentas were removed under chloroform and 'eclampsia was smartly diagnosed on the first convulsion'.[12]

There was little, if any, antenatal care. The rules made for the midwife in 1908 required her to call medical aid 'if the patient is a dwarf or deformed; when there is loss of blood; when there is any abnormality or complication such as convulsions, dangerous varicose veins, purulent discharge or sores of the genitalia'.[13]

The Chief Medical Officer of the Board of Health in 1914 noted that these conditions were often not discovered until the confinement took place. He hoped that 'in future careful inquiries would be made by the midwife as to their existence *before* the actual confinement and the patient referred to the Maternity Centre'.[14] Inquiries, not necessarily examinations; yet it is fair to assume from this that antenatal care was developing as the responsibility of midwives.

This is borne out by Dr David Hughes in his James Mackenzie Lecture of 1958, when he says that in his early years he was constantly being called to confinements that were really emergencies and he adds that he usually gave the anaesthetic as well as doing the delivery. He feared that sending for another doctor might give an impression of inexperience or even incompetence.[15]

During my first year in general practice (although this is some twenty years later) my partner once called for me to give an anaesthetic at a difficult maternity case. He handed me a mask and a bottle of chloroform. I had just come from Bart's where I had been administering anaesthetics via a Boyle's apparatus – under the benevolent eye of 'Cocky' Boyle himself. This involved pressing switches and watching bubbles in bottles. If I remember rightly, the bottles were transmitting 'gas, oxygen and ether'. Chloroform was new to me. So I put the mask over the patient's face and poured the anaesthetic on to the mask with what can only be described as careless abandon. In no time at all my partner had to neglect his end of the patient and concentrate on mine. She lived – patients really are wonderful. He asked me why I had not heard of 'one drop once, two drops twice, three drops three times' etc. An unanswerable question.

My second confession is worse. My first attempt at a forceps delivery was in Winchester. I could not have put greater effort into the exercise if I had been trying to move the Forth Bridge. But like the Forth Bridge, the baby onto whose head my forceps were now firmly attached refused to budge. After what seemed to me to be hours, although probably only a few minutes, a live and apparently healthy baby appeared, no doubt as surprised as I was at this first contact with human frailty.

Elder took a boy in a diabetic coma forty miles by car to hospital because he had heard there was some stuff called insulin and there was a chance that they might have some. He says that blood transfusions were the last rite in pernicious anaemia and leukaemia. Tuberculosis was nowhere near under control. It was common to stand by and watch a strapping young man die of pneumonia in six days 'without being able to influence it in the slightest. Septicaemia also left us helpless.'

The haemolytic streptococcus frightened doctors to death. Infected fingers, for example, eventually healed after the terminal phalanx sloughed off. Diphtheria was a killer. One in every six young people indulging in sexual intercourse developed gonorrhoea and 'tertiary syphilis came into almost every differential diagnosis in chronic conditions'.[16]

At about this time the School Health Service was being developed, a further step in the preventive field. Simple forms of treatment were undertaken only if there was certainty that it would not be given otherwise.

Maternity and child welfare services had to be established under public authorities because the family doctor service was not yet ready to accept this responsibility. The idea that a private doctor should be an outpost for preventive medicine was considered 'novel and disturbing'. Infant mortality at this time was 160 per thousand. It cost over five shillings then to feed a child per week, yet the maximum relief given was only two shillings.

The National Insurance Act of 1911 provided general medical care for uninsured workers but not for their families.[17] It was intended to cover all persons earning less than £3 per week. Some feared that it would put the GP in the same position as the man who came to read the gas meter. In fact, some of the abuses resulting from contract practices or sick clubs were eliminated by this Act. By 1911 there were between six and seven million persons provided for by contract practices, at less than five shillings per person, including the cost of drugs and dressings.

Some clubs still remained as a means of obtaining treatment for mothers and children. The GP, like his specialist counterparts in their hospital practices, still did a great deal of work for families for very little payment, if any at all, but now his panel could ensure him an adequate income. In fact, it could quadruple his earnings, and Wigg says that the National Insurance Act transformed his father's practice: 'In 1905, the practice income was £400 per year, in 1918 it was £2,000. . . .'[18]

Sadly, the Act exaggerated the division between the doctor looking after the poorer classes and the wealthy 'private' doctor. Intense hostility could build up between them as a result. However, the Act's greatest asset was that it firmly fixed general practitioners (family doctors) as a definite and durable entity within the body of society, thus consolidating the intentions of the Apothecaries Act of 1815.

The BMA deserves recognition for its work on behalf of GPs at this time. It insisted on six 'cardinal points'[19] which included an upper income limit for those entitled to benefit (£2 per week); free choice of doctor by the patient, and vice versa; remuneration to be fixed in negotiation with the profession and adequate representation of doctors on the administrative committees, both centrally and locally. There was to be statutory recognition of local medical committees and, finally, the Association succeeded in reversing the original clauses in the Bill which placed the control of medical benefits in the hands of friendly societies. Benefits were to be administered by local health committees. The method of payment chosen was a capitation fee for each person on the GP's list and patients became known as panel patients.

In 1930, under the Chamberlain Act, the duties of the Boards of Guardians (see page 38) were transferred to county councils and the parish doctor's job renamed District Medical Officer. The annual income as MO to the Board of Guardians could be somewhere in the region of £137 per annum. Another way of supplementing income was to become 'public vaccinator'. The Act aimed at abolishing the administrative distinction between the sick pauper and the sick person.

During the depression of the 1930s the maximum relief available was two shillings a week. It took over 5s 3d a week to feed a child. The result was semi-starvation and a steady decline in health of the unemployed and their families.[20]

David Hughes describes an 83–year–old doctor's surgery accommodation in the early 1930s. It was a room leading off from the smoke room. The walls were distempered a dirty, dark red. The floor was bare boards and the room ill–lit by a small gas jet (from home–brewed gas). It contained a desk which was rarely used, half a dozen chairs and on one wall a dresser–like collection of shelves for stock mixtures, tinctures and ointments. There was no examination couch and no wash–basin. The doctor had practised from the same house for fifty–eight years and it seemed doubtful whether the surgery had changed at all in that time. He was adored by his patients who would wait hours for him, either sitting on a stone bench round the pump in the yard or on chairs in the surgery.

The wage earners brought home about eighteen shillings a week in wages, yet they were private patients. The doctor's daily mileage was fifty to sixty, sometimes rising to eighty or even a hundred miles. The nearest hospital was ten miles away and until 1948 almost all the acute surgery was done by GP surgeons. The major enemies were retention of urine, hand and arm infections, quinsies, varicose ulceration, road and farm accidents. There was no ambulance service.[21]

One of my own most vivid recollections of my student days at about this time in Bart's was the septic ward, where I saw carbuncles taking up the whole of the back of the neck, big enough and deep enough to get a fist in.

Then, in 1935, came Prontosil – a breakthrough which proved to be the turning point in the treatment of infectious diseases. Insulin for diabetes and liver extract for pernicious anaemia were already available. The sulphonamides were soon to follow and the death rate from pneumonia was reduced by 50 percent between 1933 and 1944.

And so to 1938, which was a fateful year for me.

4

1938 – 1946

I reluctantly became a family doctor in 1938. Until that year such a fate had never entered my head. My interest had always been in paediatrics and my scene bounded by the walls of my hospital. GPs were regarded almost as members of another profession, and pretty inferior ones at that. I do not remember hearing them mentioned, let alone considered, during my hospital years.

Even when I went out onto the 'district' to do maternity work I never once saw a GP. The case was shared with the midwife. If in difficulty, students summoned the registrar. Not that there was much difficulty. Our patients were used to having babies and our presence was more or less a formality. I created a precedent once after one of my patients had dropped her baby into a slop pail, to join the other contents. I put BIB (born in bucket) on the blackboard. BBA (born before arrival) was a fairly usual entry. There must have been some antenatal care by the midwife, but not by us. We arrived as strangers.

Even so I can see, looking back, that there was a glimmering of the doctor-patient relationship, primitive though it may have been, and I can so well remember my surprise and delight at being invited to a christening in Peabody Buildings.

The division between hospital and general practice was of such a degree that I never thought patients had been ill before they were admitted to the ward or might continue to need help after they had been discharged. I found them all clean and tidy, neatly – if apprehensively – lying in a hospital bed. In the ward they received tender, loving care of a standard so traditional and so supreme that it was unconsciously accepted as just normal. To the sister it was *her* ward. To the nurses, they were *their* patients. To the honorary senior consultant and his medical team it was not a chore or a job but a vocation and a challenge.

I can still remember some patients' names, their agonies, their operations and even their convalescences. The hospital was geared solely to the care of the patient. Physicians might snarl at surgeons and get a fair deal of mockery in return; pathologists and radiologists might be regarded as boffins or introverted and peculiar beings almost from another world; yet individual interests mattered not a damn compared with the overall concern of the caring team for each patient.

This very excellence was dangerous. We were cocooned, we students and junior staff, from the world outside, so that when I was appointed to the children's job at Bart's, it was a natural progression towards my ultimate goal of being a paediatrician. Then came the shock. My future, hitherto apparently secure and carefully programmed, was suddenly shattered. I was married and the first baby had arrived. The income, if I remember rightly, was £80 a year and find everything. I could not live on this, and we hated continually asking for help from our families.

So I glanced through the *British Medical Journal* and found a vacancy advertised for a general practice in Winchester. What did one do in general practice, I wondered, other than treat the common cold or kids with threadworms, men with septic fingers or women with vaginitis? And sign sickness certificates, of course. Needs must, so I rang up and because it was a Bart's and Cambridge practice and I was the only candidate, I got the job. I was lucky, for it was a two-man practice in a lovely part of the country – but it was not paediatrics and I wanted to be a paediatrician.

I borrowed the money to cover a two-year purchase of a five-twelfths share of a total practice income of £1,200 p.a. I rented the house I was told to rent by my partner and thus, completely untrained for it, I joined the primary care fraternity. I could not have had a wiser senior partner than Dr G. A. Smythe. I stayed in his house as an assistant, on trial, for a month, during which time he taught me quite a lot and it helped that we were both from the same hospital. I was then joined by my wife and child who had been carefully scrutinised in the interim, and we moved into our new home.

From then on my partner practised from his own house, I from mine. We met occasionally. We each sent out our own accounts and the memory of sitting with my wife at the dining room table each month writing out numbers of accounts, only very few of which we knew would ever be paid, is still as pungent as ever. My partner's wife kept the books and I was sent a quarterly cheque.

I did not know, of course, how many patients I had. They were very few but the days were busy. It was difficult not to welcome each new patient too boisterously. Each had to be accepted with almost stern reluctance as if they had only just arrived in time before the list was closed.

I was told by my partner to call on every doctor in the city. This I did, adopting the practice of calling when I thought they were least likely to be in. I left my card and made a quick getaway. They duly returned the call, no doubt adopting the same principle, or invited us to one of their at homes. All the wives were kind to my young wife and the doctors kind to me.

The two of us had certain other appointments such as 'part-time' MO to HM Prison, St Cross Hospital and a 'dispensary' for club patients. These usefully supplemented our income.

I was very lonely in my professional life to start with, and insecure as well. I had suddenly been moved, without any preparation, from being a member of a closely integrated firm in my hospital, to any member of which I could refer if in doubt, to being virtually alone on foreign ground and in a new job.

My objective was fifty visits a day, sometimes starting at 6.30 a.m. Several patients had to be seen two or three times in twenty-four hours. I also did two surgeries a day in my house. I never knew how many people were going to be in the waiting room, ranging from none to twenty. Minor operations such as circumcisions, sebaceous cysts, boils and septic fingers were arranged for the afternoons. Simple fractures were dealt with, seemingly quite successfully, in the house or surgery, either with one's partner giving an anaesthetic or without an anaesthetic. With the coming of the National Health Service I was tickled pink to refer this type of patient for orthopaedic opinion and treatment (as a GP, I was suddenly considered no longer a fit person to deal with such specialised cases). Empires had to be built and defended!

The hardest working piece of equipment in the surgery was the steriliser, for syringes and instruments. It was almost perpetually in use. Hypodermic needles were the patients' greatest dread, being used and re-used until they bounced off the skin.

We really had to fight hard in those days. And it seems so long ago. Bringing babies into the world and trying to help patients to leave it with dignity and as little discomfort as possible involved so much more effort than today. The defeats and the victories had a far greater impact on one. I am afraid there were many more defeats than victories and the battles were much more drawn out. So much personal effort had to be put into one's work. More mental energy could be expended on a single patient in one day in 1938 than would be used up on a whole day's work in 1980.

Yet life, as always, had many compensations. I think this especially applied to midwifery. I felt an enormous pride when almost the first baby I delivered in Winchester was called Ronald. He is successfully grown up now and my firm friend. I wonder today if anyone knows who brings them into the world. It is a sad loss of a very particular and satisfying relationship.

I had a notional half day a week and every other weekend off but I would not have dared to take them for fear of losing a new patient.

Then came the biggest crisis of all, the Second World

War. I was soon called up, as one of the youngest doctors. In spite of the flags on the map moving daily nearer to the French coast we never entertained a thought of defeat. I tried unsuccessfully to persuade my partner to agree to my house becoming the practice's 'central' surgery so that it could retain a presence in the city. I had been in it for such a short time that I knew I would be forgotten if I was away for long. The practice was safeguarded by the state in that doctors staying at home were expected to hand patients back if and when those in the services returned home. In my case they did this, with the exception of a few of my precious private patients.

My wife and small child followed me around while I was in the U.K. A baby was born while I was on an anti-gas course at Porton, so she too joined the band of camp followers; but I never really got to know her, for I was soon posted abroad. I left my wife in a pub in Devon, the elder daughter with 'double' pneumonia and the baby with whooping cough. It was snowing, too. Thanks to a loyal batman (who eventually joined me on the same draft to go overseas) they were safely transported to Romsey. I saw them only once again for a few hours before returning to Glasgow and then on I went to an unknown destination, not to return for three and a half years.

So all traces of Gibson were lost to sight. And all traces of GPs like me were lost as well, some newly qualified, some well established in their practices. The upheaval in primary care that took place is impossible to describe.

Whilst we were away and even while the war was being pursued, great changes in the country's health service were being considered, but at the time those of us in the services heard nothing about them. We were under the command of the Medical Services of the Armed Forces and they were very good services. What is more, they overflowed onto civilian populations all over the world to their great benefit. Numbers of civilians in all the continents received medical care of which they could never have dreamed in peacetime. We, in turn, saw diseases of which we had only vaguely heard in the U.K. I was particularly fortunate in that I was never out of touch with clinical medicine throughout the war. Even when I became a staff officer I could wander in and out of hospital wards, out-patients and casualty departments. Moreover, one saw the wonderful work done by GP medical officers in the field units.

After three and a half years I was given four weeks' leave, quite unexpectedly. Imprinted on my mind for ever is the awfulness of that return to an almost non-existent practice, a tired partner and a neglected surgery. I spent my leave trying to resuscitate it, doing surgeries myself and getting things together again. Worst of all was being sent back to Africa for a month via a Mediterranean cruise and a well-worn Dakota that made an inconveniently false landing at Wadi Halfa. I came home slowly (almost on foot). It was all an awful waste of effort, time and money.

So it was 1946 before I started up again. All but one of us in Winchester came home safely. My good friend Hugh Noel Davies had lost his life in the navy.

This time my partner agreed to part of my house becoming a central surgery. He came to do his surgeries there. We acquired a switchboard with two switches on it. We also acquired a secretary-receptionist, Mrs Taylor, who is now the practice manager. Apart from the habit she had of putting both switches down whilst she went shopping, thus rendering us incommunicado, her only other major error was to take a medicine bottle of whisky carefully saved up for the doctor tot by tot by a loyal patient, and test it for albumen, telling me in great triumph that there was no albuminuria. The rest of the precious specimen had gone down the sink by the time I got there!

I had a growing belief that the future of general practice lay in group practice. I cannot remember what my concept of a group was, but I felt that mere treatment by the doctor was not enough in itself. It seemed, somehow, a long way from the days of the GP, the priest, the manor, neighbours and voluntary workers who, admittedly in a disjointed and rather ad hoc way, used to look after the sick and needy. All those concerned with the sick in the early 1950s (nurses, midwives, health visitors and welfare workers) were separated from each other, so the looking after was still unorganised. There was, too, a different social atmosphere. The manor had largely disappeared. Doctors and priests were widely separated. Fewer people wanted or had time to volunteer.

I was too busy settling into civilian life and being seen about to have much time for experiments in organisation. There was no question in those days of having patients handed to one on a plate. Every one had to be earned. As I said in the prologue, we had to be 'seen about' everywhere. I suppose it was advertising, except that by itself it would not have taken the GP very far. It had to be backed up by proof in his professional life that, even if not particularly clever, at least he was trying hard.

There is a legend in Winchester of a doctor in the early years of the century who used to dash around the streets in his dogcart, particularly in the evenings, giving all and sundry the impression that he was extremely busy every hour of the day. I did not go so far as this (I couldn't afford the petrol) but I found it did no harm to keep a worried and busy look on my face or to arrive and leave the patient's house in a purposeful manner, as if having little time to complete a busy round.

Talking of visiting, it is remarkable how difficult it is to gauge the time between visits. When one of my partners was new he once got up in the middle of the night to pay an additional visit to a sick baby. He was worried about it and felt he could not wait until the morning before he saw it again. A desperate error – the lights were all out and the parents asleep. This in itself should have reassured him that all was well, for parents do not sleep if they are worried about their first-born. He knocked on the door, wakened the patient and considerably frightened the parents because they thought the baby must be dreadfully ill for the doctor to call unasked at 3 a.m. He then went home. Even so, this is better than leaving too long a time before calling again. Better for families to think that you care too much than that you could not care less.

One good thing about the NHS is that the GP can visit ad

lib without having the worry of piling up expense for the family. It is private patients nowadays who tend to be under-visited for fear of hurting their pockets too much.

I was appointed to do one session in the county hospital and was 'given' a special school and two remand homes. In addition I acquired Marks & Spencer (a singular honour; their health service is incomparable) and decided that, as I had had perforce to give up paediatrics, my particular interest in future should, if possible, be adolescence. So I jumped at being given the chance to understudy a doctor at the College and St Swithun's School.

I was seen about as much as possible in both schools. Eventually I was appointed to both after some years of working in an honorary capacity. These jobs were thus mine, not someone else's I had inherited without any personal effort. What is more, they have provided me with three decades of interest and fulfilment in my professional career.

Meanwhile, the coming of penicillin and the other antibiotics had in themselves brought about a subtle and dramatic change in the GP's life. Perhaps the most significant change, and one not fully appreciated at the time, was that in a certain respect they came between doctor and patient and so, inevitably, changed the doctor–patient relationship. There was no longer need to visit two or three times a day or to make lengthy visits. Capsules left on the bedside table, to be taken two at a time every six hours, reduced the visits to one a day, if that, and the length of the illness from weeks to days. This inaugurated a change in the pattern of treatment. The discovery over the next decades of new drugs for use in other diseases immensely improved treatment and prognosis. Doctors can now do so much more to help, to their intense satisfaction. Yet this changing pattern of treatment has inevitably led to a change in the design of overall care.

It is fair to say that in days gone by untrained GPs had to strive for the excellent. Nowadays the maintenance of a low average and the exhibition of little personal initiative or effort can achieve equal gain. There is little incentive to good work – indeed, quite the opposite, unless it be inborn or compulsive.

It is no criticism of today's GPs that they can walk into a ready-made practice and do what they like with it, and the patients for which it is responsible. They have inherited the system as well as the practice.

The GP's wife and family

The sober comfort, all the peace which springs
From the large aggregate of little things;
On these small cares of daughter, wife or friend,
The almost sacred joys of home depend.

Hannah More
Sensibility

No book about general practice would be complete without a reference to the doctor's wife or husband, a figure of infinite patience and diplomacy who frequently deserves to be honoured by the state.

When I went into practice in the 1930s, complete with wife and one child, I had an income of about £600 a year. This enabled us, with intermittent and sometimes involuntary donations from both our families, to retain a cook, two maids, a nursemaid, and a gardener once a week. Since I was practising from my own house and could not afford any help in the practice, either my wife or a maid had to see patients in and out of the house during surgery (twice a day, except on Sundays) and answer the front or back door on innumerable occasions during the day. I tried to cope with night callers myself, but if I was already out, this job fell to my wife too. There were so few telephones in those days that more of the calls came via the door and a third party, usually a grubby infant or a helpful neighbour. We also, with an eye to the main chance, entertained quite a bit and I can still remember that hollow feeling of sitting as host at the head of a dinner table and wondering how on earth I was going to pay for it.

Fortunately my wife had an infinite trust in the Almighty and a certain amount of untried confidence in her husband. These two between them assured her that the tradesmen concerned would take a sympathetic view of our mounting debts. Yet even the passage of years has not dulled the worry we had in those days about keeping up the shop front and how we could continue to live in a style becoming to our station. On top of that were the interest and capital repayments regularly due on the loan taken out to pay for my partnership share.

My senior partner, Dr Gerald Smythe, rightly felt obliged to remind me from time to time that I was expected to live in a manner consistent with being a respectable GP, to live in a house chosen for me by him, to drive on my rounds in a clean car and a natty suit, to be seen with my family in church and to take part in the social events of the neighbourhood, which included the mayor's ball and the annual fete of the British Red Cross Society.

My wife, too, had to lead a very active social life. This was expected of her and, once having been assured by a discreet telephone call that a particular invitation was 'respectable', it was not done for her to refuse. She had to be seen everywhere she should be seen; she had to be well dressed, conversational and discreet. In no time at all she became chairman of this, secretary of that, organiser of the other.

Maybe I played a dirty trick on my wife. Yet it is incredible how many young wives adapt even to the strangest situations. In family medicine, if they do not adapt, their husbands soon find themselves in trouble. Even today general practice does not just consist of doctors. It includes their wives and families – and a GP's wife should be almost as much a family doctor as he is himself.

Today, in 1981, a newly qualified doctor does not have to buy a share in a practice, but he usually does have to buy a house. His wife is lucky if she has domestic help for more than two hours a week or if she has assistance with the children, other than a washing machine and a spin dryer. She has neither the time nor the money to be well dressed; she is forced to leave her dribbly young with a neighbour when she goes shopping and she is too tired to do much entertaining, with all the cooking and washing up involved. Does keeping up appearances matter nowadays? Should the doctor's personal life be his own affair? And need his wife still regard herself as part of his job?

If the way people live changes, it is illogical to expect the GP and his wife not to change too. If both of them want to go about in rags on a tandem they can do so without jeopardising their livelihood, for no matter how good or bad he is at keeping up a shop front he is assured a basic income under the NHS. As for his wife, she now combines the duties of nursemaid, cook, housemaid and gardener. She is a living example of a head cook and bottle-washer. Also, the development of group practice premises or health centres away from the GP's home has helped create a separate existence for his wife and family and enables the wife, if she so wishes, to be cut off almost completely from her husband's work and his patients.

In place of opening bazaars and supporting acceptable charities, the doctor's wife can now take on a part-time job to supplement her husband's income. She can divorce her husband or be as permissive in her behaviour as the rest of society without raising more than a handful of eyebrows or damaging the practice.

In short, society has given the GP and his family the right to lose themselves in the communal pool and to be as unrecognised or unrecognisable as any other family. No doubt the more densely populated the area in which the doctor works (and he may well live outside the practice area – preferring to commute to and from the surgery), the more his family are obscured; the bigger his practice, the more his secretary and receptionists take on the work previously done by his wife.

I have stressed all along that the GP today is basically the same animal as his forefathers, fulfilling the same role on the medical stage. I have tried to show that he is just as essential today as he has been over the centuries, if not more so. Is it possible, then, to condone an existence for him which involves cutting off his wife and children from his patients? Can we convert him from being a rather special kind of doctor whose life is intricately involved with the lives of his patients into an anonymous figure who can walk the station platform from end to end without speaking to a soul and without anyone inquiring after his wife and family, because their existence is unknown?

It cannot be done. One cannot fit the family doctor into the crowded society of the 1980s without a cross over his head to mark the spot where he stands. Even today it is not possible to leave his wife and children at home, living peaceful, uninterrupted lives in the kitchen and back garden. A GP without a sympathetic and understanding wife or husband prepared to share the load is too heavily burdened for his or her own or for their patients' safety.

Whenever I want proof of this, I remember my visits to single-handed practices in remote areas such as the north of

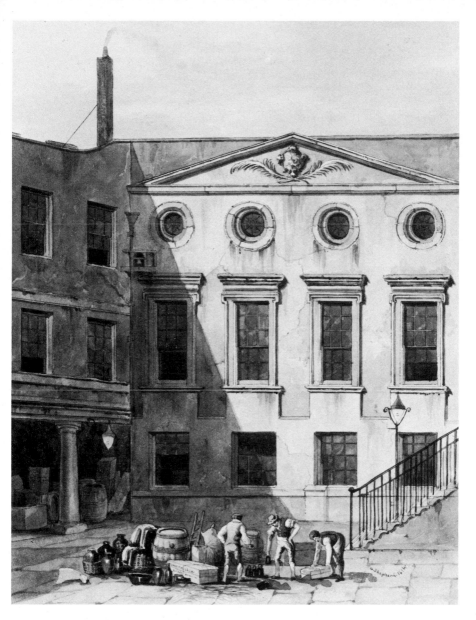

7 The courtyard of the Society of Apothecaries, from an engraving by G. Shepherd, 1814 *(Society of Apothecaries)*

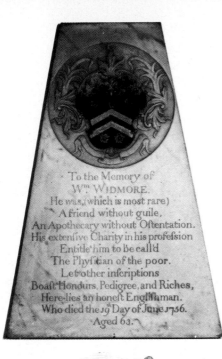

To the Memory of
Wm WIDMORE.
He was (which is most rare)
A friend without guile,
An Apothecary without Oftentation.
His extenfive Charity in his profeffion
Entitle'him to be call'd
The Phyfician of the poor.
Let other infcriptions
Boaft Honours, Pedigree, and Riches,
Here lies an honeft Englifhman.
Who died the 19th Day of June 1756.
Aged 63.

8 Memorial to an apothecary, from the church of St Swithun-upon-Kingsgate, Winchester, 1756

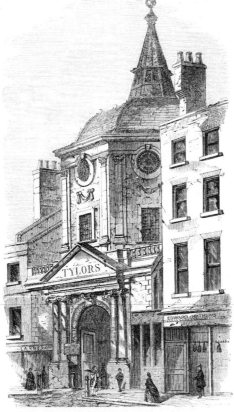

9 The old College of Physicians in Warwick Lane, built by Sir Christopher Wren after the Great Fire of London (*Mansell Collection*)

Scotland, when I was on a whistle-stop tour as Chairman of the BMA Council; or places where GPs had little scope for social life or for educating their children. I found myself full of admiration for doctors in such places, but even more so for their wives – and I gained the impression that the standard of practice in these areas was as high, perhaps even higher, then in those where doctors were working away from home, despite the amount of paramedical personnel and sophisticated equipment available to them.

There can be only one answer to this paradox. GPs today, for their patients' sake as well as their own, need special education, teamwork (with all its complicated apparatus), highly skilled techniques and even computerisation. Yet they still need to be personal physicians. As such, they cannot possibly be pictured as working in isolation from their wives and families. It is because they are known to have homes and wives and children of their own that they are felt to be family doctors (not merely because they treat other people's families). A hospital doctor, once seen, can disappear to Timbuktu so far as his clientèle are concerned. Not so their GP. They want to know where he lives and who his wife is. They want to watch his children growing up.

If he is converted into a high-powered, research-minded and academic doctor, hardly distinguishable from his colleagues in other disciplines of the profession, then it must be honestly accepted that time, circumstances and social trends have deprived him of the personal touch. The family doctor will have been ousted in favour of the general physician.

But that is not what society wants. Patients accept that their personal doctor must, of necessity, be affected, as they have been, by all the changes that have taken place over the past decades, but they still want to respect him. This is yet another paradox. How can today's GPs fit into the community and enjoy the obvious benefits accruing from it (not the least of which are the banishment of hypocrisy and the lessening of the load on himself and his family) yet still be, as it were, apart from it?

I believe that we are not dealing with an incompatibility here provided that the element of general practice inherent in the word personal remains inviolate. Provided that the very personal nature of the GP's job is recognised, with all that it entails, other desiderata can be added with impunity; he can, for example, do as much research as he likes and fit a computer into every corner of his consulting room.

All of which concentrates attention once again on the GP's wife. She can now happily lay the table in the kitchen, hang out the washing in full view of the neighbours, fetch the children from school dressed in shorts, ride a bicycle, and refuse invitations to help in charitable work, provided she is willing, in return, to accept that her husband cannot do his job properly unless she too is associated with him in his patients' minds.

But what is there left for her to do? Even stripped of all the trappings, separated from the surgery premises and relieved of most of the day-to-day professional chores by secretaries and receptionists, she still has enough left to do if she be simply recognised as the doctor's wife.

To give an example of what I am trying to say, one Sunday morning when my wife was on duty as doctors' wives inevitably are on Sundays, she had given me one unnecessary call after the other. I came home at lunch-time thoroughly fed up, but she insisted that I go six miles to see a baby who was reputed to be in great pain. No amount of argument on my part diverted her from her determination that I would go to this call, if only to soothe the mother ('After all, I know how a mother feels – and how can she diagnose what's wrong with the baby?') I loftily replied that a receptionist would have put the call in the book and the mother told to take some aspirins. But to no avail – I went.

It was as well that she was so adamant, for it turned out to be the only necessary call of the day and of such urgency that I took mother and baby to hospital myself rather than wait for an ambulance. The fact that the child is alive today is entirely due to my wife, not to me.

Similarly, I have listened over and over again to telephone conversations between anxious relatives, usually parents, and my wife in which worries have been eased simply through being sympathetically shared, and ruffled feelings calmed because it was the doctor's wife on the line and not that dragon of a receptionist. But, before there were any receptionists the doctor's wife was the dragon! Somebody has to be.

Day and night, here and there, over and over, the GP's wife is expected to act as mother, wife or friend to one patient after the other. She must never be weary, offhand, abrupt or out of sympathy with any caller. She has to understand that aggression often hides fear and diffidence urgency. She has, too, to translate her husband to his patients. It infuriates me that if my wife tells patients she has exactly the same symptoms as they have they seem delighted and readily accept her suggestions for treatment, without any longer needing a call from me; but if I say I am suffering in the same way as they are, they get quite furious. I suppose the doctor has to be above having symptoms of his own – and I noticed that even the kindest patient, if told that I was ill, far from expressing sympathy would say 'Oh, what a nuisance, when will he be back?'

I have said enough to prove what a wonderful help a doctor's wife can be to him and how, so often, she is so much absorbed in helping him unofficially that she readily comes to be regarded as part of him.

With the growth of group practices and deputising services the GP ought, in theory at least, to have more time for his family and he should have more opportunity to get away from it all.

Nevertheless, it is still rather a different existence from that enjoyed by other families and particularly in smaller practices and in rural areas. One doctor told me that he had arranged with his nearest colleague six miles away that each should stand in for the other one half-day a week. However, it proved only a paper transaction because if there was an accident outside his house or an emergency down the road no one could rationally be expected to call a doctor six miles away; another said that he always received an urgent call whenever he was about to hook a salmon; and a third was very reluctantly leaving the small town where his father and grandfather had worked as doctors before him, because he felt he just had to opt for a more settled family life.

As these examples illustrate, even if doctors in rural areas have a lighter overall workload than others, they are still tied to their practices night and day. Moreover, when emergencies happen the machinery for coping with them is more complicated, sometimes even involving helicopters.

Unless one has actually experienced it, the life of a GP and his family is difficult to imagine. Few days pass without some form of unexpected crisis. Even if they do, you tend to worry about what is going to happen tomorrow. Nights can be sleepless, plans disrupted and holidays postponed. You arrive late and leave before the end of any party – theatre, wedding, dinner or Christmas. The pattern repeats itself, so before long you tend to regard it as normal.

A doctor's wife becomes used to taking second place to the practice in her husband's life. The danger is that the children may think that they do not have a proper father and find themselves making excuses because their mother comes alone to see them playing games or receiving prizes. That is why holidays are such fun – when father is there all the time, meals are regular and conversation uninhibited.

Children also learn to forgive. One day I asked my younger daughter, who had already had the disadvantage of a father overseas for the first four years of her life and was now celebrating her husband's successful entry into the medical profession, what sort of a father I was. When she told me I was sorry I had ever broached the subject. We were much too fond of each other for it to make any difference, but it hurt and for days I cursed doctoring for jeopardising my family life.

One of the things she did tell me was that she longed to come out on a round with me, but I never asked her. I had longed to take her with me, but thought she would be bored stiff. I was not there to watch her successfully riding a horse (which, if my memory serves me rightly, took quite a time to achieve); and when she triumphantly told me about it, I just grunted instead of being over the moon with delight. I was probably deep in thought about something else at the time.

The GP's wife and family

While it is difficult for a GP to be a full-time father, it makes an enormous difference for him to have a full-time family who can cheer him up and take his mind off his patients whenever he comes home, no matter how tired he feels.

There is an important side effect to all this. The peculiar life GPs lead can put off their children from ever becoming doctors themselves. So far, there is no thought of any of my grandsons entering their father's and grandfather's profession. There is no way round it, for no matter how general practice is modernised, it is always going to be demanding. Nowadays young people can find plenty of jobs that are more regular and better paid, which is a pity, because medicine is so fulfilling.

I always worry, too, about families where the wife and mother is a doctor. There is a great need for women doctors in the community and women are so full of gentleness and compassion that they are born for general practice. Yet I cannot see how a woman can lead such a life and at the same time be a wife to her husband and, more important, a mother to her children. Dad being away is one thing, Mum is very much another. GPs' husbands must also be rather special people and they deserve a special mention here. Yet is would be disastrous if general practice were denied women doctors, even if they have to take their young with them and feed them in the health centre.

Part of the doctor's family, about whom I wish I could write more, is the lady – nowadays almost certainly part-time – who helps in the house. She, too, has to do more than sweep, dust and keep a young family in order. She has to cope with telephone calls and front door visitors and always has to give the right answers, be tactful and diplomatic, yet firm and reliable. She has to take messages and record them accurately, for I am not exaggerating when I say that one slip, even in the number of a house or the name of a street, can be disastrous. She has to learn to be discreet and to avoid potentially dangerous conversations in the village street or shop. In short, she too is a very necessary part of a GP's life.

69

Lastly, I might add what a boon the family dog can be, especially on night calls – the friendly nudge when one is feeling lonely, the warning bark when the car is left unoccupied and unlocked, and the reproachful look when a daily walk is overdue.

So much for this brief diversion from history. I hope I have proved my point that a GP needs his wife, his children and all the friends he can get, if he is to do his job properly by his patients – and stay sane. They, too, need compassion, sympathy and understanding.

5

The birth of the NHS

When I think back to those precursory days leading up to what was known as the appointed day, when the National Health Service was to come into operation, I still conjure up some of the feelings one had at the time of being just a pawn in a rather bewildering game, in which the rules were partly being dictated and partly made up from week to week. I doubt if any of us in general practice then fully realised how our discipline was to be isolated and denigrated. It is important for the reader to understand this and therefore why, in the context of history, the ensuing years were so turbulent.

If only one could adequately translate for today's GPs the turmoil and apprehensions of those days. GPs feared local authority health centres and domination by local authorities; they feared also becoming full-time salaried medical officers; direction as to where they should practice; loss of compensation for and confiscation of their practices; a tremendous increase in their work with less sense of fulfilment; increasing frustration; and direction of patients without their consent. They did not approve of payment by basic salary and they asked, amongst other things, for diagnostic facilities to be available to GPs; for improvement of midwifery standards to be obtained by special qualification through the present

71

examining bodies; for an adequate capitation fee; and above all for clinical freedom to treat their patients without interference from the state.

The concept of a national health service goes back as far as 1920, when a committee, chaired by Lord Dawson of Penn,[1] recommended a comprehensive health service provided through primary (GP) and secondary (hospital) health centres. From 1930 onwards the BMA was considering plans for developing the National Health Insurance scheme so that it included the whole community, giving free treatment by both the family doctor and hospital services.

In 1933, the BMA published 'Essentials of a National Health Service' and it continued throughout the prewar years to recommend that a comprehensive service be introduced with the least possible delay.[2]

Undiscouraged by a world war, the association's efforts continued and in 1942 a Medical Planning Commission (set up by the BMA and the Royal Colleges in 1940) published a draft interim report, the most important recommendation of which was to 'render available to every individual all necessary medical services, both general and specialist, and both domiciliary and institutional'.[3]

Shortly afterwards, the Beveridge Report was published.[4] This was an immensely important document, which concerned itself both with health and the wider issue of social security. It was accepted in principle by the coalition government and a White Paper was published – 'A National Health Service'.[5]

By 4 May 1945 the BMA was committed to a 100 per cent medical service for the nation and, passing over much debate and argument between the profession and the Minister of Health, Sir Henry Willink, the election of July 1945 carried a Labour government into power with Mr Aneurin Bevan as the new Minister of Health. He proved to be a man of determination and the 'builder who managed to get his tender accepted'. Almost certainly the greatest of this country's health ministers, he would brook neither delay nor lengthy negotiations. His White Paper was published in 1946[6] and became law in November of that year. The appointed day was fixed for 5 July 1948.

GPs were to come under the control of new bodies known as Executive Councils, similar to the 1911 Insurance Committees. The bulk of preventive and social medicine was to remain in the hands of local authorities, including maternity services, child welfare, health visiting, home nursing, home helps and ambulances.

While Lord Dawson had tried hard to bring the GP closer to the hospital, Bevan deliberately drove a wedge between hospital consultants and GPs, making the divorce between them absolute. Cottage hospitals were to be taken out of the GP's hands, except in rural areas; he could be retained in hospitals in a kind of second-rate consultant grade known as SHMO (Senior Hospital Medical Officer) but he would be gradually phased out. Bevan thought he had done well by the hospital doctor (including merit awards) and he said he had 'stuffed their mouths with gold'. So it was fair to ask what, if anything, was left for GPs and it was understandable that there was a justifiable fear for their future.

The government, in 1945, anticipating the National Health Service, instructed a committee chaired by Sir Will Spens to determine, amongst other things, what ought to be the range of total professional income of a registered medical practitioner in any publicly organised service of general medical practice. The committee concluded in 1946 that the majority of doctors had been grossly underpaid. On the translation of 1939 values to those appropriate in 1948 the report said:

> We leave to others the problem of adjustment to present-day values of money, but we desire to emphasise as strongly as possible that those adjustments should have direct regard not only to estimates in the changes in the value of money but to the increases which have in fact taken place since 1939 in incomes both in the medical and other professions.[7]

The government and the BMA disagreed over the adjustments and, pending the outcome of negotiations, GPs were paid, from 5 July 1948, at rates representing an increase of about 60 per cent on the figure of £1,111 derived from Spens.

It all started for me in June 1946, not long after my return from Africa, when our senior ophthalmic surgeon, Mr R. H. Balfour Barrow (Baffer) rang me up and asked if I would succeed him as Honorary Secretary of the Winchester Division of the BMA. I was callow and foolish enough to be honoured by this suggestion, once I had persuaded myself that he was talking about British Medical Association and not the British Military Administration which I had just left.

Like all secretaries desperate to find anyone to take over such a traditionally thankless task, he told me how little work was involved – just arranging meetings and writing minutes, he said, and there was nothing to it. What Baffer failed to tell me was that Winchester at that time contained a shoal of the most energetic, far-seeing and responsible doctors in the country (of which he was one). It proved to be tremendous fun and as near to a full-time job as anyone already fully committed to a busy life in general practice could possibly wish. The activities of the Winchester division and the impact these had on the BMA are still remembered today.

We issued memoranda on reorganising the association to fit the needs of the day, we circulated these to every division in the country, tabulating the replies on the back of a roll of wallpaper – on the top of my grand piano – and dramatically unfolding it in front of a startled Organisation Committee sitting at BMA headquarters. We achieved the necessary support to command a special meeting of the Representative Body, at which we lost practically every resolution we put up, but caused sufficient commotion to stir many doctors throughout the country into attending BMA meetings.

We then set about the association's public relations, demanding, amongst other things, a special department with a press officer at its head. We must have been a menace to the staff at headquarters but they were very patient with us and even agreed to cover the costs of our campaign!

The relevance of this to the health service's impact on the GP is that in helping to build up interest in and loyalty to the BMA a greater number of doctors became involved in formulating some sort of comprehensive policy to set against Aneurin Bevan's determined will.

The Winchester division meetings at that time read like an agony column. We reached a peak when the chairman, the indefatigable Dr C. J. Penny, instructed me to send, at his expense, a telegram to every doctor in the division under-lining his expectation that they would be attending a general meeting in the nurses' home of the Royal Hampshire County Hospital the following Sunday morning. My recol-lection, supported by the attendance book, is that some 99 per cent of them did that very thing, one in a wheelchair. We did not know it then, but this was to be our finest hour! And all, as will be seen, for very little.

There were two plebiscites by the BMA. In February 1948, of 84 per cent of doctors who answered, 90 per cent disapproved of the Act and 88 per cent would not accept service within it. Fewer than 4,000 doctors were prepared to accept the terms offered. In April, after further negotiations and an assurance that there would be no full-time salaried service, only 77 per cent of doctors replied. Resistance was crumbling and fewer than 10,000 doctors opposed service.

So the appointed day arrived and a service came into being in which each type of doctor was compartmentalised from the other. In other words, three separate and distinct services were running within the overall umbrella of the Act. GPs should with confidence have been practising from premises, owned or not owned by the state, together with nurses, health visitors, midwives, social workers and others. This was necessary for the satisfaction of each particular discipline and, more important still, for the most efficient total care, as opposed to mere medical treatment of the patient – and, one can add, for economy of effort and finance. Yet they were separated in function and administration.

Similarly, GPs should have had their own particular place in hospitals, and particularly cottage hospitals, so that they could treat patients up to the level of their training and ability, leaving the specialist to concentrate his time on patients in need of his special skills. Hospital consultants should have been encouraged to hold some of their clinics in practice premises within the community. Yet these two services were also separated in function and administration.

In 1950, the BMA published a report on *General Practice and the Training of the General Practitioner* (the Cohen Report).[8] This detailed the daily round of the practitioner in the urban and rural areas and showed how the range of work of any particular practice was affected by its locality; how the type of practice was affected by a particular GP's habits, outlook, temperament, knowledge and equipment and how GPs differed in the time and effort they devoted to individual cases. Yet, in spite of all the variants one could clearly see that the GP's commitment was total. He was part doctor, part social worker and part priest.

The report concluded that

Such responsibilities which cannot be assessed or classified demand not only medical knowledge and experience but also personal qualities which defy analysis and yet which have so important a place in General Practice.

Lord Cohen and his colleagues were defining someone who could not be just a doctor. He (or she) had to be something else as well, even to the extent of being all things to all men. The committee was confirming what history had already shown to be true.

In a comprehensive health service, therefore, this particular doctor should have been rated as a very important person and as the hub around which, for an effective service, the hospital and the paramedical services would revolve. Yet a contrary view had prevailed. The hospital was to become the most important unit, with the family doctor and community services playing a secondary role.

There were three major reasons for this upside down approach. At that time GPs were wandering in the wilderness with no royal college of their own and the BMA was as yet comparatively untrained in the hurly-burly of high-powered medico-politics. Secondly, no Minister of Health could hope to get a service off the ground without the support of the Royal Colleges of Physicians and Surgeons and no matter how benevolent and sympathetic these powerful bodies might be to general practitioners they could not be expected to give primary health care services priority over hospital care. Thirdly, during these years there had been a remarkable series of discoveries of the greatest importance to medical science. Together with new and complicated instruments for the diagnosis and treatment of disease, these promised an exciting new life for the practising doctor in the middle years of the century. Every advance in science has always overflowed onto the GP service, making it more complex perhaps, yet at the same time adding to its quality and interest, upgrading primary health care and reducing the load on hospitals.

Those in the corridors of power disagreed. They thought the GP outside the hospital would be increasingly isolated and only fit to deal with rudimentary diagnosis and treatment. Thus the family doctor who entered the health service did so as a filter for and signpost to the hospital. He was described as the Cinderella of the service and the one who had fallen off the hospital ladder. His patients had a different picture of him, yet it was to take him decades to achieve his rightful place in the NHS. The intervening years were tragic from the point of view of trauma to the GP and wasted years to the service, to say nothing of wasted money.

The NHS was described as little more than a comprehensive scheme for National Insurance. It was also called a 'National Sickness Service'. The service worked because of inherited good will and because, as ever, the welfare of the patient took precedence over everything else. Yet it was not long before the good will started to run out and doctors became frustrated. Fortunately, this increasing disenchantment was not allowed to overflow onto the patients who were (rightly) enjoying a free GP service for the whole family, free treatment in hospital and state welfare services from the cradle to the grave, all as a right.

GPs were paid out of what was known as a central pool. The Medical Services Review Committee, appointed in 1958 under Sir Arthur (now Lord) Porritt, described this as the total sum of money set aside for the payment of General Practitioners in the National Health Service, based upon the number of doctors taking part and upon an agreed amount for practice expenses but having no regard whatever to the amount or quality of the services they undertake, whether in general practice or elsewhere.

The committee recorded its firm view that both the capitation method of payment and the pool system fell far short of providing the best incentives and encouragement to good general practice.[9]

In this comment the committee was generous for, in my view, the pool was an almost iniquitous invention. It afforded no incentives at all and no encouragement for anything other than a miserable standard of practice or for GPs to operate anything better than a mere basic 'service'. The profession has to take its share of the blame for ever agreeing to it.

The constant claims by GPs for an adequate income were vindicated by Mr Justice Danckwerts in 1952.[10] His award, given within a month, provided that the 'betterment' which should be applied to the 1939 remuneration to bring it up to date, for the year ended 31 March 1951, should be 100 per cent. This was a triumph for the BMA negotiators, Dr Wand and Dr Stevenson, and it led to the first serious attempt to reorganise general practice within the service. The working party which followed it reduced the maximum list from 4,000 to 3,500, provided a special loading of the capitation fee in the middle range of the lists (so as to favours GPs with a moderate list), set aside £100,000 a year to establish a Group Practice Loans Fund and established an Initial Practice Allowance to help doctors to open practices in under-doctored areas.[11]

After this there was peace for a time but the undercurrent of discontent flowed on, exacerbated by the intrusion of politics into the doctor's life, and it was not slowed down by the increases in income. In fact Danckwerts, having helped with the money problem, helped also to highlight the clinical frustrations; the overwork due to lists which were still too large and incessant patient demand, these two leading to inadequate time to spend with each patient; isolation from the hospital service; and an overall lack of incentive to improve the service.

So morale went down and down. Something had to happen. Slowly and at first imperceptibly it became clear that general practice must be rescued and the first overt and exciting move to achieve this was the founding of the College of General Practitioners on 19 November 1952.[12] Much work had gone on before the foundation day. In September 1951 two members of the BMA (the late Dr F. M. Rose and Dr J. H. Hunt – now Lord Hunt of Fawley) had a discussion with the General Practice Review Committee. A steering committee was set up under the chairmanship of the Rt Hon. Henry Willink, QC, Master of Magdalene College, Cambridge and Minister of Health, 1943–5, and its unanimous report was signed on 19 November. Two quotations from the report's conclusions are relevant:

It is being increasingly realised that this development and emancipation of general practice is not only a question of professional pride and status but an urgent economic need – to keep patients out of hospital whenever they can be investigated and treated at home. . . . A golden opportunity now presents itself for general practitioners to found an organisation of their own, to watch over their academic interests and their education.

The college was divided into faculties. General practitioner members of the college, attending meetings through their faculty areas, discovered that they were in good company in wishing to raise the standard of practice, to take an active part in undergraduate and post-graduate education, to encourage research and generally to concentrate on the medico-scientific, leaving the medico-political to others. Hope began to replace despondency and to encourage them further they found enthusiastic advice and support, backed by finance, from their colleagues in other disciplines, through colleges, associations, societies, journals and the pharmaceutical industry.

It was not long before advances in practice administration and organisation were receiving support through the college, such as designs for group practice premises, the concept of appointment systems, encouragement to those already engaged in unofficial attachments of students and vocational training for the newly qualified, research proposals and the founding of travelling fellowhips – too much activity to swallow at one go yet, in no time at all, enough to change the whole face of general practice.

In 1954, the County Medical Officer of Health for Hampshire, Dr Ivor MacDougall, suggested to my practice that we should agree to a health visitor attachment. This was accepted with some reservations. Health visitors in those days were unseen women who we thought tended, without consultation, to disagree with our treatment of young mothers and their babies. After a few weeks, reservations became willing acceptance. There was wonder as to how the partners ever worked without her, the now famous Mrs Noble. Patients were soon ringing her for advice and saving the doctors' time. Yet she was also, in her care of the elderly, uncovering hitherto unknown and unintentional areas of neglect. So she saved work but also added to it, but since she and the doctors now knew and understood each other and worked from the same premises the concept of total care came nearer to realisation. This was so much so, that she was soon followed by a district nurse and a midwife.

Although progress was being made, step by step and area by area, in upgrading general practice – by GPs themselves it will be noted, not by any government Act – worries about money continued. In February 1957, 'against a background of controversy', a Royal Commission[13] was appointed. The terms of reference were:

> to consider how the levels of professional remuneration from all sources now received by doctors and dentists taking part in the NHS, compared with remuneration received by members of other professions, by other

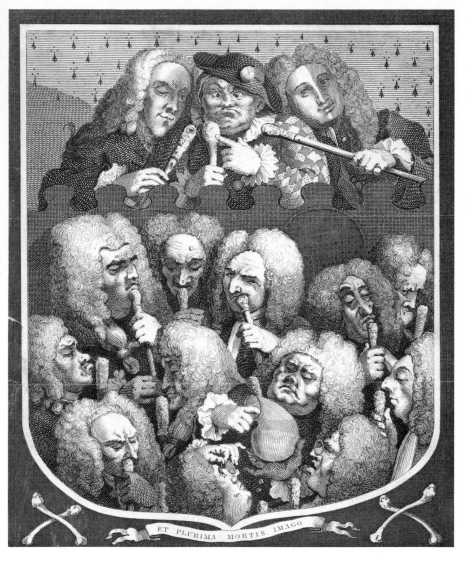

10 'Consultation of physicians', an engraving by William
Hogarth *(Mansell Collection)*

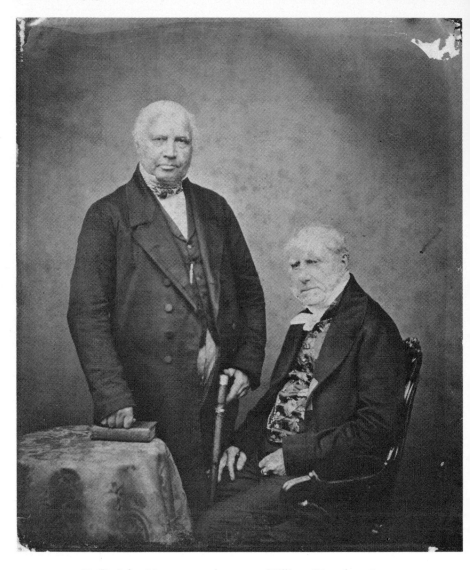

11 Dr John Nussey, apothecary to William IV and to Queen Victoria, with Dr Michael Este, his successor *(Society of Apothecaries)*

members of the medical and dental professions, and by
people engaged in connected occupations; what, in the
light of the foregoing, should be the proper current levels
of remuneration of such doctors and dentists by the NHS;
whether, and if so what, arrangement should be made to
keep that remuneration under review; and to make
recommendations.

A step of great significance in 1958 was the setting up by the
Royal Colleges, the College of General Practitioners and the
Society of Medical Officers of Health, of a Medical Services
Review Committee under the chairmanship of Sir Arthur
Porritt[14] with the following terms of reference:

> to review the provision of medical services to the public,
> and the organisation, in the light of ten years' experience
> of the National Health Service, and to make recommen-
> dations.

The committee first met in November 1958 and reported in
1962.

Needless to say, the daily round and common task of the
GP amidst all the change and turmoil of 1948 was more than
a little disturbed. Business had to be carried on as usual, the
sick did not cease to be sick for a few weeks to enable GPs
to settle into their new role. I had no idea how many
patients, or potential patients, I had and it would be foolish
not to admit to excitement as every day more patient cards
came in via the letter box, or a call at the front door, until it
seemed that I was suddenly the possessor of nearly 4,000
'registered' patients. At first, neither I nor my patients knew
the rules and regulations, nor the extent of the free gifts on
the Christmas tree. We had to learn as we went along and
the snag was that everything required, or thought to be
required, now had to be channelled through the GP. 'I
certify that' became the order of the day.

Yet the benefits to the community of a free service were
obvious from the first. Seeing patients who should have
been seen ages before, usually wives and mothers – with

prolapsed wombs, varicose veins, flooding periods, lumps in the breast and so on – who had had, for financial reasons, to put husbands and children first, confirmed that we could never go back to pre-NHS days. Hell though it might be, if we were to be able to do our job properly in the future, money could never again be allowed to come between us and our patients.

Even if we were driven from time to time, through sheer desperation, to think in terms of 'payments for items of service' or some other deterrent to lessen the workload on the GP, those of us who went through the agony of the first few years would find it difficult to approve of any alternative scheme involving payment by the patient in the first instance. Hotel charges in hospital fall within a different category.

As a side effect, too, those patients who elected to stay private, not just to queue jump as the bigoted politician suggests, but for several other perfectly acceptable reasons, actually paid their bills and bad debts disappeared.

From the beginning it was clear that the patient-demand, the workload, would soon break any doctor who tried to keep up his standards. Many patients could not be properly examined (if at all); too many left with a prescription no longer composed by the doctor – more and more consisting of 'Mist' this and 'Tab' that according to the whims of the National Formulary or the persuasive ability of the drug firm representatives.

The workload was really appalling. It was not as though we were just dealing with more patients for a far greater number of reasons. There were new forms to learn about and a wider range of prescribing for which we were responsible. Eye-testing forms alone took up a great deal of time and it was clearly going to be necessary to try to streamline the administration and organisation of the practice, by such means as installing new methods of record filing and converting the old fashioned surgeries into appointment sessions. There were, in addition, fringe activities, with meetings here and there to talk or argue about this, that or another facet of the new service.

I doubt whether the Minister of Health and his staff realised the pressure that was suddenly to be forced on to GPs by the new service. At least, I hope they did not. They too were learning as they went along. We, on the other hand, had no time to learn. The doors opened on the appointed day and only we were there to cope with the sudden overwhelming load on general practice.

So it was that I was sitting wearily at home after supper one evening when 'Baffer' Balfour Barrow came in and asked if we were thinking of taking on another partner. Up until then I had had no such thoughts but I suddenly realised that unless we soon expanded to three one of us was going to crack and crack badly. The same problem must have applied to many general practices at that time.

Baffer had had a letter from a Dr Robert Forbes, then Secretary of the Medical Defence Union, to say that his son, James, would like to practise in or near Winchester. I thought there was no harm in us seeing him, even if we could offer him only the now traditional blood, tears, toil and sweat, and he duly arrived for interview. He had been trained at St Mary's (he was an excellent rugger player) but had done his house jobs at Bart's. He also wore an old school tie with which I was familiar. It is extraordinary how life so often provides a rescue service in the nick of time and when it is least expected.

By mutual consent Jimmy Forbes joined the practice and in no time at all the three of us had moved to roomier accommodation. We found a four-storey Georgian house down the road, in which, by an incredible coincidence, the practice had been before. Each floor became a separate consulting unit with waiting and consulting rooms; reception and filing were on the ground floor but we soon had to move the filing upstairs away from the gaze of the patients; and the secretary's office, the nerve centre of the practice, was on the first floor with a common room on the second. We learned as we went along – common rooms, for example, must be on a working floor and not sited in isolation up a flight of stairs.

In retrospect, this was exciting too. Patients queued down

the passage and out onto the pavement so, as I have said, an appointment system was forced on us, nor could we have ever done away with this once it was established. The sight of a queue to a tired doctor and a sick patient is heavily demoralising. Those who have never known queues of patients for an evening surgery should think many times before advocating the demolition of appointment systems.

We decided to spare no expense on furniture and equipment. Looking back, I do not know how or why, we did it. It all came from our own pockets. We were poor and money which we could have spent on our families was put into the practice. These are not the words of a martyr, but they are those of one who will never forget the bitterness against governments who initiated and encouraged a service geared to a basic standard, thus battening on the good will of GPs to provide a better and more acceptable service at their own expense.

It is not to be wondered that some did not bother and others, in trying, became too cynical to continue for very long and emigrated. Nor is it surprising that 'Please see and treat' increasingly became a method of introducing a patient to hospital.

I lost my hospital job, of course, and other doctors were downgraded in their hospital work because they had no higher degrees. GPs went into hospitals now as visitors, in no way considered capable of treating their patients. Paradoxically, they were not stopped from looking after patients in nursing homes.

The domiciliary consultation was a boon, so long as it was a consultation and not a home visit by a consultant on his own. Later, open access to laboratory and X-ray departments helped tremendously and through this service we were able to keep many patients at home who otherwise might have been in-patients. Antibiotics, with the appearance of disposable syringes and needles, were time-savers and much welcomed.

The duplication, or even triplication, of such services as maternity, inoculations and vaccinations was irritating. More so was the separation of the patient from the family doctor and home midwife when taken into a maternity department for confinement. Hospital confinement was right; exclusion of GP and midwife was wrong.

So the family doctor service in its origins was faced with a number of deficiencies and omissions, mainly resulting from the sharp tripartite divisions of the NHS but in great part due to orienting the service round the hospitals with the consequent denigration of the GP. Practically every positive step enabling the GP to do a worthwhile job had to be initiated by GPs themelves and then fought for again and again, through the BMA, the College of GPs, evidence to committees and working parties, lectures and seminars throughout the country. If only (and what is the good of saying 'if only') the true value of a top–class primary health care service had been recognised on the D-day of the NHS we might have started in 1948 where we are today in 1981.

We would also have had a health service based first of all on prevention of disease and then on the community services, the latter being geared to cope with the majority of items involved in the total care of the whole patient by an all–embracing primary health care team, thus enabling hospitals to be used economically and effectively for only those patients truly in need of specialist investigation and treatment. The money, the physical and mental effort, the frustration and the arguments which would have been saved are incalculable. But this was only the beginning. The arguments were to continue for many years.

6

1960 – 1964

During the 1960s primary care in the NHS nearly broke down, and the frustration and despair of GPs mounted to the climax of threatened resignation and the launching of a charter.

Three very important reports were published between 1960–63. Each of them, in due time, was to have a profound effect on the life of the family doctor, so that historically these four years may prove to be the most significant of any. They were, too, constructive years in that they laid the foundations of a future family doctor service on which others could build, so I must describe them in some detail.

The first report, in 1960, was that of the Royal Commission on Remuneration.[1] Although this was in general a vindication of the profession's case, it was in some respects disappointing to GPs, particularly as it approved continuance of the pool system of payment (though somewhat amended) and indulged in some wishful thinking by hoping that more would be done to make the pool system intelligible 'to those whose living depends on it'. It offered no suggestions as to the reduction in the number of patients on GPs' lists and made no change in the general system of allowance for practice expenses.

The amendments the Commissioners suggested included a recommendation that private earnings should be taken out; that Exchequer contributions to superannuation should no longer be deducted in arriving at the sum payable to doctors;

that all GPs over the age of seventy should be eliminated from pool calculations and that group practice loans should be paid as a separate transaction and no longer taken out of the pool. Clearly these were helpful recommendations but they still left the doctor who was bent on raising his standard of practice to pay for improvements out of his own pocket. There was a proposal that £500,000 should be set aside per annum expressly to recognise distinguished general practice by additional remuneration but this, on the surface at any rate, smacked of the 'merit awards' paid to consultants and was quite unacceptable as such to family doctors. Nevertheless, it was additional money.

The main recommendation was, and still is, of great significance. It was designed to avoid recurring direct confrontation between government and profession on the subject of remuneration and it proposed the setting up of a Standing Review Body to keep medical and dental pay under review, to make specific recommendations and to report direct to the Prime Minister.

Members of the Review Body were to be of such distinction that it would be regarded as a better judge than government or representatives of the profession on proper levels of remuneration and in forming its conclusions three basic factors were to be considered: changes in the cost of living; the movement of earnings in other professions; and the quality and quantity of recruitment in all professions. These three factors are of major concern in this book, right up to the end.

Furthermore, the Royal Commission thought that the recommendations of this Review Body would be of such weight and authority that the government 'should be able to feel bound to accept them'. The caveat (or let out) was that it would be an advisory body only. This could, and did, react to the disadvantage of the profession. The other handicap was reporting direct to the Prime Minister; there was no provision that he need tell the profession when he had received the report or, indeed, what was in it and in chapter IX we shall see the unfortunate consequences of this restriction.

Lastly, the commission did not recommend that the profession could give evidence direct to the Review Body. Professor John Jewkes, in a Memorandum of Dissent, said there should be a right of direct access to the Review Body and, in the event, this opinion prevailed.

Government and the profession accepted the concept of a Review Body which, after consultation, was set up in 1962, under the chairmanship of Lord Kindersley. In addition, one million pounds was set aside *from the central pool* for the purpose of improving standards in general practice.

Close on the heels of this report, in 1962, came the report of the Porritt committee.[2] This was not a statutory committee but had been set up by the Royal Colleges and the BMA. Insufficient recognition and commendation has been given to this committee's report which recognised and categorically stated that a good GP, with a broad outlook and widespread interests, was still a basis for good medicine and that a sense of vocation, the satisfaction of doing a worthwhile job and a sense of professional responsibility still played a large part in his life.

I will list some of the committee's recommendations so that they can be followed through in ensuing chapters: the formation of group practices and the building of primary health care teams; attachment of health visitors from the local authorities to family doctors; appointment systems; planned post-graduate courses for GPs; direct and unrestricted access to consultants in charge of radiological and pathological departments of hospitals; encouragement of special interests in general practice and the siting of GP maternity units as close as possible to consultant staffed hospitals; properly organised deputising services.

Three recommendations merit special mention: the first, that there should be close co-operation between GPs and skilled ancillary or paramedical workers, including family case workers, psychiatric social workers, probation and children's officers, mental welfare workers and various voluntary bodies. We shall discover in chapter VIII what actually happened six years later to this very necessary ingredient in the total care of the whole patient.

The second, that a GP should be encouraged to look after his own patients in hospital. This was in line with the Platt working party's view (1961)[3] that 'GPs will continue to be employed at cottage hospitals in which they maintain responsibility for their own case, with advice available from consultants visiting regularly.' So also said a Royal Commission in 1977, fifteen years later.

Finally the third, that 'both the capitation method of payment and the pool system at present fall short of providing the best incentive and encouragement to good general practice.' In this the committee was more successful, for the Government agreed to the abolition of the pool in 1965.

The next very significant report was published in 1963 and came from a sub-committee of the Standing Medical Advisory Committee of the Department of Health. Its terms of reference were to study the future scope of general practice and it was chaired by Dr (now Dame) Annis Gillie.[4] Its main recommendations tallied almost exactly with those of Porritt – quite coincidentally, one imagines – but Gillie went even further. There was to be no financial obstacle to research in general practice; there was a need for trained secretarial staff, specially taught in communication with patients, and accommodation for local authority staff on practice premises, which should be central, with separate examination rooms; there should be a common room for all.

This committee, too, had recommendations of particular importance. The first was that medical centres should be developed in all district hospitals (for use by doctors of all disciplines; a centre in which they could learn and talk together as one profession).

This proposal was first implemented by doctors, with the encouragement of the Nuffield Foundation. The second proposed that a general practice or practices should be part of each University Department of General Practice and these should be active in undergraduate and post-graduate education and research. Every entrant to general practice should have specific training for this work and many teachers and trainers throughout the field of general practice should themselves be GPs and there should be two years' vocational training for general practice. This latter concept has been implemented by stages over the years. Its purpose is to ensure that young doctors will no longer be thrown in at the deep end of general practice without first having been taught to swim. It represents tremendous progress from the days when the newly qualified left their hospitals to work in a discipline about which they knew very little, if anything at all. Such vocational training is to be enforced by statute in 1982.

Gillie completed the picture so admirably painted by Porritt, and put the varnish on it. Government and the profession now had in their possession a potentially first-class family doctor service. With the Royal Commission's proposal for a Review Body on remuneration and the enterprising proposals of Porritt and Gillie all that seemed necessary was to translate these ideas into practice so that doctors and their patients could benefit from them. Sadly, this is an over-simplification. A great deal of debating and negotiation had to follow.

The chief reason for the delayed reaction to these reports is, I think, that Porritt and Gillie were way ahead of both government and the main body of the medical profession in their thinking. They were too forward-looking to be swallowed at one gulp, with the result that, instead of implementing the recommendations in the 1960s as one package, and producing a top quality and uniform service throughout the country there and then, the Porritt-Gillie ideals have been introduced into the service piecemeal over the years with some, even now, not yet fully activated.

Putting it another (and kinder) way, what may seem obvious in 1981 was very novel – in parts almost revolutionary – in 1963. Even though opinions expressed in the reports must have resulted from verbal evidence given to the committees and from methods of practice actually seen by them during their visits round the country, the time was not yet ripe when any government or the representatives of the profession could agree to the introduction of such a service in its entirety, without further time for indoctrination and education. This democratic process, as always, takes time, but it is preferable in the long term to the dictatorial alternative – though Mr Aneurin Bevan might not have agreed with me.

The chronic inadequacy of financial resources must be taken into account here too. Yet the fact remains that there have been those in the Department of Health and in the profession who have had no doubts, since the 1960s or before, of the way in which the service should evolve and no body set up to investigate it since then has been able to suggest any variations on the original theme or any development of it, except to comment on the need for such items as more health education, audit of GP services, a more radical approach to GP prescribing and a streamlining of the NHS structure. These would hardly be earth-shattering in their impact on the family doctor service and in no sense an argument against the recommendations enunciated by the three now historic reports of the early 1960s.

That the Minister of Health (Mr Anthony, now Lord, Barber) was on the right lines in 1964 is indicated in a letter he wrote to the then chairman of the General Medical Services committee (the late Dr A. B. Davies), in which he considered that the Annis Gillie report had focused attention on many of the discontents in general practice and the time had come to consider these in detail. He suggested therefore, and it was agreed, that a working party should be set up between his department and the profession under the chairmanship of the Permanent Secretary, Sir Bruce Fraser, to consider the report and recommendations of the Annis Gillie committee and any other matters relevant to the work of the general practitioner in the NHS – a possible reference to the non-statutory Porritt committee – apart from remuneration. His object, he said, was to foster good medicine. The working party met for a whole day each week amidst high hopes that great good would result. I was a member of it and, in spite of its rather ignominious end, it was one of the best developments that ever happened, because it brought general practice, hot and first hand, bang into the department.

The department received, and returned, straight talk with

no holds barred. I remember particularly an implied criticism that the stress and strain of night calls on top of a day's work was somewhat exaggerated. One tired GP, who had just come off night duty during which he had had four calls, only one of which could be considered justifiable, spat out a reply with no regard for the usual diplomatic niceties. After a short silence an under-secretary said 'Do you really mean to say that actually happened?' He did, and it was most impressive.

On this sort of governmental working party it is customary for the two teams to sit on opposite sides of a very long table. In this case the department representatives stretched along one side and some six feet away the GPs were arrayed along the other. The very width of the table seemed to accentuate a disunity, yet we were all striving for the same objective.

I mention this arrangement, and will do so again later in relation to the Review Body, because I believe that this incident of the night calls, and the genuine anguish in the GP's voice, suddenly brought us all together. General practice burst explosively into the Department of Health, and the artificial gap between us disappeared.

So the Fraser Working party (later Fraser-France, when it was taken over by Sir Arnold France) deserved to succeed. It had decided to produce interim Commentaries and had issued four (in July 1964) on the distribution of doctors; on absences for holidays, sickness and study, and the employment of locums; on the employment and training of ancillary staff and the attachment of local Health Authority staff; and on the patients' demands on the doctor's time – this underlining for the first time that doctors were *not* obliged to see a patient whenever and wherever he or she thought fit.[5] It would, no doubt, have issued others, but time was running out.

In 1963 the Review Body recommended an increase of 14 per cent in doctors' pay. This was intended to last three years and was accepted both by government and profession. In fact, GPs received 6 per cent. Although they had not realised it at the time, they had already received part of the

14 per cent – due to the central pool and confusion between net and gross income.

This was the last straw for the family doctor and so, not for the last time, a Review Body report triggered off an explosion, and terms of service were to take precedence over conditions of service for the next few years.

7

1964 – 1968

In 1964 I became chairman of the BMA's parliament – the Representative Body. I doubt if anyone envied me such promotion, coming at this time.

The profession had submitted a new claim, for an increase of something over 30 per cent, or an average of about £900 a year for each GP, to be back-dated to 1963 and paid in addition to the 14 per cent recommended. This was the first time the Review Body had been approached about only one section of the profession. The first Special Representative meeting I had to chair (on 25 March 1964),[1] therefore, was about the Memorandum of Evidence submitted to the Review Body by the BMA.[2] The Porritt and Gillie reports were relevant to this, as were also the profession's concern about the shortage of doctors in the service and the career earnings of GPs compared with those of doctors in the hospital service.

After this there was an Annual Representative meeting in Manchester in July, which was described as a 'highly successful meeting which brought to an end one of the most turbulent and eventful years in the long history of the Association'.[3] Representatives emphasised that family doctors had reached the end of their tether and nothing short of a radical overhaul of general practice would enable them to practise medicine as they would wish – under proper conditions. This may seem to be an over-reaction. To see it in its right perspective one has to take into consideration all the stresses and strains I have described in chapter V and add to

94

these the sudden shock of what seemed to GPs (in my view, rightly) to be an inadequate Review Body report, seemingly unresponsive to the intense burden of work general practice had been carrying in the early years of the NHS.

Unfortunately, in its frustration and fury the meeting passed two resolutions: that charges for prescriptions should be retained and the policy that there should be no financial barrier between doctors and those who used their services 'should not be interpreted to preclude any form of charge to the patient for the doctors' services.' This was unfortunate wording and suggested that doctors were advocating a return to the days when patients paid for their treatment.

The BMA's apparent change of policy was regarded by the press as an attack upon the innocent patient (also an over-reaction. Some patients are certainly not innocent in their demands on the doctors' time). Mr Paul Vaughan, the Association's press officer, said that the press was bitter, discouraged, dismayed and angry [4] and *The Times* (20 July) had a leader in which it said that the change of policy was arrived at with the scantiest attention to the possible consequences. 'The BMA,' it said, 'must do better than this. . . .'[5]

In fact, some 500 doctors at the meeting were not trying to penalise the patient. They were interpreting the desperation of family doctors in the only way they could find, but they left their representatives to cope with a very difficult crisis, summed up by Dr. J. S. Happel at a BMA Council meeting, when he said that GPs were so overworked they were prepared to consider anything – even charges – to alleviate the burden at the present time.

The crisis overflowed into the House of Commons on 27 July, when there was an important debate on the family doctor service – note, family doctor, not general practitioner.[6] I must give a full account of the debate which was opened by Mr Kenneth Robinson, then in Opposition, later to be Minister of Health. He said that in his view the troubles of the family doctor were by no means entirely concentrated around the subject of pay. For many of them pay was very much a secondary issue. The reason for the acute malaise in the profession was that the GP was feeling frustrated in his wish to do a better and more significant job, to give a better service to his patients than present arrangements allowed him to do.

The anxieties were much more concerned with the method of pay than with the current level, and especially with the very much criticised arrangements for the central pool, which were so complicated that few doctors fully understood its workings, and many had hardly an inkling of them.

He then described how a general practitioner who spent more on giving a better service to his patients, on administration, on maintaining his surgery premises, on employing ancillary staff and a receptionist, on running an appointment system, and so on, got back substantially less than he spent. But there was another kind of GP, who did not worry about functioning from a shabby surgery in a back street, did not employ help, did not use an appointments system, and so on. He got back a great deal more than he spent and made a handsome profit on the deal. Mr Robinson said he had often described the situation as ludicrous.

He went on to talk of the advantages of group practice but he noted that those building their own purpose-built premises did so by subsidising the NHS out of their own pockets or could not afford to build them at all. He urged that government should accept responsibility for producing premises for group practices.

He then spoke of the threat to the GP's status within the profession. In future, he suggested, general practice must be regarded as a specialty which required special post-graduate training, which would include actually working under supervision in general practice for a period. It was an enlightened speech from one who was very soon to be in the seat of power.

Members then went on to debate certificates, prescription charges, refresher courses, the attachment of health visitors, a review of the basis of remuneration, unnecessary calls on GPs (television was accused of playing an important part in bringing people to the surgery), help with rent, rates, wages and running expenses, general practitioner annexes to new hospitals, a salaried service, the refunding of the cost of equipment, the need for more general practitioner beds in hospitals, direct access to X-ray and pathological services and one partner in a group specialising in midwifery.

It was urged that GPs should realise that their services were not being devalued and one member, Miss Joan Vickers, described doctors in the GP service as the most selfless human beings in the whole of the welfare state.

This was all good stuff and my reason for reproducing it in such detail can now be seen, for it is nearly all accepting the Porritt-Gillie recommendations. A high level of debate in which the general tone from both sides was of concern and a wish to help. But, as Mr Laurence Pavitt said, there was 'plenty of talk and plenty of tribute, but very little action'.

Mr Anthony (now Lord) Barber, Minister of Health, wound up the debate for the government. He pointed out that finding solutions to the GPs' problems was no easy matter. He had no intention of imposing a salaried service against the wishes of the profession. He was appalled at the intolerable attitude of a small minority of patients whose actions and lack of consideration suggested that they had no conception of a family doctor as a highly trained man whose hours of work and devotion to duty should of themselves invoke particular consideration. He was considering television and other ways of bringing this home to the minority of patients. He wanted to change the system of payment (the pool) so that, for instance, those doctors who employed the staff they wanted should not be at a financial disadvantage compared to those who did not.

He wanted to ease the burden on some doctors by encouraging more of them to go into what were known as under-doctored areas and fewer to go into other areas. He was leaving the question of amendments to the terms of service to the Fraser working party.

He was willing to look at any suggestions relating to interest free loans to group practices for the building or purchase and conversion of practice premises, thus encouraging doctors to co-operate by working together in group practices. Considerable progress was being made in providing direct help to GPs by attachment to them of local authority staffs, such as health visitors, district nurses and midwives. He mentioned that in Hampshire 160 family doctors had such workers attached to them. He had been told that the results were excellent.

He wanted to increase the number of GPs – the actual number required was difficult to assess; 350–400 British doctors were emigrating each year for good but only a minority of these were GPs and other doctors were immigrating from overseas. It had been decided to provide at least one new medical school, at Nottingham, together with expansion of existing schools. And so the debate ended, with the minister putting forward these seven ways of easing the burden on GPs. Ten years of Conservative government were coming to a close.

But, sadly, the nadir had not yet been reached for the Review Body's reply to the GPs' request for a pay award amounting to £18 million a year was a report recommending only £5½ million. Dr Derek Stevenson, Secretary of the BMA, said that he had never known 'such a spontaneous upsurge of resentment and anger' (11 February 1965)[7] and the General Medical Services Committee (a committee of the BMA and at the same time a statutory committee of the NHS, responsible for GP affairs) unanimously decided to ask the 23,000 GPs in the NHS to resign. The resignations, collected in bulk, were to be ready for use if negotiations with the Minister of Health (now Mr Robinson) failed. Press reaction swung right round to the side of the doctors. On 12 February the *Daily Express* called on the government to stop exploiting doctors' skills and abusing their spirit of service: 'Respectable and dedicated men are being driven to desperate action . . . they have the support of the public . . . let Mr Robinson announce immediately a new and fairer deal for British doctors.'[8] The *Daily Telegraph* pointed out that the average doctor, under the new award, would get no more than an extra penny for each consultation[9] and the Bart's hospital *Journal* said: 'Seventeen years of rumbling discontent and confused negotiations. It is hardly surprising that the general practitioner has had enough.'[10]

Nothing less than urgent action now was going to stop the family doctor service from crumbling into chaos. I was sharing in the general dejection and frustration. I felt that it was up to the profession to take the initiative and one night, alone in the house and with the help of a dog and a superb bottle of brandy recently donated by a grateful patient, I drafted what I called a Charter for General Practice which contained four basic Rights. First, to practise good medicine in company with doctors in other branches of the profession from suitable, up-to-date and convenient accommodation, properly equipped and adequately staffed by trained medical and non-medical personnel; the remuneration should be adequate to meet both the capital and current expenditure involved and should come with the minimum of interference to the independence of the contracting doctor.

Second, was the right to practise one's art to the best of one's ability, with the least possible intrusion by the state, with protection from abuse of one's services by patients and safeguards against unjustifiable and punitive litigation.

The third and fourth rights concerned a guaranteed minimum income and guaranteed financial security for the GP after retirement.

I hoped this would be a charter for the patient as well as the doctor for I stressed that our services to patients must be improved as a result of it. The BMA Council met on 27 February 1965. [11] The draft Charter was debated and, with suitable rewording of the four Rights, it was passed to the General Medical Services committee which set up a working party to consider it. Cutting an intense and exciting story very short, an approved Charter was published in the *BMJ* on 13 March 1965[12] and on 16 March the minister said he was prepared to negotiate on every single item in it except the level of remuneration. [13]

On 2 June a joint report was published of discussions between the profession and the minister. [14] The government had agreed to establish a General Practice Finance Corporation to make loans for purchase, erection and improvement of premises to be owned by doctors; to make additional finance available for employment of ancillary help (in the form of direct reimbursement of expenses incurred in the employment of staff, 75 per cent up to £500 p.a. and 50 per cent of the remainder) but excluded from this the employment of doctors' wives – and much was to follow from this restriction which GPs felt was particularly unjust; to a relaxation in sickness certification and to the negotiation of a new contract involving mutually agreed methods of payment which would enable the government to agree to the abolition of the pool. There were some additional proposals, including making deputies responsible for their own actions and the urgent necessity for incentives to encourage more doctors to practise in under-doctored areas. All the above takes us back to Porritt and Gillie. The mills of the NHS were grinding slowly towards the desired objectives.

It was mentioned in the last chapter that the Fraser working party came to an ignominious end. It was overtaken by the crisis I have just described and it passed peacefully away. Nevertheless, the profession owed a lot to it.

Twenty-eight million pounds was estimated as being necessary for the full implementation of the Review Body's recommendations in its next (seventh) report, [15] involving about a one-third increase in aggregate net income. This precipitated the next crisis for the government. Whilst agreeing that special consideration of workload and manpower in general practice justified an exceptionally large increase in remuneration, in the light of economic difficulties and its current policy on prices and incomes, it could not implement an increase 'of such magnitude' in a single step. It therefore proposed an immediate payment of half the full amount retrospectively from 1 April 1966, increasing net income by rather more than 15 per cent, with the full amount being paid with effect from 1 April 1967. This was known as 'phasing' and a scheme was devised (reluctantly approved by the profession) of how it was to be done.

Although GPs in all good faith and, mindful of the economic situation, had agreed to the phasing of their award the money had not been paid by 20 July when – exactly eleven weeks after this agreement – the Prime Minister, Mr (now Sir Harold) Wilson, called for a six-month standstill on wages, salaries and other types of income, followed by a further six months of severe restraint.

It takes severe restraint on my part, even after a decade, to describe what followed this announcement. We were well and truly caught, with no award at all. We literally demanded an interview with the Prime Minister and he agreed to see us on 1 August (1966). I had now been translated to the chair of the BMA Council and I knew that part of this job was going to be to head various delegations to see ministers about the problems of all types of doctors, but I had not bargained on an intensive argument with the Prime Minister so soon after my appointment.

He took the whole weight of our attack upon himself and, to my recollection, did not once refer for help from the Minister of Health or any of his other advisers. When we accused him of treating doctors worse than anyone else he sharply came back with three others who were worse off. He forgot the third for a moment but, refusing help, remembered that it was the electrical engineers. We charged him with not giving a thought to young doctors and he said that only that morning he had told young seamen how much better off they were than young doctors.

Our experts, chairmen of committees responsible for hospital doctors, GPs, Medical Officers of Health and others, each threw questions at him yet he seemed to have all the answers. Our case was too strong for us to be defeated, but he had everything to lose for it was vital that we should not be allowed to breach the pay standstill, because if the doctors did others would follow. He could not stop any action we might take but he could – and did – make it clear to us how dangerous the situation was.

He said that it was not the intention that anyone should suffer a net loss as a result of the freeze but he was determined that none should be excepted from it. He did, then, make one very important gesture to us for he said that if we would accept the standstill he for his part would ensure that after the six months the award would be honoured. This we were not to tell the profession. I asked how he thought I and my colleagues could sell the freeze to doctors and not be able to tell them of his assurances. He was adamant.

When we left the Prime Minister we went with the Minister of Health, Mr Kenneth Robinson, to his room. During the course of the meeting I said that if the PM did not keep his word at the end of six months the Minister's position would be 'somewhat difficult'. Mr Robinson said he would resign. It was this assurance that helped us to come to our eventual decision, but this took hours and hours of worried discussion.

Following the acceptance of the freeze by the profession, a meeting Dr Stevenson, secretary of the BMA, and I had with the Minister on 22 September was widely reported in the press.[16] Doctors were particularly furious that Clydeside shipworkers had been allowed to break the freeze on the grounds that a 'substantial proportion' had already received rises. We asked for similar action for doctors. It was denied us. In a confidential letter sent to 70,000 doctors after this, Dr Stevenson said 'It must now be apparent to every doctor that as a profession we are increasingly subjected to political considerations.'

The details of the new pay structure from 1 October were issued at the end of the month and on 22 November the Minister confirmed that 1 April could be the operative date for the second phase of the new pay scheme.

Meanwhile, GPs still waited for the implementation of improvements in the service first mooted ten years before. This was bad enough for the GP in his surgery. For those who, in addition, were everlastingly struggling to attain our objectives, it is a wonder to me that we were able to fight on without doing ourselves permanent mental or physical damage (or both).

To be fair, Mr Kenneth Robinson, the Minister of Health who had to bear the brunt of government actions and the profession's rage, deserved (and had) our sympathy. He genuinely wanted the improvements we were seeking and must have shared our frustrations.

Now for some other important activities of the 1960s.

Owing to the generosity of the Nuffield Foundation, money was made available to the Wessex Regional Hospital

Board for building post-graduate medical and dental centres in certain hospital groups in the region. Centres were flourishing in Kingston and Portsmouth when, in 1963, it was decided to build one in Winchester. We were asked for subscriptions to help to provide the library and 'certain internal furnishings'. This was, of course, to prove an immense boon, particularly to GPs who could meet all their colleagues from other disciplines there and join them in social parties, at clinical meetings or in the bar. This was the professional centre first mentioned by Gillie. With it went the appointment of clinical tutors in all hospital groups where centres were being built.

In the same year I asked the Nuffield Provincial Hospital Trust to support a scheme for training receptionists and secretaries in general practice. Eventually they turned me down but I was rescued by the regional advisor to the Postgraduate Medical Federation, Dr Donald Bowie, who suggested I should try the Hampshire education authority.

To my delight, the Education Officer, Mr R. M. Marsh and the Principal of Eastleigh Technical College, Mr F. Bloor, strongly supported the idea, so we set about arranging a three-term course for receptionists and a four-term course for secretaries, under the guidance of the head of the household arts department, Miss E. M. Malpas. Dr Michael Drury was working on similar lines in Bromsgrove and we linked up. The BMA Council then agreed to a loan of £2,000 to help inaugurate an Association of Medical Secretaries.

There are four particular points to note here: first, that this was done without any state backing; secondly, too many girls opted for working in hospitals, presumably because of shorter and more fixed hours; thirdly, we hoped by getting trained non-medical staff into practices we might raise the standard of service to patients, if only by teaching GPs how to organise or, perhaps, how NOT to organise their work; and lastly, that although I have described this effort in a few sentences, I had two heavy files full of evidence, memoranda and correspondence.

In other words, no matter how many committees and

individuals support a concept which is increasingly seen to be necessary, its practical application involves months of painstaking effort and prolonged debate, most of which has to be repeated if, later, a government department is involved.[17] [18] And then, of course, one has to sell it to a profession of individualists which is traditionally suspicious of any innovation, fearing that it may come between them and the treatment of their patients.

In 1965 a Royal Commission was set up under Lord Todd to review undergraduate and post-graduate medical education in Great Britain. It reported in 1968, after over a hundred meetings.[19]

The BMA set up a committee to prepare evidence for the Royal Commission under the chairmanship of Sir John (now Lord) Richardson.[20] I was on this committee and, with Dr John Happel (a rural GP and also a member), wrote a paper on vocational training for general practice and continuing education for the family doctor.

The bibliography we quoted ranged from 1948 (*The Training of a Doctor* – Cohen)[21] to 1962 (*Training for General Practice* – RCGP),[22] seventeen references in all. Yet we were still only writing about it, although since 1948 an increasing number of practices were accepting a voluntary teaching role, unpaid. The BMA evidence to the commission (published in 1966) included forty-three recommendations.

Two years later, in a 404-page report, the Royal Commission gave general practice a great deal of what it wanted: it commented on the fact that group practice within general practice was becoming increasingly common, enabling doctors within the group to develop a personal interest in a particular branch or aspect of medicine; that general practice will be (note the tense!) a satisfying and challenging *specialty*, aided by proper diagnostic services, ancillary staff and efficient practice organisation; that the GP would play a responsible part in the hospital and other health services and be recognised as a specialist in his or her own right by virtue of unique and essential contributions to medical care; that every undergraduate medical student should be given an insight into general practice when he or she should see patients presenting new symptoms to the doctor for the first time and learn how decisions have to be made at this stage; that universities should offer senior academic appointments in general practice, and GPs teaching students should be properly paid and given university status.

The four years from 1964 to 1968 came near to cutting the ground from under the constructive efforts of the Royal Commission, the Porritt and Gillie committees and the Fraser-France working party. The reason was, of course, that few of the recommendations of these bodies had yet been translated to practical effect in helping the over-burdened GP in his surgery. While committees were sitting, doctors were working – and it was not until the fateful Review Body report of 1963 was misconstrued that tired doctors found a peg on which to hang their frustrated weariness.

8

1968 – 1970

As we approach the 1970s it is impossible not to dwell for a while on medico-politics (defined very simply as 'money and Terms and Conditions of Service'). The professional life of the GP since the National Health Service Act has been so much at the mercy of medico-political forces that digressions from the consulting room to the corridors of power in London are inevitable, particularly since every decision made in London has had some impact, good or bad, on doctors, nurses and patients throughout the country.

Previous chapters have shown that during the early years of the NHS it was by means of self-imposed and voluntary adaptations to their methods of practice that some doctors were able to improve their service to patients and this had two distinct disadvantages: it brought about a varying standard of practice from area to area and it involved the more forward-looking GPs in having to dip their hands into their own pockets to pay for the improvements they needed to give them greater satisfaction in their work and be of benefit to their patients.

Examples of such initiatives include the up-grading of group practice premises, the employment of receptionists, the setting up of appointment systems, the attachment of health visitors, nurses and midwives to particular practices from the local authority and the acceptance of medical and para-medical students for training in general practice. To this incomplete list can be added the provision of relatively ex-

106

pensive office and medical equipment at no cost to the state.

General practice can, of course, be carried on from premises akin to mud and wattle huts with corrugated iron roofs and Yale locks to limit the hours of service. I have seen such premises. Patients can be admitted by the doctor's wife, seated on wooden benches in the hall and treated in a dining room boasting a saucepan, one syringe and a virtually non-existent filing system. This, too, has been described and cynics would say that nothing better was required of doctors by the state under the NHS Act.

If this truly had constituted an adequate primary health care service this book would not have been written and the service today would be the disappointment it threatened to be in the 1950s. The fact that it is not is due to the determined initiative and enterprise of a number of GPs who refused to accept such conditions and set out *on their own* to raise the standard of their practices, even though this involved them in a considerable sacrifice.

Yet they could not be left on their own. If everyone throughout the country was to gain from new projects of proven value and if doctors were to be able to graft them permanently onto their pattern of practice, statutory recognition and support was necessary. Hence the need for the medico-politician.

It is naïve, indeed, to believe that improvements in the service are achieved by a single visit to the Minister of Health. On the contrary, new concepts have to be referred to committees, submitted to conferences, discussed with civil servants and only then negotiated with whoever happens to be in the seat of power, right or left of the political centre. At any stage along this tedious and frustrating journey there may be a hold-up, set-back or even flat rejection of what up until then had seemed a wholly desirable proposition. Moreover, after all that, an outcome unacceptable to the profession can result in a situation verging on mutiny and a collapse of the service (as will be seen in chapter 9).

Medico-politics is a dirty word to most doctors and some even go so far as to hold in contempt those who dabble in it. A successful achievement of their aspirations is accepted as an act of God. Failure is due to the amateur and ill-conceived efforts of those doctors who, in a moment of weakness, were mistakenly elected to represent them.

I do not resent this attitude. I think it is healthy for academics and practising doctors to be able to go peacefully about their business without being troubled by extramural arguments. Yet, dirty word or not, the history of family doctoring since the beginning of the NHS is in great part medico-political in content and, much as I regret the possibility of boring some of my readers and losing the attention of others, I am forced to immerse myself more deeply in the interface between government and the profession, for we are now entering an era in which crisis followed crisis – each in turn threatening the life of the GP in his surgery.

The turmoil began in 1968, for it was in that year that a committee set up by the government in 1965 under the chairmanship of Mr Frederic (now Lord) Seebohm to review the organisation and responsibilities of the local authority personal and social services in England and Wales, and to consider what changes were desirable to secure an effective family service, produced its report,[1] and it was also in 1968 that the Secretary of State for Health and Social Security published a Green Paper on the reform of the NHS administration.[2]

The Seebohm Committee, on which health was grossly under-represented, recommended a new local authority department, providing a community-based and family-oriented service which would be available to all.

The new department will have responsibilities going beyond those of existing local authority departments, but they will include the present services provided under the National Assistance Act 1948, educational and child welfare services, the home help service, mental health social services, other social work services provided by health departments; day nurseries and certain social welfare work currently undertaken by some housing authorities.

So health was to be divided from welfare as by a brick wall. Far from the whole patient being cared for through one department and by one unified caring team, there were to be two departments, each with half a whole patient and with one calling its particular half a client. The committee wanted a 'unified provision of personal social services' but based their recommendations on the premise that health and welfare were two separate entities, with little overlap or common interest, although they conceded that there was a need for a good health service.

This could not be taken lying down for it was completely at variance with the concept of total care of the whole patient by a closely integrated, caring team working under one roof and under the overall umbrella of one authority, thus requiring local authority social workers to work as closely as possible with family doctors and certain services to be provided by the area on a domiciliary basis at the request of the family doctor (to help him in his care of the patient), including the ambulance services, nurses and midwives, health visitors and medical social workers, social and mental welfare officers, psychiatric social workers, physiotherapists and home helps.

Mr Crossman was now the Secretary of State for Health and Social Security and he was darting about like a young trout in the best of chalk streams. If he knew where he was going we certainly did not and I doubt whether his own staff did either. We had to re-orientate our whole approach in trying to anticipate his next move.

We saw him weekly at the Department of Health, negotiating for what we knew doctors needed in the health service and what could not be lost to the proposed new local authority social service departments. We were seeing the Associations of County Councils and of Municipal Corporations too, in an hotel somewhere in London – so was he, in the DHSS. It was all supposed to be very secret. We were probing around trying to get their agreement and seeing how far they would go to help us. I suppose he was trying to work out how much he dare give us without offending them (and vice versa).

In particular, we fought to keep health visitors, home helps, psychiatric social workers and other vital people within the health service. Once the Permanent Secretary, Sir Alan Marre, asked me why I was so hot under the collar about having everyone under one roof. I could not persuade even him that if they were only next door they might as well be miles away from the point of view of total care.

In spite of our efforts, we lost on nearly all counts, although it was agreed that nurses, midwives and health visitors should not be transferred to the social service departments. I think we knew we had lost when Mr Crossman said plaintively, 'But I *must* give the local authorities something.' We were not thinking of it in terms of gifts (or even votes).

I was feeling increasingly bitter and disenchanted; after all, five minutes after I left the train following each visit to him, I was in a patient's house working as a family doctor; I knew what I, and I hope all doctors, needed for that patient. I could not reconcile this with using the patient as a sort of gift voucher to be torn in two pieces – one bit as a client of local government and one as a patient of the NHS. If ever there was a time when our wish for a health service divorced from politics was fully justified, this was it.

The saga did not finish here for later I shall describe the practical effects on the family doctor of the implementation of the Seebohm report, with some belated comments on it by Mr Crossman in 1973.

At the same time as we were discussing Seebohm we had to cope with the minister's Green Paper on the reform of the NHS. A Green Paper, as opposed to a White one, is a consultative document which all concerned in running the service can debate amongst themselves and then submit their comments to the minister. A special working party was set up to bring the report of the Medical Services Review Committee (Porritt) up to date and to study all other relevant reports on the structure of the NHS. This reported to the BMA Council in June 1968.[3]

A Special Representative meeting of doctors of all disciplines was called for 31 January 1969.[4] Thirteen major principles were presented to the meeting for debate. These included a reiteration of precepts unchanged since the NHS was first mooted: service to the community had first priority; the family doctor's independent contractor status, with freedom of choice between patient and doctor, and absolute confidentiality between patient and doctor must be maintained and the clinical independence of the family doctor ensured. Repeated references in this book to these cardinal principles may seem unnecessary but a tacit acceptance of them is not enough. They need to be constantly underlined, for an attack on any one of them would have a profound effect on the status and working conditions of the GP.

In addition, the conference considered that there must be satisfactory provision for medical education and research, especially in areas where medical schools were located; it emphasised that the chief administrative officer must be medically qualified and it urged that adequate finance be provided for each branch of the service. In other words, so far as general practice was concerned, it must be ensured a fair share of the financial cake.

With particular reference to the Seebohm report, it resolved that there must be medical supervision of all social work with a predominantly health content and purpose – sadly, a pious hope.

Since the objective of the Green Paper was to produce a service in which there was administrative unity, the doctors affirmed that providing adequate safeguards on their major points of principle were obtained, they would support unification of NHS administration but they considered that the main proposals enunciated in the government's Green Paper were unacceptable. So ended the short life of the first Green Paper. We were promised a second one and Mr Crossman arranged a working party to prepare an alternative set of proposals.

In 1968 the Standing Medical Advisory Committee of the Central Health Services Council set up a sub-committee to review the working and organisation of group practice, with particular reference to health centres. The chairman was Dr Harvard Davis, Senior Lecturer in General Practice at the Welsh National School of Medicine.

In February 1970, the Report of the Royal Commission on Local Government in England (the Redcliffe-Maud Report) was published.[5] This contained a suggestion that reorganised local authorities might become responsible for all aspects of the NHS in their areas. This had always been absolutely against our declared principles. We could not view with any confidence the possibility of the health service becoming a pawn in the local political game and we feared the creation of different standards of service between one authority and another. Also, with money for the health service included in the bulk grant to local authorities we suspected that they might succumb to the temptation of giving it a place on their list of priorities below education, housing and roads – especially when local elections were imminent. Fortunately, we need not have worried, for the government failed to implement this part of the Redcliffe-Maud Report.

In the 1960s there were other important developments which had an impact on general practice, including: therapeutic abortion; cervical cytology; metric medicine; the drinking driver; drug dependence, linked with irresponsible prescribing, and Britain's entrance into the EEC.

All through the decade there had been calls for the retention of cottage hospitals and for GPs to play a part in the care of their patients in hospital. In our practice we had clinical assistantships in the district hospital which were of great value to the individual doctor and, through him, to the group. They were a help too in keeping us in touch with our hospital colleagues, and vice versa.

There was also a continuing cry for GP maternity beds in district hospitals or in any new maternity hospitals, with open access to physiotherapy departments.

So far as my practice was concerned we were bulging at the seams. We had come a long way since 1960: six partners plus vocational trainees and student attachments; helping to train receptionists, entertaining overseas visitors, holding regular seminars with psychiatrist colleagues; acting as hosts and working with nurses, midwives, health visitors and their students. All this led to the inevitable, yet sad, conclusion

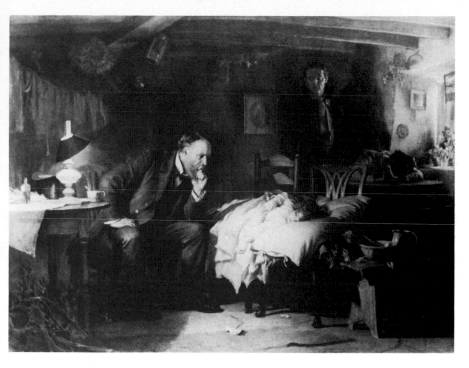

12 'The Doctor', painting by Luke Fildes, R.A. *(photograph loaned by Dr Trevor Hughes)*

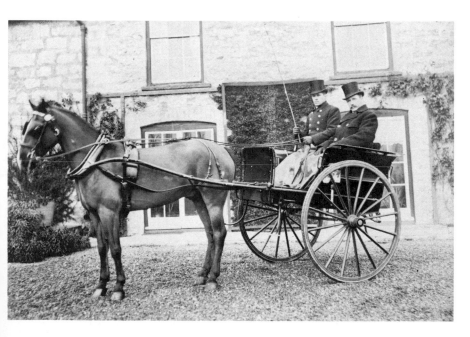

13 A country doctor's carriage, with coachman in livery *(photograph loaned by Dr Trevor Hughes)*

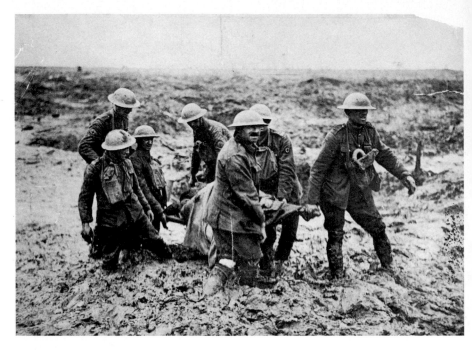

14 A stretcher party in World War I *(Mansell Collection)*

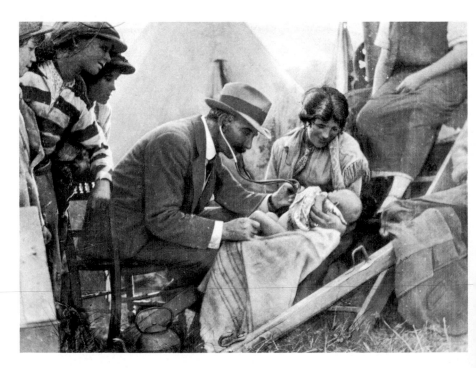

15 A doctor examining a baby in a gypsy camp *(Mansell Collection)*

that we must find new premises. There was no suitable site in the city on which we could build. Eventually, during a Sunday evening party, I asked our County MOH (Dr Ivor MacDougall) if he would consider building us a health centre. He said of course he would, for all doctors who wanted to work in it. And he did – but that, too, with all its complications, comes into the 1970s.

A great deal had been achieved in this decade. General practice was now established as an important discipline in its own right. The service was now geared to encouraging a high standard, with special training being considered for those opting for family doctoring as their life's work. So we could move into the 1970s with a certain amount of confidence for the future of family doctoring, but I am afraid there is considerable medico-political activity still to come.

Some patients and problems

God and the doctor we alike adore
But only when in danger, not before;
The danger o'er, both are alike requited,
God is forgotten, and the doctor slighted.

John Owen
Epigrams

When a young recruit to general practice sees the crowd waiting for his first appointment session, he may find it necessary to glance out of the window to make sure there are still some healthy people walking about in the streets. His first impression may well be that the entire available population has turned up in the surgery to welcome him.

At this point he can comfort himself with the thought that not everyone in the waiting room is necessarily sick, at least not in his sense of the word. The alternative is to take one look at his list and make a dash for freedom!

The first group of patients he will learn to recognise are the 'club members'. They are there for various reasons: because they are lonely and have nowhere else to go, have been shopping, are exchanging symptoms with another patient or are part of a self-appointed welcoming committee, there to see whether they approve of the new recruit to the practice. Such approbation, incidentally, will not be given until he has been fully tried and tested, although good looks and a pleasant smile may, of course, help to create a favourable impression. The fact that they are club members and there mainly for social reasons should in no way diminish the attention they receive or be viewed as a source of irritation. Often they will leave with a prescription for some medication which both they and the doctor know is quite unnecessary and they will usually expect to be invited back for a further appointment. Club members should not be discouraged. Any nuisance value they have can be minimised by a good receptionist, who will give them an appointment on a slack day or at the beginning of a session, and the amount of time they take can be gauged to the half minute, for they have a keen sense of custom and know precisely how long their appointment is to last. Being quite capable of reading the appointment book upside down, they rarely overstay their welcome.

The occasional suggestion that they should undergo an examination comes as a welcome surprise to them – and the results sometimes not so welcome a surprise to the doctor. It is usually kind to give notice of an examination, so they can be freshly bathed and appropriately arrayed.

Similar to this category, but not necessarily of it, are the chronic hypochondriacs, the tireless grumblers who genuinely think they are sick, though no one else believes them. These are a menace – they know no rules and would not obey them if they did. They have to be on some doctor's list and to reject them merely invites a neighbouring doctor to reject one of his in retaliation – a swop that may be a relief at the start, but is pointless in the long term.

The one consolation is that relatives and neighbours are on the doctor's side and sympathetic towards him. In return, he has to realise that whilst he suffers for ten minutes or so once a month, they get it all day long. If they recommend that the patient comes to see him from time to time, it is usually a sign that they need some time off. Here again, a good receptionist will wangle as long an interval as possible between their visits.

Next are the genuinely chronic sick, who need to be seen regularly for assessment and for topping up or monitoring their medication. It is amazing how many of these there are, but appointment sessions can be shortened if the partnership team runs special clinics for diabetics, hypertensives, the young, the elderly and the handicapped. If no such clinics are available, up to three-quarters of a session may have to be given over to chronic patients.

There is an understandable tendency to resent the amount of time patients of this kind take up on a busy day. I have sometimes been guilty of resentment myself, but young doctors should beware of any such feelings and must always encourage rather than deter visits from the truly chronic sick.

A monthly list is an important part of primary care, whether it involves surgery or home visits. I sadly admit that with increasing pressure of work the first appointments to be postponed were the chronics, particularly the elderly. Yet I have no doubt at all, and never had, that one of the most useful jobs I did in general practice was to keep a regular watch on the chronic sick or those who by reason of age or infirmity were most at risk.

Just seeing them was quite often sufficient, for their

appearance or their conversation almost always indicated whether there was or was not any need for a fuller examination or for closer and more frequent supervision by the practice nurse or health visitor.

No one busy GP is able to keep tabs on every patient 'at risk', but he can at least try. It is a sign of failure when a patient who should have been seen regularly presents a condition that might well have been avoided. The growing tendency to let chronic, 'at risk' patients decide for themselves when they should next come to see the doctor or to leave it until a crisis makes a visit essential is to my mind retrograde and regrettable. It goes against the basic principles of primary health care. It may be time-consuming and tedious to keep a regular eye on chronic patients, but in the long term it undoubtedly justifies itself over and over again.

It is necessary for doctors to be ill themselves for them to realise the true value of a family doctor. Even if he only sits and talks or is able to bring in the right specialist, he is unique and there is no one who can replace him. From the patient's point of view, with the burden of chronic illness, advancing years or loneliness it becomes even more imperative to have on call a doctor who is known and trusted. There is never a stage when a GP can 'do nothing' to help them. Just being there accounts for much.

Next comes the group of psychiatric patients. There will be at least one, possibly two, at each session. As with other patients, their illnesses vary in degree, but they have two particular features: they need more time than other patients and their problems are, in the main, insoluble.

The GP shares the care of these patients with the psychiatrist. If the GP has the time to spare he can frequently do well for this type of patient on his own, especially if he can manage to avoid some of the powerful drugs to which these patients are sometimes exposed. But time to talk is essential, a great deal of time coupled with patience, sympathy and understanding.

Although these patients can be helped so much by GPs with the right disposition and dogged determination, enough time for them cannot be found within the normal working day. I have described how in our partnership we co-operated with three psychiatrists and a psychiatric social worker, all acting in an honorary (unpaid) capacity. The patients were seen after hours; the overall problems were discussed by the team once a month in our common room after 8 p.m. with the result that the patient and family were all under care. It was ideal. We learned an enormous amount from the psychiatrists; they seemed to enjoy seeing patients at our level and, of course, the benefit to the patient was immeasurable. There was an unexpected spin-off too. With members of the team working so closely together it was easy to talk about other patients not under team care, even if it was only to ask advice over the phone or beg a visit from a specialist at a particularly awkward moment, followed by a second visit without question of fee.

Yet it all petered out, partly because of our embarrassment at taking up so much specialist time without being able to offer any reward (although no complaint came from them). But more particularly, I fear, because the GPs were just too tired to go on giving up the very little spare time they had even for such a worthy cause.[1]

What the scheme really taught us was how much time these patients needed and by comparison how inadequate our normal treatment was. Yet, short of having one partner doing little else but psychiatry and referring all our cases to him there was no alternative but to revert to the ten-minute surgery appointment, occasionally augmented for new patients by special timeless appointments on a Saturday or Sunday morning or a half day.

Although we each had our 'special' interests (skin diseases, adolescence, physical medicine), to give over whole days to one group of patients would mean ceasing to be a GP and becoming a sort of pseudo-specialist, and that was not why we were in general practice.

This experiment of ours demonstrates clearly how even the most well-meaning and industrious GP cannot expect to cope adequately with all his psychiatric cases. As a result the GP finds himself referring them to the specialist not so much because he needs to or wants to, but because he has to. And nothing can be worse for this kind of patient than this sort of treatment.

A very important group of patients which must be allowed to take up a great deal of the GP's time is those who are suffering from stress and strain. They are not psychotics, hysterics or, necessarily, inadequate personalities and they are not to be confused with those who come in for a certificate to back up absence from work in favour of bed, the races or a grandmother's funeral. Not even the GP can remove the cause of their symptoms, which could be summed up in one word as worry, and the young doctor may wonder if his medical degree is not being wasted by spending hours dealing with the effect on his patients of having to live in a 'developed' country.

Certainly in the short time I was in practice before the war I do not remember having to deal very often with what I call the stress syndrome, but nowadays it is too much in evidence. I mention this group for two reasons: to plead that they be given as much of the doctor's time as possible, spread over more than one visit, and to emphasise how necessary it is not to be put off by the initial presentation, which is rarely straightforward.

A few will frankly admit at once that there is nothing wrong with them except that they are worn out or 'can't go on' and they are visiting the doctor, somewhat ashamedly, because they hope he may have some miracle cure to help them. The majority, however, will present any one of many possible symptoms, ranging from a headache to pain in the chest, dyspepsia before or after meals, irregular periods, skin irritation or insomnia, to mention only a few. That is why a second visit is so necessary, and a simple question such as 'what is really wrong?' or 'why have you really come to see me?' can open the floodgates.[2]

These patients, usually middle-aged, represent the main reason why doctors are so often accused of prescribing unnecessary sedatives, tranquillisers and hypnotics. Whilst it is wrong to prescribe such drugs in vast numbers or continuously over many months, how else can they deal with these patients? The doctor can talk, advise, issue a certificate for a period of rest, contact other members of the team to see whether anything more permanent can be done to help and remind the patient that he is always there if needed. But he cannot change the scene outside the surgery in which his patients are living and working. He may not be able to do anything more than remove them temporarily from it, but he has a tremendous responsibility because there is no one else to help at this stage. If GPs ignored the needs of this group, the effect on society as a whole could be catastrophic. Neither the government nor the public are fully aware of how much work of this type a GP has to do. Since no one can effectively act as a substitute for him and no one can remove the cause of the symptoms, he deserves all the support society can give him and some recognition of why so many of his patients are being doped with tranquillisers or sleeping tablets.

Then there are adolescents. They are not often seen in the surgery. If they are, it must be assumed that it is only after hours of worry on their part or persuasion by the family. A sudden impulse may have urged them to come to see the doctor, who represents to them just another form of adult discipline. Most adolescents, even though their appearance may sometimes be off-putting, are very good patients once they get to know the doctor. At first they may be incoherent and sometimes seem aggressive or unco-operative. The doctor needs to have time to spare to talk to them and to explain what he thinks is wrong and what he proposes to do about it.

A few are antisocial and badly behaved. They give their age group a bad reputation. These are more likely to become involved with the police, the welfare or probation services before they reach the GP. If, by good fortune, the GP gets to them and their family first, he can do a lot to prevent further trouble, even if only in a supporting role. It is sometimes difficult to arrange, but if young people can be seen out of turn and have time spent on them, the result may be singularly rewarding and the GP can find he has made a friend for ever. To keep them waiting or send them away too soon may result in never seeing them again.[3]

The final group is made up of acute patients, sometimes rare visitors to the doctor with textbook diseases.

These are the GP's life-savers. He may go several days before he sees one. When he does, he lavishes all his enthusiasm and expertise on them. Time ceases to matter. A five-minute appointment can stretch to thirty or forty minutes. The waiting queue fades from conscience. At least, for a few minutes, he feels like a real doctor.

Nothing is too much trouble for the patient who is in obvious need – full examinations, every conceivable investigation, visits from specialists to the home, jealous guarding from colleagues in case they sniff out that he has an interesting case and sneak in a visit when he is off duty. He deserves such a patient from time to time. He works so hard as a priest and social worker that he feels he merits the occasional opportunity to act as a doctor.

It is the sheer variety of patients that makes general practice so exciting. GPs, more than any other section of society, know that no two people are alike. No two people ever deal in the same way with similar symptoms. If there were only one type of patient or if they all arrived with a diagnosis already attached to them, half the fun would have gone.

It is such a responsible job too, caring for the whole patient; and, if help is needed, steering them to the right second opinion in time. In my own practice, even in the few groups I have mentioned, I have come across diseases varying from the non-existent right through the whole spectrum to the disguised and neglected – and have prescribed all sorts of treatment, from the orthodox to the entirely unexpected and unrecorded.

The variety of different types of specialist and hospital is so bewildering that, but for referral from general practitioners, specialists would largely be unemployed and hospitals uninhabited. It is a sobering thought: one man with all that choice to make – and he is wide open to criticism if he makes one mistake, from 'My dear, he never even looked at me' to 'I can't think why he didn't refer you to me before.'

The variety of people he has to deal with also makes

tolerance an essential quality in any doctor. There is no place in medicine for politics or class distinction.

What I mean by politics is easily illustrated by my own experience when it was proposed to build a hotel near Winchester Cathedral. One half of the population deplored the near-desecration of this ancient building; the other half applauded the replacement of an untidy car park by a well-designed hotel. During this local civil war visits to patients became fraught with danger. Wherever I went on my rounds I found myself obliged to listen but I was careful never to nod or shake my head at the wrong moment, nor to give the impression that I agreed or disagreed. To disagree erects a barrier between patient and doctor. To agree may please one patient, but upset the next who has heard on the grapevine that the doctor's views are contrary to his. Personal friendships can be destroyed by this sort of crisis. It is not worth risking the doctor-patient relationship as well.

As to class, good health cannot be bought and disease is no respecter of persons. It is the patient's approach to illness that matters. The true man (or woman) emerges when fighting illness. The duke and the dustman look much the same without their clothes on. A doctor needs to know his patient's character and personality. Indeed, knowledge of a patient's character can be crucial in determining how to handle a disease.

I recall the dignity with which a patient in a gardener's cottage coped with pulmonary TB, helped by a loving and untiring wife who relied on relatives to do the cleaning and shopping. At the top of the long drive in the big house his employer had inoperable cancer. There was a butler to admit me, a sweeping staircase, a vast bedroom and nurses in attendance night and day. But that is where the difference stopped, for the squire and the gardener were equally trusting and uncomplaining. They had different political views and were poles apart in terms of social class, but if they had been in adjacent beds you could not have told one from the other.

Like lightning, illness and misfortune strike everyone, without distinction. One day the new GP may get blasted out of her Ladyship's house because she has contracted shingles and cannot be cured in time for Ascot. Next day he may be threatened with a knife by an illiterate and aggressive labourer for suggesting that his girlfriend's pregnancy cannot be terminated in two days.

When I entered general practice, it was usual to talk to relatives downstairs before going up to the patient and to have another chat before leaving. It was expected and much valued. Nowadays, it can be up the stairs hoping one will not see anyone on the way, a quick examination accompanied by the minimum of conversation, down the stairs at top speed, out into the car and straight on to the next patient. Relatives, cowering in the sitting room not daring to interrupt this lightning assault, have no recourse other than to ask the patient 'what did he say?' If shortage of time makes the five-minute visit necessary, the doctor should be prepared as an alternative to make himself available to relatives if they phone or ask to see him at the surgery.

Patients much prefer the old-fashioned approach and do not understand the breakneck steeplechase that has replaced it. Some, even if they cannot really afford it, pay to see their doctor privately, not because they want to jump the queue, but because they value a precious ceremony not available on the NHS.

The question is, should patients and relatives be taught not to ask questions – or should young doctors as part of their vocational training be taught the importance of courtesy and concern? Nowadays it is a rewarding experience to find a young trainee doctor who does not have to be *taught* about the traditions of patient-visiting and who has that inborn instinct for caring, giving the appearance of having all the time in the world for each patient no matter how far away they live or how busy he is.

I must mention two more aspects of a GP's life – both very important and complex ones.

The first is the care of the dying, a subject which deeply affects the GP. When talk is of the dying, thoughts at once fly to the elderly. But young and middle-aged people can die and the emotional strain on the family and the family doctor is infinitely greater in these cases.

The subject of Euthanasia is relevant to the care of the dying. The Shorter Oxford Dictionary defines it as 'a quiet and easy death; and the means of procuring this'. A working party of the BMA's Board of Science defined it as meaning 'a good death' or 'gentle, easy death', but Euthanasia nowadays has unfortunately come to mean the deliberate termination of the life of a person suffering from a distressing irremediable disease. 'Voluntary Euthanasia,' the BMA report says, 'implies that an adult person of sane mind has expressed an informed wish for Euthanasia.' Euthanasia, therefore, means killing.[4]

Every doctor in his time has helped patients to die. Doctors do not talk about the subject even among themselves, and that is how it should be. Nor can non-medical people fully understand the complexity of a problem which highlights more than any other the danger of trying to persuade two and two to make four in a medical situation.

The thoughtful and sensitive debate in the House of Lords on 12 February 1976 (following previous debates in 1936, 1950 and 1969) acknowledged that the care of the dying is one of the most emotive and complicated subjects in which the medical profession is deeply involved.[5]

The definition of incurable, the fallibility of medical diagnosis and progress in the treatment of diseases previously described as hopeless all have to be considered in this context. No two cases are alike and no two cases follow the same course.

It is the doctor, and only the doctor, who must take the ultimate responsibility for each stage in the achievement of a quiet and easy death. I cannot accept that there is any place or any need for legislation. However, there is a case for more understanding, for the education of undergraduates and vocational trainees specifically in the care of the dying and for family doctors and their caring teams to be prepared to accept the intensive and often harassing programme of care involved.

My advice to a young doctor is, first, do not take on the care of a dying patient (especially a young patient, where the grief and stress is so much greater) if you believe you may not be able to give the case the attention that may be demanded; assess the whole situation carefully before agreeing, do not become so emotionally involved with a patient that your own judgement may be disturbed and, once having embarked on a programme of care, do not be deflected from it except after close consultation with the caring team – which should include the family.

Considerations must include the environment, the make-up of the family, the voluntary help available and the agreement of other members of the caring team – nurses, in particular, should be fully consulted. The ideal is a situation in which the patient, the relatives and the caring team work together from day to day, coping with each new symptom as it arises, supporting and helping for as long as necessary. And it must be accepted that the whole process may break down at any minute. The relatives may be the first to crack, particularly if there are children in the house; any member of the team may find it impossible to carry on; the household may break down – the home help, the friends who are doing the shopping, the cooking, or sitting in from time to time. So hospital care may suddenly be needed and this is not difficult to arrange if a hospital consultant is already in close contact with the team.

Nevertheless, if ill patients who know that they are dying want to end their days in their own bed under their own roof and surrounded by their own family, they have a *right* to do so and to expect help from their doctor. Indeed, the care of the dying, more than anything else, can test and prove the value of the concept of total care.

The second question to confront the new GP, often to be repeated during the course of his professional life, is 'should a doctor tell?' This particularly applies to patients who are suffering from an incurable disease or are dying.

Here again, there is so often an oversimplification of a very difficult problem by non-medical authorities, who tend to answer yes or no without qualification. Discussions, articles in the non-medical press, talks on television or radio – some misguided and ill-informed, some responsible and

126

well-intentioned – tell doctors how to cope with these patients. None of these people are dying themselves and they have rarely had the experience of caring for a patient or his family other than in a non-medical capacity. They may acknowledge that doctors are dealing with an extremely complex and difficult decision, yet they expect his answer always to be either black or white for they are unaware of the vast grey area in between.

The truth is that there is no easy answer. But there are useful guidelines and well-tried procedures that can help a doctor decide what or how much he tells a patient. To start with, assessment and diagnosis in hospital can be a great help – subject to certain important provisos.

First, the decision to tell or not to tell a patient in hospital that he is dying should not be made without full consultation with the family and the GP. This takes time, of course, but it is vital, and once the decision to tell has been taken, it should *not* be left to the ward sister or a junior doctor to break the news. That is the responsibility of the senior member of the team and, ideally, he and the GP should visit the patient together, since the latter can be very helpful in advising how best this particular patient can be told.

If the GP is not at the bedside, it is essential that he should be told exactly what has been said to the patient and the family *before* the patient is discharged home. Nothing is more humiliating to the home doctor or disastrous to the management of the case than the patient and family knowing more about the diagnosis and management than he does. What could be worse is that, in his ignorance, he gives the patient an emphatic opinion and is then told that the hospital has given one to the contrary. When asked to visit a dying patient, a GP should first ensure that he has received a letter from the hospital appraising him of the full facts of the case. If he has not received such a letter, it is vital that he contact the hospital before, not during or after, his first visit.

Assuming that everyone concerned with care is kept in the picture from the first, what are the main points in assessing whether the patient should be told or not?

First, a preliminary consultation with the patient's family

may clearly direct the doctor to the approach he should make – and as often as not the family's attitude is helpful and decisive. However, the advice or instructions given by the family can sometimes be completely contrary to the doctor's own convictions. Their attitude may, for example, be based on religious convictions, on cowardice, indifference or a completely disordered approach to or failure to grasp the significance of the disease or its likely prognosis.

Almost as difficult is the family who may give no advice at all. With pathetic trust in their family doctor, they say, 'We leave it to you, doctor. We are sure you know best.' The doctor is then on his own and must, with the nurses and health visitors in his team, make his own decision and run the risk of breaking up the last weeks or months of happiness in a family and of jeopardising his relationship with the patient and the family in the process.

Next, the patient's social responsibilities have to be considered – his business or professional commitments, including the need to put his personal and family affairs in order, and the attitude of his employers. Then it may be necessary to give a patient reasons for continuing treatment or for embarking on new and highly sophisticated therapy, together with the comparative prognosis with or without it.

Above all, the mentality and personality of the patient are of paramount importance and one of the most difficult items to assess. So often 'Tell me doctor, I can take it' means 'For God's sake don't tell me.' On the other hand, an apparent demeanour of complete ignorance or indifference to the diagnosis can boil down to a wish on the part of the patient to spare relatives and doctors the agony of telling.

It is sometimes said that the doctor's decision must be based on a variety of factors which include the intelligence, social status, religious faith and personality of the patient. Although each of these is important, is the doctor supposed to allot marks for each and, according to the result, tell or not tell?

Again, older GPs will probably accept what younger men and women may find unbelievable: that often a curtain descends between the patient and reality, and one has the

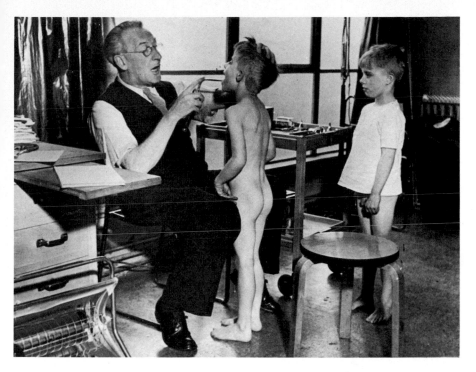

16 The first school health service *(Mansell Collection)*

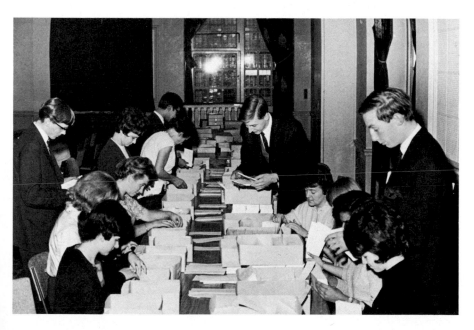

17 Doctors' mass resignations from the NHS being recorded at
BMA House 1965 *(British Medical Association)*

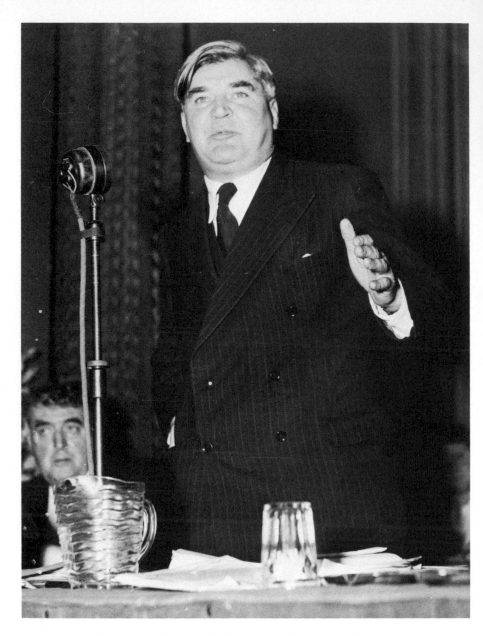

18 Aneurin Bevan, as Minister of Health, speaking at the Socialist Party Conference at Margate in 1950 *(Keystone Press Agency)*

amazing situation of an intelligent patient (even, on occasion a doctor) not giving even a passing consideration to the diagnosis which to the onlookers stands out a mile. Yet I have witnessed this too often not to mention it here. It is, moreover, a factor of vital importance in deciding when to tell the truth to a patient. It favours delay, for if a patient is prepared to live with an incurable illness and to die from it without any sign of recognising his condition (and I am sure the lack of recognition, though incomprehensible to us, is genuine) intrusion by a doctor with a damaging prognosis is unwarrantable.

Two reasons compel the truth. The first, when relatives can tolerate the situation no longer and for their sakes the direction of management has to be changed. The second, when an incompatibility or even hostility arises between doctor and patient, a loss of confidence is born and grows, the patient's condition deteriorates and the doctor is blamed for this and for not taking action to arrest it. If, even under this strain, the opinion of doctor or relatives rebels against telling the truth, the only resort is to call on a second opinion, hopefully the consultant whom the patient knew in hospital. Finally, the age of the patient must influence the doctor. An elderly patient may expect to die; a child certainly will not.

There is also a further complication to this so-called simple yes or no. Until a patient has actually been told it is impossible in every case to anticipate his or her reaction. There may be unexpected co-operation, collapse, disbelief, resentment or actual relief that there is no longer any need to struggle. The GP has to be prepared for any reaction and try his best to support and understand it. A patient may turn his face to the wall and die, or may decide to fight to the last ditch. In either case the doctor must accept the decision and give whatever help he can – and his ability to do so is tremendously reinforced when care is in the hands of a primary health care team.

What is the true answer to this problem then? Telling or not telling a patient that he has an incurable disease is part of the treatment of his illness. In the same way that some patients in pain require sedatives and others do not, so some dying patients will require to be told and others will not. No rigid rule could, or should, be applied. No textbook or misguided, if well-meaning, expert should be allowed to dictate to doctors that in every case it is part of the treatment to share the hopelessness with the patient. It is not a question of yes or no. Later in his career every doctor finds that the long list of factors to be considered is so firmly implanted in his mind that subconsciously he reaches his decision comparatively quickly and with little overt consideration. And he will nearly always make the right decision.

In contrast, I believe he will nearly always be wrong if his decisions do not rely on his own judgement and experience, but are based on no other factor than advice given to him by professional theorists.

I would add one additional plea. I have talked of 'management' or 'care' and not 'treatment' because these days the narrow concept of 'treatment' is not in itself enough. No cases demonstrate this more clearly than the ones we call hopeless. What I want to stress to the trainee GP is that he should not regard the case as closed when the patient dies. He has a duty, too, to the bereaved. Caring for the bereaved is part of caring for the dying. At first, as with the patient, a curtain will come down between the family and reality, and they will carry on as if nothing had happened. It is here that the doctor and the nurse need to advise and help, aware that one day, sooner or later, the curtain will go up again, the play will go on, but the leading actor or actress will be missing.

It is at this stage, soon after the patient has died, that the bereaved are most likely to collapse and one or two visits by the doctor and nurse can be an enormous help, together with the assurance that they are always there if needed. It is not doctoring or nursing in the strictest sense and probably not covered by their official terms of employment, but it is an integral part of compassion, sympathy and understanding.[6][7][8][9]

There is another topic not unrelated to the above that I

cannot ignore, namely medical ethics. It is far from being a favourite subject of mine and most doctors have no need to spend their day worrying about the ethics of their job. Yet a basic knowledge is vital. There are two major books of reference on medical ethics, one published by the General Medical Council[10] and the other one by the BMA.[11] Both are excellent and very comprehensive, and every GP should have a copy of each in his consulting room.

The Hippocratic oath was probably written in the fifth century BC and many fundamental principles of professional behaviour have remained unchanged throughout recorded history. The World Medical Association in 1947 produced a restatement of the oath which became known as the Declaration of Geneva. This was further amended in Sydney in 1968[12] and the Commonwealth Medical Association, meeting in Jamaica in 1974, confirmed an ethical code.[13] The code states in simple and succinct terms that a doctor's primary loyalty is to his patients; that a doctor shall respect human life and studiously avoid doing it any injury; that he shall respect the confidence of his patients as he would his own; shall by precept and example maintain the dignity and ideals of the profession, and shall not permit any bias of race, creed or socio–economic factors to affect his professional practice.

The General Medical Council says that good medical practice depends on the maintenance of trust between doctors and patients and their families and on an understanding by both that proper professional relationships will be strictly observed. I hope that in this book I have shown that this is the essence of family doctoring.

One intensely difficult aspect of the GP's life is professional secrecy. Particularly today, when he is under pressure from so many sources, this is an area in which the trust between him and his patient can often be at risk. It is therefore of paramount importance that young doctors and students should understand that it is a doctor's duty – some would say a duty more important than any others – to observe the rule of professional secrecy, to refrain from disclosing voluntarily to any third party information learned directly or indirectly in his professional relationship with a patient. It is important also to understand that the death of a patient does not absolve the doctor from his obligation to maintain secrecy.

There are certain exceptional circumstances in which a doctor is permitted to break professional secrecy. If there is any doubt in his mind, then he should telephone or write to either his Protection Society, the GMC or the BMA. These three bodies are there to help him and all three would much prefer to help him before he makes an irreversible decision rather than deal with the possible consequences afterwards.

Other ways in which a doctor is deemed to have broken his professional trust are by exerting improper influence on a patient to obtain a loan of money and by entering into an emotional or sexual relationship with a patient, or a member of a patient's family, which disrupts the patient's family life or otherwise damages or causes distress to the patient or his family.

In relation to this last, even when a doctor is busy, there is no excuse for dispensing with chaperones during an examination of a patient. It is so easy to become lax or to shrug off such a refinement as inapplicable in the 1980s. But an embarrassing situation can occur in the most unexpected circumstances at no more than a second's notice. If alone with a patient at home or in the surgery, it is well to postpone the examination. Nowadays male doctors need to remember that this applies not only to female patients but also to males.

In my view, and there are some who think differently, the fact that we live in a permissive society does not in any way change the special relationship existing between doctor and patient. For the sake of both, this relationship must be protected and not abused.

The freedom of doctors to treat their patients without interference is now a well-established principle. Doctors may also freely take on patients or remove them from their list. These are further examples of trust, on the part of the state and the public. Doctors should guard them jealously.

It is in prescribing and certification that doctors are

perhaps most often tempted to break this trust. GPs are expected to exercise care in the compilation of certificates and similar documents and should not certify statements they have not taken appropriate steps to verify.

On more than one occasion while serving on the disciplinary committee of the General Medical Council I thought 'There, but for the Grace of God, go I.' On other occasions when doctors had clearly abused their terms of service I found it difficult to subdue my distaste.

There cannot be any excuse for lax prescribing and certification. The careful compilation of notes is essential, including details of drugs used and the dose and quantity prescribed, together with the diagnosis entered on the certificate and the date on which it was issued. Over and over again, in my experience, good doctors have put themselves at risk because, although their prescribing and certification were in all probability above suspicion, there were no records to prove their integrity. No one is perfect and it would be ridiculous to suggest that every set of notes should be comprehensive in every detail – but blank, or nearly blank, notes are inexcusable.

Nor should the employment of trained receptionists and secretaries, who write prescriptions and certificates for doctors to sign, be used as an excuse for doctors to relax their vigilance. Yet, in spite of many warnings, some doctors are still issuing certificates and prescriptions without seeing the patient or being in contact in any way. They risk their own reputations by doing this and, worst of all, put the whole profession at risk (to say nothing of patients) because they are in gross breach of the trust placed in them by the government and the public.

While discussing ethics, I should also mention that doctors may, of course, decline to provide any treatment they believe to be wrong. There is a distinction between treatment believed to be detrimental to a patient's best interests and treatment to which a doctor has a conscientious objection – but in both cases a full explanation should be made to the patient and a second opinion offered, given by another GP or, preferably, by a consultant.

Some idea of the ethical dilemmas facing doctors today can be gleaned from the 1981 *BMA Handbook on Medical Ethics* (Section Five, pp. 30–37). The list is terrifying and includes pre-symptomatic screening, the termination of pregnancy, the care of severely malformed infants, artificial insemination by donor semen, genetic counselling, euthanasia, brain death and tissue transplantation . . . . Those who guard the ethical behaviour of doctors have a tremendous responsibility too. As each new problem arises they have to judge its impact on doctors and patients and inevitably on occasion they find themselves learning as they go along.

Nevertheless, as I said at the beginning, the fundamental principles of professional behaviour must remain inviolate. Other principles need to be built onto them, but cannot replace them.

Last of all, I want to end this chapter with two pleas to young doctors. First, once you have signed an agreement with your partners, put it in the drawer and forget it. It is very necessary to have an agreement, and preferably one approved by the BMA, but to live by it and be constantly alluding to it is hardly conducive to a happy relationship. Secondly, even when you are worked off your feet remember that, in the main, you are not dealing with 'ordinary' people. Many of the patients waiting to see you are worried or scared for some reason or another. Often, they have been full of apprehension while waiting for their appointment and are terrified of what may be going to happen to them. So, come out and meet them in the waiting room, call them by their name and not by a number, a green light or a shout of 'next' from the depths of the consulting room. It makes a tremendous difference.

Even the most weary doctor must learn to smile at the end of the consultation. He will be forgiven if he does not get up to shake hands.

9

1970 – 1972

GPs were pretty weary at the beginning of the 1970s, having had to cope with a vicious epidemic of what was known as 'Mao flu'. . . .

Not having any particular impact on general practice, but taking up a lot of time and stirring up a great deal of emotion, was a sudden urge for an inquiry into the structure and function of the General Medical Council (GMC). It was stimulated by the possibility of an annual retention fee for doctors to retain themselves on the medical register. A committee was formed under the chairmanship of Sir Brynmor Jones to consider the composition of the GMC, with a view to achieving a majority of elected members over those nominated or appointed. Its report was published in March 1971.[1] I was on this committee and it was whilst on my way back from one of its meetings that news was given us that the Review Body's twelfth report,[2] received by the Prime Minister, Harold Wilson, on 2 April 1970, was to suffer a delay in publication. We had always recognised the inherent danger in the Review Body reporting direct to the Prime Minister.

Dr Derek Stevenson pressed for publication (on 11 May) but the Prime Minister wrote on 22 May to say that in the light of the decision to dissolve Parliament the government had concluded that it would not be right to continue with the consideration of the Review Body report during the election period.[3] He regretted that this would mean a delay in announcing a decision and publishing the report. He hoped we would agree that there was now no point in his meeting us.

We did not agree, and there now followed a most intense period of activity which I must describe in some detail because GPs were at the centre of the turmoil. Mr Crossman in the third volume of his diaries gives his side of the story.[4] He starts off by saying that 'Stevenson and Gibson were blowing the thing up into a sensation.' He then describes how he first persuaded the Prime Minister not to publish the Review Body's report, although the PM thought publication should not be delayed. Then, under pressure from Mrs Castle and others, Mr Crossman reversed his decision and decided to publish the report and the government's reaction to it. At the end of this meeting he told his colleagues that he must be able to say to doctors that the Prime Minister would see them. The PM agreed to this. He also reached an agreement that 'if we were going to have this during the election we would have to give the junior doctors the full claim'.

Five minutes after the Cabinet meeting he saw us, 'having decided to have a long row' with us. I agree that he was angry but we were too. On the lighter side, he ended up by saying that he had been angry with us, but as friends. The only response I could make to this was to get up and walk out without comment. Not so the representative of the junior doctors, Julian Elkington, who said, 'It is not reciprocated.' When, later, Julian was due to see the PM with us he expressed a rigid determination not to shake hands. I persuaded him that he must do this even if he proposed to do some throat-cutting, or its modern equivalent, later.

We went to No. 10 Downing Street on Thursday 28 May.[5] To our surprise when we went into the Cabinet room only Mr Crossman and the Prime Minister were present. After a brief introduction, the PM took to his pipe and left his secretary of state to take the brunt of our wrath, which included me telling him to resign. (I did not know it, but he had already done so, to become editor of the *New Statesman!*)

The Prime Minister then announced that he would concede publication of the Kindersley Report, but not until 'next week'. We argued against this delay and, in addition, asked that his decision should include nothing less than the whole Review Body recommendations. They refused to accept this and we were left wondering why there was all the difficulty and mystery.

One evening, Derek Stevenson and I heard, quite off the record, that it was the government's intention to refer the Review Body's report, or part of it, to the Prices and Incomes Board (PIB). This was almost unbelievable, but it did explain the mystery. We had to keep the information to ourselves, but because of it we were given time to prepare action if the rumour proved to be true.

We were summoned to meet Mr Crossman and his entourage on the morning of 4 June. We were given a short time in a room by ourselves to read the Review Body report and the government's reaction to it, including the proposed reference to the PIB. In one stroke the government had forfeited the trust and co-operation of the profession.

We were furious and sent in a message to say that if we were not seen without further delay we would leave.[6] As soon as we sat down I said that there was no point in our staying and we were off (I can't think why he describes me as a nice fellow!). Crossman says in his diary that we were hostile and violent. This is an exact description. We made it clear that we could not collaborate with him in any way and we knew, though he did not, that thanks to our useful piece of intelligence we were prepared for action.

My notes on this meeting in the Cabinet office include such sentences as 'Even if doctors don't resign they will play hell with the Health Service'; 'You are offering us what we should have had two years ago and have referred any new pay to the PIB − this is a confidence trick'; 'This is dishonest. I must warn you that if you make this statement (about reference to the PIB) we cannot hold the profession'; 'Our impression is that you don't care about the health service.' Again, a measure of our discontent.

We asked for the 'compelling reasons' why the whole

award could not be implemented. He gave them as the sheer bulk of the award, the impact on the economy in view of the repercussions it was likely to have on others and the backlog of claims coming up. He used the words 'in a period of extreme economic peril'. A note I have says this was withdrawn and the words 'in the possible case of a period of extreme economic peril' substituted.

Somehow these last words leaked out to the press in the form that the reason why the government could not accept Kindersley in full was because the instability of the economy had put the nation in peril. In his diary, Mr Crossman describes his conversation with us, but he adds, incorrectly, that we went off and immediately gave the information to the Tories.[7] We were not interested in party politics – only justice.

Having made it clear to him that we would not collaborate in any way we tried to leave the door open by offering to see him again that evening. He did not send for us and we later knew that, that afternoon, the Review Body itself had resigned after Lord Kindersley had seen Mr Crossman.[8]

The following day the committees representing the hospital doctors and the GPs met, followed next day by an emergency meeting of the BMA Council.

I had worked most of the night with Dr Stevenson on the speech with which I had to open the debate. The atmosphere was tense and the mood a mixture of anger and anxiety. We were reaching the climax of a situation which was not of our choosing, was without precedent and might lead to action the results of which could overflow onto our patients. Yet we could not turn back.

I will quote the last paragraphs of the speech, for I hope they sum up the whole imbroglio:

I would say to Mr Crossman from this chair, as I have already said to him, that it is he and not us who has put the NHS and the care and treatment of our patients at risk. All we wanted – and still want – is to go about our calling in peace, uninterrupted by the machinations of politicians of any sort or at any time – election or no election.

This is now *not* a question of money or of politics, it is a matter of principle, of integrity in public life, of honest government. Our confidence in government has been destroyed and our hands are clean. We did not ask for it, we did not expect it. It is a national disgrace that a noble and dedicated profession should have been mishandled and insulted in this way.

What has happened to us could happen to others. So in taking action we are not only protecting ourselves but our patients in all other sections of society.

We collected resignation forms from doctors and held them at BMA House (and my goodness, how well and loyally the headquarters staff worked). Our action was to include a withdrawal of all certification by GPs and a refusal by doctors to sit on any committees. There was no question, therefore, of any interruption of or interference with the treatment of our patients.

The point, so far as GPs were concerned, was that the Review Body recommended an increase in remuneration of 30 per cent. The government accepted a direct reimbursement of 70 per cent of the whole of the salaries of ancillary staff and an increase in the reimbursement of practice expenses. They were not prepared to accept the increase of 30 per cent without further advice but agreed an increase of 15 per cent from 1 April, bringing the total increase in fees and allowances to 20 per cent. The chairman of the Prices and Incomes Board was to report (by 15 July) as to how much of the balance of the 30 per cent should be paid. This was a monstrous injustice.

In presenting the profession's case to the Review Body, we did not just think of a number and then go along to the Cabinet office for a cup of tea. The exercise took months of preparation.

Although originally set up by the government with membership approved by the profession, the Review Body was completely independent and jealous of its independence. Its members were selected for their expertise in the relevant subjects involved in the determination of the level of remuneration of doctors and dentists, having in mind the terms of reference within which they were required to work. We had great respect for their neutrality and integrity.

It was natural that where a particular report of the Review Body did not match up to the aspirations of the profession, there should be demands from some quarters for its abolition and a return to direct negotiation with government. To us this would have meant the loss of a most valuable arbitrator. It was naïve indeed to expect that each report had to satisfy the doctors' expectations in full or else the Review Body had to go. The whole point of such a body was that it was an unbiased arbiter between government and profession, whose fully deliberated report was to be accepted by both sides.

The BMA's mechanism for producing evidence was complicated, but effective. It involved the committees representing hospital doctors and general practitioners each preparing their own case with expert help from actuaries, accountants, economists and statisticians, over and above the BMA's own expert staff. The two then came together to form a joint evidence committee under the chairmanship of the Chairman of Council and this committee included senior and junior counsels and solicitors. The objective was to produce agreed evidence on behalf of the whole profession.

The evidence was submitted in writing to the Review Body and in due course we were summoned to meet them in the Cabinet office. They were courteous and friendly but we had no illusions. We were talking to people who knew as much about doctors' and dentists' remunerations as we did. We had to ensure, therefore, that our evidence was complete in every detail, down to the last decimal point, and that it was skilfully presented. They were there to consider the professions' and the government's evidence in depth and having done so, to come to a determination without fear or favour.

Usually, after an opening address covering the whole subject, each case was heard separately, dealing with hospital doctors at one session and GPs at another. Sessions were lengthy, intense and wearing from start to finish. After that, all we could do was to await the result and hope that we had done well. Then we started all over again preparing the next year's evidence. The exercise used to cost us something like £50,000. I dread to think what the financial burden must be today.

We had every right, therefore, to be enraged when we were callously told by government that our level of remuneration, already having been under the microscope of our own independent Review Body, was now to be re-examined by yet another body, the Prices and Incomes Board.

On 9 June I wrote a letter to *The Times* in which I said that doctors, whose desire was to be allowed to get on quietly with treating their patients, found themselves at the centre of a storm of controversy. I made an appeal to the Prime Minister to call us round a conference table before further damage was done to a public service in which doctors had loyally served for so many years.

On the same day there appeared a letter signed by presidents of six of the Royal Colleges. The surgeons and GPs did not sign it. We had prior knowledge of this letter and we were able to persuade them to omit one paragraph. Although this could have created an atmosphere akin to 1948 all over again in fact, thanks to the far better understanding between us, this particular letter was dignified and constructive and could only have helped us in our efforts.

The press did not like my letter. They thought we should have approached the Prime Minister direct and not via *The Times*. Mr Crossman made remarks on the BBC news about the health service *vis-à-vis* the playing fields of Winchester and the row boiled up. Fortunately we had the overwhelming support of GPs – and, indeed, the whole profession – in our actions. Mr Crossman persuaded Mr Wilson that there could be no question of him initiating negotiations or seeing us whilst we 'behaved in this way'.[9]

Then the Conservatives won the election. There can be no doubt that the fracas with the doctors must have gone against Labour, particularly Mr Crossman's comments on the state of the economy. A grave situation faced the new government. We saw the new Secretary of State, Sir Keith Joseph, on 26 June. He said he understood that the conflict was about a matter of principle. We agreed. He accepted the principle and the fight was over.

Whilst Derek Stevenson and the permanent secretary retired to compose a letter which Sir Keith would sign and give me to read to the Representative Body which was meeting in Harrogate and waiting for our return,[10] I think I missed an opportunity for he said he was surprised we had not decided to press for the permanent elimination of certificates. In point of fact, this would have been immoral, to achieve our objectives and then to say that, in spite of this, we were never going back to certificates again. But it was a mouthwatering thought!

We had won. We had to win, but it had been immensely wearing. Trying to keep my practice going, with the utmost help from my partners, and at the same time doing a full-time job in London, was not easy. I kept my sanity by constantly reminding myself that my BMA work in London was in the nature of an insubstantial pageant and that my real joy was when I was back in a patient's house in Winchester. Yet would I, or any of my colleagues, have been still caring for our patients as family doctors if we had allowed the constant haggling in London to overcome us, resulting in unresisted dominance by governments?

The strain was even greater on Mr Walpole Lewin as Chairman of the Consultants and Specialists Committee and Dr (now Sir) James Cameron of the General Medical Services Committee. They had to obtain the approval of their committees before they could make any move and the two committees had to agree with each other. I do not know how Julian Elkington got so much time off to represent the junior doctors, but he did and he fought like a hellcat for them.

There is an opinion that the profession should not be represented by 'amateurs'. From the point of view of the workload it would be easy to accept this but the advantage of representation by those in active medical practice far outweighs any other consideration.

The profession accepted Sir Keith's letter. In the event, GPs accepted a further increase of 5 per cent, making 20 per cent in all, and we proceeded to the election of a new Review Body.

At the same meeting, on the initiative of Dr Frank Wells of Ipswich, it was decided to recommend a voluntary ban on the prescribing of amphetamines.

At a further meeting with Sir Keith Joseph he said that he disapproved of the Review Body, in the consideration of its reports, opting back to Pilkington (the Royal Commission of 1957). So he had conceded one principle only to throw a bag of nails at another, even more sacred one.

Here was a threatened move against a principle which we had thought to be inviolate and we reacted violently. We were successful, for the Review Body in its tenth report (1980) reiterated the principles under which it was set up and its intention to adhere to them. This gives some idea how we could not relax our vigilance for a moment. It seemed that there was never to be peace, whichever government was in power.

There could also be crises at field level. On 5 October 1970, my partnership, together with two single-handed GPs and one partnership of two doctors, moved into our new health centre. The first mistake we made was to agree to a design which fitted our current requirements, including consulting and examination rooms for our trainee, for which, of course, we had to pay rent, but made no allowance for future expansion. Secondly, we did not wander round from time to time during the building stage to see how things were going. Had we done so, we could have avoided some elementary mistakes such as positioning all the electrical points for desk light, telephone, intercom and bell to reception area at our feet instead of on the wall. We might also have made sure that the wiring provided for our intercom sets fitted them. As it was, we had to discard all of them, though recently purchased, and pile them in a cupboard. Thirdly, we had not realised the extent to which we could be 'administered'.

We moved in over a weekend and, as the administrators

were off duty from Friday night to Monday morning, we were able to put up the shelves for the patients' notes behind a wall in the reception area, so that they would be out of sight of the patients (whereas it had been planned that they should be in the open area behind the counter). The side effect of this was that there were now no points available for typewriters, the telephonist was exposed to view and the room on the second floor we had planned as a quiet room for us, for undergraduates and vocational trainees, with three study bays, audiovisual aids and a small library, had to be given over to typists.

Nevertheless, we were pretty happy. So long as we could retain the comfortable doctor-patient relationship we had had in our small premises, we reckoned we were well off. We soon learned, and had to accept, that we were only renting parts of the building. The 'landlords' were very discreet; our common room lunches on Mondays were undisturbed and we enjoyed being able to practise in such surroundings. We had each chosen a particular colour scheme for our rooms and furnished them at partnership expense. This was a very worthwhile luxury, as were the treatment room and separate rooms for nurses and health visitors.

It was the administration, however, that was to prove our undoing. Meanwhile, we looked out on a quiet stream running underneath the building (very tempting for anglers!) and luxuriated in such capacious premises.

Implementation of the Seebohm Report reached the statute book during the last week of Parliament. In 1973, nearly three years later, the twenty-fifth anniversary of the NHS, Mr Crossman said:

Quite candidly I wasn't terribly enthusiastic for implementing Seebohm before we'd got Local Government reform done . . . I am not sure I was wise to do it. Because you then set up this new self-perpetuating oligarchy of these great new social welfare departments which are rapidly expanding and are really creating jobs for themselves – in the office – very very fast. I think we're in grave danger now of getting another, rival, hierarchy, possessed by a desire for professionalism and status in a much more dubious profession than doctoring. . .

Logically speaking, the psychiatric social workers should have gone to the Health Service – they didn't want to – there was a very weak case for their not going.[11]

He was giving our case, in a nutshell – but too late.

He had agreed to implement Seebohm because Baroness Serota, Minister of State for Social Services, wanted him to. Our arguments against it were to no avail, except that we achieved quite a few modifications, but it is not pleasing to know that he agreed to psychiatric social workers leaving health and going to welfare because this is what they wanted, irrespective of the fact that it was not necessarily to the good of NHS patients.

In such manner and for such reasons is the care of patients determined. Helpless pawns in a political game. Those caring for them and working with them can have their opinions set aside at the whim of ministers.

As an active GP, like others, I was now to suffer the consequences. Happy relationships built up over the years were replaced by strained communications with strange people, strangely titled and working from a spacious new building. Home helps and meals on wheels became suddenly only obtainable after exhaustive inquiries as to their genuine necessity, and an assessment of this had to be made not by us but by others. We were talked to, over the phone, about patients we had known for years, by youngsters who had met them for the first time and were prepared to tell us all about them. We were *told* to go and visit patients as emergencies. We were refused admissions by people who disagreed with us and called our patients 'clients'. Everything was reputed to be so much better than it was, yet nothing was so good. And it was all incredibly expensive.

Clearly, we had to be as understanding as we could. I vividly remember a gentle and kindly GP roaring into our secretary's office, stamping his feet in a rage and saying, 'Ronald, you must do something about this.' I told him I had spent months and months trying to do something about it and I was sorry that I had failed. There was no pleasure, only misery, in experiencing the result of failure.

However, there was no point in giving vent to bitterness and taking it out on innocent people. It was too late. Only time could help and the task now was to pick up the pieces and try to put them together again, even if it took years, in the hope of regaining the original pattern of care we knew to be right.

Eventually, we managed to get a social worker attached to the centre, in that he came in every other Tuesday, sat in the secretary's office and waited to see if we had any problems. He could not attend our common room lunches on Mondays, with nurses and health visitors, because he had to attend case conferences. But he was a useful contact and we could ring him if we were getting frantic. He would help to find, or direct us to, the right person in his department. We greatly appreciated the help he gave us.

I finished my five years as chairman of the BMA Council in 1971. In 1972 I became chairman of the Standing Medical Advisory Committee of the Central Health Services Council of the Department of Health, of which I was deputy chairman. I was also a member of the newly formed Personal Social Services Council. SMAC was a very exciting and rewarding committee; and I enjoyed being freed from 'money and Terms and Conditions of Service'.

I wanted to get a working party going on collaboration between health and social services. The Central Health Services and Personal Social Services Councils agreed to this. A committee was duly formed under the chairmanship of Dame Albertine Winner, and it was reinforced by a request from the Standing Nursing Advisory Committee to take part in the project.

We undoubtedly looked at each other sideways to start with, sizing each other up and wondering what to expect. We decided at an early stage to concentrate on collaboration at grass roots level ('Collaboration must never exist for its own sake, only for the good of those we serve').

The report was published in 1978.[12] I quote a few comments:

It is now self evident that the health and social welfare of individuals are inextricably interwoven. Despite this, there is often a lack of contact between health and social services and there are gaps in the knowledge which each has of how the other functions. . . If individual patients/clients have related medical and social problems, then clearly there is a need for collaboration.

There are circumstances in which no amount of collaboration will solve all the difficulties which complicate the delivery of health and social services, nor is collaboration an absolute virtue in itself.

Inadequate resources are clearly a great obstacle to providing an adequate service of any sort.

Collaboration may be less likely to occur at field level if there is ineffective co-ordination at the level of strategic and operational planning. *The various reorganisations of the personal social services in 1970, of local government and of the National Health Service in 1974 did not take sufficient account of each other. . .* (my italics).

The working party emphasised the value of examining different types of collaboration in relation to needs and expectations. Although, it said, it could be argued that there was a need for the two services to be administered by one authority a further reorganisation could not be recommended at this stage. It stressed the need for interprofessional contact in the early years of basic training, for the encouragement of a multi-disciplinary team approach and for someone within the team to take on the role of a co-ordinator for each patient/client.

Finally, the working party emphasised the special responsibility of specialists in community medicine, area nurses and health service liaison officers in fostering collaboration, encouraging joint initiatives, taking a mediative role and breaking down barriers. This was a courageous attempt to rebuild and cement together the broken fragments of the structure of total care, shattered by those who were too far away from the grass roots to appreciate fully the damage they had done.

Meanwhile, the GMS committee had established a useful contact with the British Association of Social Workers. Doctors were, not unnaturally, particularly concerned about the confidentiality of medical records.

Another item on the SMAC agenda which pleased me was community hospitals. This was good news: recognition of the cottage hospital, under a new name, and of the principle of the small hospital within the community as a stage between the patient's own home and the large district hospital. Is is surely ideal if some patients can be adequately treated without needing to move from the community hospital in their own neighbourhood, and if others reach a stage of convalescence when they can be transferred back from the district general hospital to their 'own' smaller hospital and their GP.[13] Yet it was not so easy as all that, there had to be negotiations about the admission and discharge of patients and the proportion of beds allocated for geriatric patients.

Mr Crossman's second Green Paper on the recognition of the health service came to nothing. Sir Keith Joseph published a consultative document in 1971.[14] This was followed by a White Paper in 1972.[15] [16] The new health service was to be more integrated within itself but more segregated from other services. (So much for the concept of 'functional and administrative unity'.) Expertise in health care was concentrated in the NHS and expertise in social work with social service departments, and there was tremendous emphasis on management and cost effectiveness. In a speech I had the temerity to suggest that 'hospitals are about sick people and real management starts at the bedside'.

There were frequent meetings with the secretary of state and officials. On some issues the government itself agreed to move amendments to the Bill, on others the BMA Council prepared amendments which were moved by medical peers in the House of Lords. The main points were the preservation of clinical freedom in the NHS; doctors were accountable in ethics and law to their patients for the care they prescribed; they could not be held accountable to the NHS authorities for the quality of their clinical judgement; and all NHS authorities should include a significant proportion of elected medical members.

Executive Councils were to be replaced by Family Practitioner Committees (what's in a name, except that FPC to GPs could mean Family Planning Committee). Local Medical Committees were to continue, with the same relation to FPCs as previously to Executive Councils, but the BMA was concerned that health centre provision was to be the function not of FPCs but of Area Health Authorities. And how right they were! An amendment was urged to contain in its text the main functions of FPCs. The BMA took the lead, in consultation with the Royal Colleges, in ensuring that advisory committees would be statutory and health authorities under an obligation to consult them, and model constitutions were drawn up for the new medical advisory committees at regional, area and district levels.

This was all that could be done to try to humanise an Act which should never have reached the statute book. Far from creating integration it seemed to emphasise separation; it took the grass roots even further away from administration and imposed a new administration that was incomprehensible to the doctor in the field and even to those working within it. It also involved practising doctors in a spate of extra committee work. Fortunately GPs, by insisting on retaining their independent contractor status and their Local Medical Committees, were shielded from the worst effects of the reorganisation. Unfortunately, at the same time their very insistence on this independence disrupted the integration of the profession which reorganisation had hoped to achieve.

10

1972 – 1976

We were not yet done with government. Seebohm, the re-form of local government of the NHS had created a seething cauldron of activity. Mr (now Lord) Carr and Sir Geoffrey Howe now joined the scene, with an Industrial Relations Act 1971[1] which had far-reaching implications for doctors.

The objective of the Industrial Relations Bill was to canalise negotiations on terms and conditions of employment; 'organisations of workers' had to be registered under the Bill. The wording made it clear that its provisions would apply to doctors in salaried employment generally. There was some doubt whether GPs would be covered by the Bill. The government stated that it should apply to *all* doctors.

Other professional bodies, notably the Royal College of Nursing whose royal charter was also at risk, faced similar problems in registering as an organisation of workers, yet registration was essential if doctors were to be left with any negotiating power. Eventually, largely due to a brainwave on the part of Dr Elston Grey-Turner, then deputy secretary of the BMA, a Special Register was introduced which enabled organisations which were limited companies or chartered bodies to register in a special category without changing their existing constitutions.

All GPs, and all hospital staff engaged in the NHS, could now continue to be represented as separate bargaining units for the purposes of the Act and the BMA was recognised as the sole bargaining agent for these two bargaining units.

150

'Eminently satisfactory,' it was said. (The Industrial Relations Act 1971, was repealed by the Labour government, but the Special Register was preserved in Sanctions 2 (2) and 30 (1) of the Trade Union and Labour Relations Act 1974.)

In 1971, amongst all the turmoil, the Harvard Davis report on the organisation of group practice was published.[2] The GMS committee received it favourably as 'a comprehensive compilation and restatement of current thinking about general practice'.

There were several constructive suggestions, amongst them that there should be experimental schemes of arranging specialist consultations in group practice centres; that social workers should be attached to group practices for case work and to make assessment of psycho-social problems; that home helps should be part of the group practice team and that the aim should be to keep sick people at home unless specialist services within the hospital were necessary.

'Substantial numbers of patients are inappropriately using costly hospital services,' the report said, and GPs knew this only too well. When they visited wards they saw a high percentage of elderly people in hospital for social rather than medical needs and, in fact, not requiring any greater medical or nursing attention than could be given within a properly organised community, geared to total care, by a primary health care team.

In January 1973 my partnership received revised charges for salaries and services at our health centre. It was suggested that the net charge to doctors should be increased from £579 p.a. to £741 p.a. per suite, an increase of 42.7 per cent. We could not accept this. We appealed to the minister in October of that year, our appeal being in two parts: the first, about these charges; the second, detailing items which singly and together represented a failure by the landlords to implement the agreed wishes of the partners, either in time or at a reasonable cost. We also laid stress on the teaching role of the partners and hoped this too would be taken into account.

Local authority estimates for items of work were wildly in excess of our own and this does not take into account the persistent appeals by us to get the work done, against constant delays, or the arguments and differences of opinion, largely based on differences in outlook and methods of working. When we had been in our own practice premises and some work had to be done, one of us agreed to arrange it and within days, usually and conveniently over a weekend, it was done and well done, almost certainly by a patient and at acceptable cost. Now, in the health centre, we agreed in committee what needed doing. Either nothing happened or when it did surface again it was accompanied by a monumental estimate and we had no control at all over how the work was done, or by whom.

After much delay we felt, with the utmost regret, that we must appeal to the Ombudsman via our MP. In September 1975 therefore, Part Three of our Memorandum was issued, in the form of an Appeal to the Parliamentary Commissioner. I will quote one sentence of this lengthy document:

> It is clear to the partners that in the running of a Health Centre the local Health Authority is not sufficiently conscious of the fact that any expense it incurs has to be paid for by the doctors who are its tenants. There is, therefore, no incentive to the authority to run the Centre as economically as possible, since only the doctors will be the losers if money is not well spent. The doctors cannot accept this state of affairs so complacently – or any longer.

In fact, the partners had shown more patience, though certainly not complacency, than many might think reasonable and we noted with apprehension that the pattern set by the County Council was being matched by the new Area Health Authority.

In December 1975 we appeared before a tribunal appointed by the minister – somewhat belatedly, one might think. In June 1976, the Ombudsman sent his report to our MP. He considered our complaint was fully justified. There was a satisfactory result to the tribunal's hearing, the increases payable by us were less than those originally proposed and the revised charges were to take effect from April 1972 rather than October 1971. This brought to an end three years of bickering. Outstanding throughout was the understanding and help given to us by the clerk to the Family Practitioners Committee and his staff. The BMA's stand for Family Practitioner Committees *vis-à-vis* Area Health Boards in the reorganised NHS was vindicated. We had been beating our heads, apparently fruitlessly, against a bureaucratic wall and sadly comparing this with our own organisation and administration in privately owned group practice premises.

This is my justification for including such an unhappy episode in a history of general practice. The lessons to be learned from it are that there should be an agreement drawn up between landlords and tenants, checked, rechecked and approved by General Medical Services Committee experts; plans should be made for a health centre building adequate in design and size for the probable demands of at least two decades ahead; every stage in the building should be supervised by the would-be tenants; on occupation, responsibility for the hiring and firing of staff should be under the control of the GPs who should also be responsible for the maintenance and redecoration of the building, as are normal tenants of rented buildings.

Every effort should be made to divorce the control of the centre from the 'administrators', most of whom have no idea of the workings, the needs and the philosophy of general practice. I accept, of course, the overall supervision of the landlords, as in normal buildings, but not constant niggling or petty and expensive interference. Although we could be said to have won, we obtained very little consolation from it. We went into the health centre to care for our patients, not to fight a running battle with administrators.

In 1970, Sir John Peel's committee on Domiciliary Midwifery and Maternity Bed Needs reported.[3] The General

Medical Services committee's comments on this report stressed the need for all intending GPs to obtain, without difficulty, experience and training in obstetrics in hospital posts, early in their post-graduate career. The committee accepted integration of the maternity services as a goal with a focus in the district general hospital but underlined that the service in the community must be fortified; general practitioner units, elsewhere than in the district general hospital, must continue; domiciliary midwives must be able to practise to their professional satisfaction, employment in hospital not being allowed to interfere with attachment to GPs, and GPs must be able to play their full part in an integrated service, the strength and effectiveness of which would depend upon mutual recognition of the proper responsibility and status of its members.

Sir John came to see me at one stage. His understanding was most encouraging. He did not want segregation of beds in units so that, for example, GPs were in one ward or one one floor, separated from consultants; but he was not yet ready to accept domiciliary midwives in the units. I, for my part, hated the idea of them leaving their patients at the back door and collecting them, and their babies, from the front. Full satisfaction for all concerned could only come from an integrated team, known to the patients and working together from A to Z. In the event, this last principle was accepted and, due to the determination of all concerned (led by Sir John), total care within the maternity services was achieved.

Meanwhile, GPs were being assailed by other potential troubles, originating from inside and outside Parliament. In 1971 I referred to the 'ever present threat of legislation on Euthanasia'.[4] (The 'right to live' was defined legally by the European Convention of Human Rights. This was accepted by the United Kingdom and has been in force since 1953. Section 1, Article 2 reads: 'Everyone's right to live shall be protected by law. No one shall be deprived of life intentionally save in the execution of a sentence of a court following his conviction of a crime for which this penalty is provided by law.')

Since I have already discussed this subject in the second interlude, all I want to add here is that potential GPs and all students should have terminal care included in their training syllabus. Terminal care units are a most commendable innovation but I continue to hope that community care will be planned, in all areas, so that those who wish to die in their own beds can do so with as little trauma to their relatives as possible.[5]

The Abortion Act of 1967 had come into effect on 27 April 1968. It had a continuing impact on general practice. GPs were concerned at the differing facilities and attitudes from area to area. It was very necessary for them to be able to get prompt appointments and to know which obstetrician was sympathetic and which not. We once discussed with Mr Crossman the delays in obtaining terminations. He asked why we were picking on this subject in particular; why not tonsils, for example? We pointed out that tonsils were not necessarily delivered in nine months. This conversation underlined the difference between the glass house and the grass roots.[6]

Another extra task for GPs was in the field of family planning. The department agreed that no GP would be obliged to provide contraceptive services. Those who wished to do so would have their names included on a contraceptive services list, either for their own patients only or for other patients as well. I remember the argument about GPs not providing condoms (the GMS committee emphasised that doctors would not be involved in this) and I gained some light relief by commenting on the apparent impression that health visitors could be called 'in an emergency' to provide them, presumably from a machine in their cars. As GPs are independent contractors the government could not assume that this extra work would be carried as part of the NHS obligation, and it quickly agreed to extra remuneration. It was not so easy with consultants.[7]

Deputising services were becoming increasingly popular throughout the 1970s. The BMA Deputising Service, originating in 1966[8] and overhauled in 1970, now operates in most urban centres outside London and there are other services. One of the aspects of the service that I, and others, thought would be difficult to implement was to obtain an adequate supply of deputies. This, to my knowledge, has never been a problem, although always in one's mind must be concern at overtired young doctors coping with a day's work after a night's deputising.

What impact has this service had on the traditional doctor–patient relationship and what part has it played in the current popular game of knocking the doctor? The workload and long duty hours taken together with the decreasing workload and shortening hours of other sections of the community make it inevitable, and reasonable, to expect GPs to look for support in the shape of deputies to take over from them for certain hours. The burden lies on the GPs themselves to ensure that the service is not abused and on the organisers to maintain the highest possible standard. One suggestion voiced in responsible quarters is that deputies visiting patients should properly be armed with medical notes, for their own sakes as well as the patients', and this is not possible. It may be, in years to come, with computerisation.[9]

In the mid-1970s there was a mounting concern amongst doctors, social workers, probation officers and the police, about the overprescribing of barbiturates. As a member of the Home Office Advisory Council on the Misuse of Drugs I was asked to chair a working party to consider methods of reducing the use of these dangerous drugs. On my visit to certain centres, and at one memorable meeting of the Pharmaceutical Society, I was appalled at the prescribing methods adopted by some doctors. At first I refused to believe that pads of signed, blank prescriptions were left with receptionists for them to fill in, mainly for 'temporary' patients asking for barbiturates. Nor could I believe that prescriptions were being given for a hundred or more tablets at a time, with repeats as requested. How could the general public maintain its respect for a profession indulging in this sort of activity?

Clearly, dealing with a profession traditionally wary of any apparent attempt to interfere with its clinical freedom, it would have been unwise to recommend an outright ban. Yet to do less would be to leave social workers, the police and others to continue to deal with the, sometimes lethal, results of our lax prescribing. In the event, it was agreed that we should launch a campaign extending over two years, to achieve a voluntary ban on the prescribing of barbiturates.

From my knowledge of the BMA's Representative Body I calculated that it would take at least three annual meetings to achieve the necessary understanding and support: the first would greet the idea with suspicion; the second would need to have its downright opposition gently quelled; the third would accept the idea and be grateful that it had thought of it in the first place. All this happened to plan. The more I see of the Representative Body the more I am full of admiration for its wisdom and, above all, its standard of debate when considering clinical and scientific matters. Fewer barbiturates are now prescribed but it is alarming that, to compensate, the use of tranquillisers is increasing.[10]

Doctors have usually done quite well under Labour governments. I may not have shared their political views but I admired the efforts of, for example, Aneurin Bevan and Kenneth Robinson during their years in office. The former may have set one group of doctors against the other in order to get his way, but his way was my way when it came to providing a health service for the people, free of financial constraints. The latter set out with a dedicated determination to do his best for the NHS.

Mrs Castle had succeeded Sir Keith Joseph, so it was now her turn to see what Labour could do for the NHS. 'Health' was excluded from her title and she took office at a time when there was a definite lowering of morale and an increasing cynicism within the medical profession.

The first major argument with the profession was about 'pay beds' and Part Two of her *Diaries* (headed 'I fight with the doctors') as published in the *Sunday Times*, 14 September 1980, describes her confrontation with the consultants and specialists over the pay beds dispute in Charing Cross Hospital in 1974.[11] In January 1975 she skilfully defused the anger of both GPs and hospital doctors in order to prevent further industrial disruption of the NHS, following the rejection by the Review Body of the profession's claim for an 18 per cent interim pay rise. She told the General Medical Service Committee negotiators that she hoped they could stop talking the language of confrontation or she feared the NHS would really face collapse, and she thought her plea 'did the trick'. With peace maintained within general practice she was free to concentrate on her Health Services Bill. Her diaries provide valuable insight, however, into the vulnerable personality of a woman who fought hard for the interests of the NHS and against those whom she believed could do it harm.[12] [13]

In August 1975, just when consultation and conciliation were needed to bring everyone together in a constructive effort to refurbish a failing service and abate the mounting unhappiness of doctors, a consultative document was published on the Separation of Private Practice from the NHS.[14] This proposed to take powers to control by licensing the extent of private practice outside the NHS. The threat to the independent practice of medicine was clear: it was a policy to abolish private practice altogether and it brought things to the boil. There was an inevitable confrontation between government and profession. To make matters worse, the Prime Minister Mr (now Sir) Harold Wilson decided in October to set up a Royal Commission on the NHS but refused to refer the question of the private sector to the commission. It was not until Lord Goodman had been brought in to advise and the Prime Minister had guaranteed to preserve a viable independent sector that the BMA agreed to exploratory discussions on the Goodman proposals. This was after the Central Committee for Hospital Medical Services had conducted a ballot of consultants, which showed two to one in favour of the Goodman proposals being incorporated in legislation and an overwhelming majority against Mrs Castle's consultative document.[15]

It is sad that there is such a paranoid and irrational approach to private medicine in some quarters. People opt for private treatment for several reasons: they cannot bear the noise and suffering in a hospital ward; they are self-employed and have to time their stay in hospital to fit their work; they do not wish to have something for nothing – and there are still some who feel this way – or they want to jump the queue. The latter exist but are a small minority. Another factor, completely ignored, is that in some practices remuneration from private patients enables the doctors to afford an extra partner who helps also with NHS patients, at no cost to the public sector. The introduction of such political dogma into a caring service which, by its very nature, is forever under stress, creates wholly unnecessary and inexcusable turmoil which can only act adversely on patient welfare.

There were other petty annoyances, such as a proposed reform of the GP complaints procedure. With Service Committees, the General Medical Council and the civil courts, there was no need to add to the list of bodies dealing with accusations of negligence against GPs. Altogether, doctors felt they had a low priority within the service, and when they, or any other group within the NHS believe – rightly or wrongly – that they no longer have the understanding, co-operation and support of 'their' Secretary of State (the father or mother figure) they are bound to lose heart.

Of course, no government to date has been able to afford to pay NHS employees adequately, hence the constant playing around with Review Body awards and the recurrent bickering. Health ministers have done their best with the money available – and Mrs Castle was probably more successful than most in extracting money from the Cabinet for the NHS – but GPs can be forgiven if they wonder where they would be now but for the permanent battle with the Establishment.

In 1974 I was elected to the General Medical Council. I wanted to get on it for two reasons: to see whether it was as bad as it was painted and to check on how interested it was in the welfare and future of general practice. I found it to be a most efficient body. Work on it is hard and concentrated.

One was always conscious of the responsibility of membership. Regulating the profession sounds very cold and mathematical. In fact, the disciplinary side of its work is enacted with a genuine consideration for the accused doctor coupled, of course, with a consciousness of the necessity to maintain a high ethical standard, and the two are not necessarily easy to correlate. The educative side has an immense responsibility, with all its ramifications throughout the Commonwealth. It requires continuous concentration combined with an expertise which only the GMC can command.

So far as general practice is concerned, I am content that the council is on the side of the angels! On some occasions when, for example, an application by an overseas doctor for registration in Britain was being considered, a member might comment that 'Training is adequate for general practice', but this was rare and confined to only one or two members who were not yet fully indoctrinated. GP members of the council were quick to quell this sort of comment.

The GMC is deeply involved in the EEC. Recognition of general practice as a specialty in the medical directives has its active support, as also of the BMA. There will be a long haul ahead – defining the role and function of the GP in health care and vocational training for GPs – but we can be satisfied that the GP's cause is being energetically pursued.

The president of the GMC sits on his podium on a higher level than any other doctor in the U.K. The problem in the past has undoubtedly been that he has failed to lift his telephone often enough to communicate with the profession. This has given an erroneous impression of a sort of demigod sitting in autocratic isolation – hence the misunderstandings of the early 1970s which, under the present regime, could never be repeated.

The Brynmor Jones Committee (set up by the profession) had reported in 1971 and been superseded by the appointment by Sir Keith Joseph, in 1972, of a Committee of Inquiry into the Regulations of the Medical Profession.[16] It reported to Mrs Castle in 1975 (the Merrison Report). The report was excellent in every respect but one: to meet the

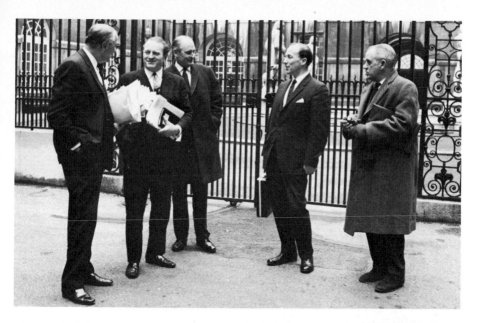

19 B.M.A. delegation en route
to talks with Richard Crossman
on immigrant doctors, 1969
(British Medical Association)

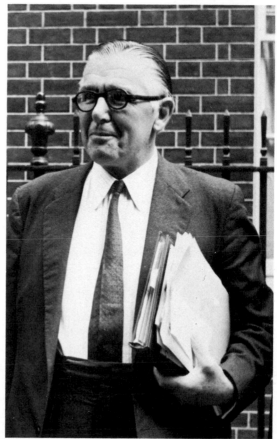

20 Richard Crossman, Secretary of State for Social Services,
during crisis talks in 1969 *(British Medical Association)*

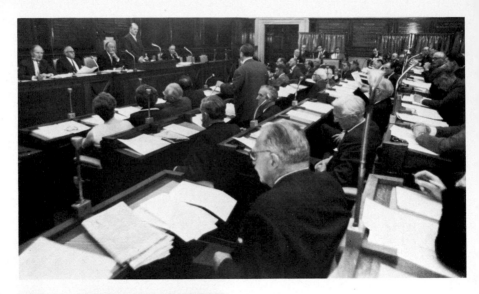

21 B.M.A. Council in session during the 1969 crisis *(The Times)*

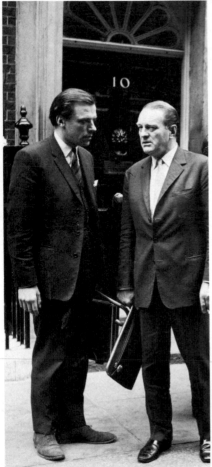

22 The author with Mr Julian Elkington, Chairman of the Junior Hospitals Staff Committee, outside 10 Downing Street after seeing the Prime Minister during the 1971 crisis *(British Medical Association)*

demands of the profession for a majority of elected members on the GMC (as opposed to those appointed by the universities and Royal Colleges, and nominated by the Privy Council) it proposed a total of a hundred members. After some delay, due to lack of parliamentary time, the new GMC emerged in 1979.

The pity of it all was that, once in Hallam Street, no one considered who was elected, appointed or nominated. It seemed irrelevant. Each member had the same purpose. But this was not seen by the whole profession and the opinion was that the council was unrepresentative of the profession and controlled mainly by academics out of touch with reality. The Merrison Report effectively brought all the functions of the GMC up to date. How a hundred members will cope is another matter. Apart from the additional cost of such a large body, the major difficulty will be to get as many members as possible involved in committee work, and not just attending three times a year for council meetings. It is worth noting, too, that the controversy took a decade to sort out.

11

1976 – 1979

In response to a demand from general practitioners for a new charter, a working group was set up in 1977 under the chairmanship of Dr John Ball. The profession was suffering from the government's pay policy[1] [2] and considered that quite disproportionate sacrifices in the national interest had been made by the medical and dental professions.[3] A delegation saw the Prime Minister (Mr Callaghan) but their arguments provoked little response.

In 1976 the report of a Special Committee on Child Health Services, chaired by Professor Donald Court, was published.[4] When it was set up I wrote to Professor Court urging him to ensure a more adequate representation of general practice on his committee. His reply did nothing to cheer me. The result, to my mind, was that an otherwise excellent report was spoiled by one recommendation: that there should be general practitioner paediatricians (GPPs). This concentrated the minds of GPs so much that it diverted their thoughts from the rest of the report. One partner in a practice, it would appear, was to be set aside and widely known as the doctor who dealt with children. Any partner spending 70 per cent of his time in child health would be no longer a GP, but a paediatrician spending 30 per cent of his time as a generalist. I could not imagine his other partners happily and willingly handing over all their babies and children to him. Attempting to promote such a concept is to unveil an almost complete lack of understanding of the GP, even today. Similarly, the idea of health visitors, attached to general practice, reverting to being workers in a geographical field and becoming specialist child health visitors was another *faux pas*. How could they be attached to group practices yet be responsible for a different group of patients? What a pity.

But the Court Report uncovered a wide gap in medical care. It suggested a child–centred service including adequately trained and experienced staff; involvement of parents; one service following a child's development from early pre-school years to adolescence; primary and specialist care as one co–ordinated service, with at every level both developmental and educational medicine as well as the treatment of acute illness. All these demanded support for a proposed service based on general practice, with 'child developmental centres' in district general hospitals. The Court report well merits implementation, but cannot, and I am sure will not, be allowed unwittingly to disturb inter-doctor and doctor-patient relationships within general practice.

In 1976, the first Southampton-trained doctors emerged (the school was inaugurated in October 1971). By the time they qualified these young doctors had seen more of general practice than any from other medical schools. In building up a curriculum for his students the Dean of Medicine, Professor Acheson, had acknowledged that 60 per cent of the permanent medical jobs were in general practice and he set out to ensure that doctors trained at Southampton would have a better understanding of medicine outside the hospital, including general practice, and a deeper insight into the relationship between hospital and community care. To this end, 10 per cent of the students' clinical training was done *outside* the hospital and the clinical programme allowed third year students to devote half a day each week to the community aspects of subjects they were studying in the wards.[5]

At last we were seeing students exposed to the rough and tumble of life outside the closed hospital community so that they gained an understanding in their early years of how their academic training could be translated to practical effect in a primary health care service. This was good news indeed. We saw the beginning of this enlightenment with the birth of the Royal College of General Practitioners, the voluntary attachment of students to some general practices and the Nuffield pilot scheme for vocational training in Wessex in the 1950s. Southampton set the seal on all this.

The General Medical Services Committee supported post-graduate training in general practice and the introduction of mandatory requirements.[6] So the objective towards which so many of us had been striving over the years was now in sight.

A worry remains in relation to continuing education. Doctors are perpetual students and because of this they must be provided with adequate facilities for continuing education. The facilities are undoubtedly there in abundance, including post-graduate courses, the provision of medical libraries in every region, weekly and monthly medical journals and regular visits by representatives of pharmaceutical firms to individual practitioners. Already, too, the computer is adding its expertise to all these other educational aids and it will not be long before the GP will not even have to leave his consulting room to keep himself up to date. The problem (unresolved by a special panel on medical research and information set up by the British Library) is how to persuade doctors to make use of all the excellent opportunities available to them. This book would be dangerously incomplete if it omitted any reference to this aspect of family doctoring, even though an acknowledgement of it inevitably involves adding to the doctor's burden of work.

The Charter Working Party surfaced in February 1979.[7] Its report contained many recommendations on the structure of and variations in the method of remuneration of family doctors. A special conference of GPs on 12–13 June 1979 supported the objectives set out in the report and welcomed the opportunities it offered to improve the quality of care and range of services they could provide for their patients with greater satisfaction to their work in primary care. The conference proposals included separate fees for all doctors providing out of hours service and for counselling work where they had a special expertise; an optional salaried service in remote rural areas; unrestricted access to a full range of investigations; therapeutic services in hospital by right and not discretion and financial incentives to buy certain appropriate equipment for use in health centres or private premises.

Perhaps the most important recommendation was that there should be a system of clinical audit maintained by the profession and of service audit, with the profession exercising responsible control over its own activities.[8]

Another worry for GPs was a Private Member's Bill (Mr John Corrie) before Parliament in June 1979 to amend the Abortion Act. It reflected the continuing opposition to 'abortion on request' among some MPs and members of the public. Its recommendations included changing the upper limit for termination from twenty eight weeks to twenty, altering the words of the clause on conditions from 'risk' to 'grave risk' to the life of the pregnant woman, widening the conscience clause and licensing pregnancy advisory services.

This received no support from the major medical organisations. The BMA considered no amendment to the Act was necessary. A *BMJ* leading article on 28 July 1979 (p. 230) said that 'An ideal law should surely reflect clinical realities, and requires that the criteria for termination should become progressively more stringent with the length of pregnancy';[9] and *BMA News Review* said 'What is more frightening than the very slim possibility that a viable life will be snuffed out, is the very real probability that if Britain goes back to the pre-Abortion Act days, the lives of many distressed women and girls will be in the hands of back street operators for whom little is precious, other than money.'[10] Fortunately, this Bill came to nothing.

In July 1979 the Report of the Royal Commission on the National Health Services was published.[11] It was a 491-page document containing 107 recommendations. Its membership of sixteen included one general practitioner (Councillor Dr Cyril Taylor) from Liverpool and one retired general practitioner (Dr Christopher Wells, OBE, TD) from Sheffield.

Although, as the Commissioners acknowledged, the

Report contained no 'blinding revelations' and a number of its recommendations merely reiterated those of Porritt and Gillie (such as the provision of health centres, an acceptable standard of surgery premises, a closer working relationship between the caring professions, the monitoring of deputising services and the training of receptionists – all old stuff that should have been activated long ago), it drew timely attention to new problems building up within the service over the past decade or more which called for discussion and action. These included a more radical approach to GP prescribing, the feasibility of introducing a compulsory retirement age for GPs and an expansion of health education.

Two others in the same category were of great importance: the need for government to attract groups of doctors to work in declining urban areas. The provision of services in these areas constituted a major challenge to the community and a much more flexible and innovative approach to the improvement of services was indicated; and positive progress in the development of community hospitals so that patients not requiring the full, specialised facilities of the district general hospital could be looked after in smaller units nearer home under the care of GPs.

The Commissioners chanced their arm in a big way when they suggested that Family Practitioner Committees (almost sacred to GPs) should eventually be abolished; and meanwhile Community Health Councils should have the right of access to Family Practitioner Committees with many more resources made available to them to act as the patients' friend in complaints and that GPs should make local arrangements specifically to facilitate audit (examination) of the services they were providing with health authorities checking progress into their development. In addition, they advocated the establishment of pharmacies in health centres.

The government's response to the Commission's report took the form of a consultative document on the Structure and Management of the NHS in England and Wales. This was published in December 1979[12] and is undoubtedly an attractive document which, having reminded us that the needs of the patient must be paramount (without which comment no NHS testament would be complete!), accepts that morale in the service has suffered as a result of a failure to make quick decisions and a general wastage of money. Although we have seen in this book that more than a wordy acknowledgement is needed to mend the rift between health and welfare created by Mr Crossman, it is reassuring to read that the Government considers that those in the NHS should be willing to work together with the social services, education and housing. One can only hope that the intention is to support this pious hope with a decisive, practical policy.

Other encouraging news is a concession that there are too many tiers in the NHS and too many administrators. To adjust the present structure the government proposes to strengthen management at local level with a greater delegation of responsibility to those in the hospital and county services; to remove the area tier in most parts of England and Wales and establish district health authorities; to simplify the professional advisory machinery so that the views of clinical doctors, nurses and the other professions will be better heard by health authorities, and to simplify the planning system in a way which will ensure that regional plans are fully sensitive to district needs.

These proposals, taken in conjunction with an avowal, against the wishes of the Royal Commission, to retain present arrangements for the administration of family practitioner services and to invite views on whether community health councils should be preserved or not, should add up to a much more effective and happier service. They have gone a long way to meet the needs of the service and those working in it at field level.

Meanwhile, the Review Body's eighth and ninth reports had been published in May 1978 and June 1979.[13] The tenth report appeared in May 1980.[14] The fees and allowances recommended in the tenth report were designed to increase the intended average net remuneration for General Medical Practitioners, after allowing for practice expenses, to £16,290 a year, assuming no change in the level of workload or responsibility. It was estimated that GPs 'would, in addition, receive an average net income of some £665 from contraceptive service fees and £495 from hospital work and other official services.' The government accepted these recommendations.

I want to end this chapter by underlining that the Review Body agreed with the Royal Commission of 1957 (Pilkington) that it is wrong for doctors and dentists to occupy a fixed position in the general pay hierarchy or for their remuneration to be determined by an automatic formula. Its recommendations continue to be based on informed judgement which takes into account not only remuneration outside the medical and dental professions but also 'such matters as changes in the cost of living, the level and quality of recruitment to these professions, the need to retain highly qualified men and women in the service of the community, and changes in workload and responsibilities or in the working environment.'

In other words, they are still 'jobbing back' to Pilkington and our fight to retain this had been justified. This is reassuring. The whole profession must strongly defend it if it is threatened by any further assault in the future. With the acceptance by government of this tenth report, the remuneration of GPs is up to date. The agony of constant deferments, arguments and confrontations is abated – for sometime to come, I hope.

One last glance at Pilkington (1957–60) is instructive. I quote from paragraph 436 (p. 147):

Seven people such as we have in mind will make recommendations of such weight and authority the Government will be able, and indeed feel bound, to accept them. This procedure will in fact, therefore, give the profession a valuable safeguard. Their remuneration will be determined, in practice, by a group of independent persons of standing and authority not committed to the Government's point of view. In the interests of preserving confidence and goodwill it is moreover essential that the Government should give its decision on the Review Body's recommendations very quickly. . . .[15]

1976 – 1979

We have seen that the years that followed the writing of these words, with all their bitterness and frustration, have proved only too forcibly the wisdom of the Royal Commission's intentions and the folly of repeatedly attempting to set them aside.

12

Primary health care in the 1980s

One of the advantages of researching and recording the history of general practice is that it is now possible to marshal the factual evidence to help frame a plan for its future.

First, there are three incontrovertible precepts which form the bedrock of any health service. Without them, such a plan would be impossible:

1 Any truly effective system of care must be organised around service to the patient, the service taking precedence over those who serve in it.
2 There is historical justification for the continued existence of the GP, the man or woman whose vocation is to act as a family doctor and *care* for the whole patient. With all the travail, changes and chances of the past centuries, and particularly the last thirty years, his position within the hierarchy of care, supported as he now is by his own Royal College and an experienced General Medical Services Committee, is stronger than ever.
3 Successive governments have resisted the temptation to interfere with the clinical freedom of the GP and have accepted the preservation of his independent contractor status.

170

This is encouraging groundwork. The rest may not be so easy.

The initial disorganisation of care, noted in the first chapters, has been replaced, if anything, by over-organisation and by repeated state interference involving changes of policy and running battles over money, known as 'diversionary activities of restless governments'.

After thirty years of the NHS, although there is much to be praised in it (enough for it to be preserved at any cost), some weaknesses have been exposed. Among these is too heavy a concentration on treatment, too little on prevention and far too little on health education, too much central control and a service top-heavy in administration. The years have proved that there should be an absolute minimum of political interference in health care.

Doctors and nurses now work in a service in which, with the ancient traditions and ethics of their calling, they are expected to go hand in hand with others who are in the painful process of proving their worth and establishing their role in care.

Some of these co-workers sadly, and not necessarily through their own fault, have drawn the patient into their struggles with government and taken a sideswipe at doctors in the process. As the service has priority over those who serve, this is regrettable. Moreover, doctors, since they have the ultimate responsibility for care, cannot ever allow their leadership of the caring team to be successfully challenged.

Workload in general practice, though changing in nature, is still a problem and this must be taken into account in planning. Fewer people in the surgery and fewer visits to patients' homes do not necessarily denote less work. Quality of care takes more time than quantity, and quality includes the replacement of time spent in visits and consulting rooms by time spent on such items as special clinics for children, the elderly, the diabetic and the hypertensive. In fact, every timesaving device, from the computer to the receptionist and the appointments clerk, has been planned to enable a busy man to find time to cope fully with the sum total of his work, and not to shorten some items of service and eliminate others.

171

In deprived and declining urban areas where there is high unemployment, poor housing, high population density, and concentrations of the homeless, it is almost impossible for a GP to act as a true family doctor, and where they are most needed doctors are frequently in short supply. In these areas, too, GPs tend to be older, single-handed and with large lists, so that comprehensive care is difficult to promote, and will be even if new health centres are provided and incentives given to encourage close teamwork between members of the caring professions. In 1980, one in seven doctors (14 per cent) in Kensington, Chelsea and Westminster was over seventy. The figure for Camden and Islington is one in eight. In the rest of England and Wales two out of 100 doctors are seventy or more.[1]

A health service is a voracious consumer of money and there is no limit to the percentage of the gross national product which it could consume if all its needs were met. Yet there is a limit in every country to the amount that can be allocated to health and social security. What is required is a united and determined effort to reach as many as possible of the essential objectives within the available budget – and this will involve an assessment of priorities. Such an evaluation will never be acceptable to all sections of the profession but if it is reached by everyone co-operating and understanding each other's needs, at least some sort of agreed programme ought to evolve, to replace the present rather *ad hoc* and random method of evaluation.

Poor communications corrupt a good health service and general practitioners in any area are far more likely to accept deferment of a new health centre if they are properly informed that the money has been diverted to meet a more urgent medical need.

No plan for a health service can be viable unless it can be guaranteed that all those working in it will be adequately remunerated, cushioned against inflation and assured of security in retirement. I hope, therefore, that the 1957 Royal Commission's definition of the Review Body's decisions will be respected and accepted by government and profession alike. Thus, recurring crises should be reduced to a minimum. The state has, over and over again, laid itself open to the charge of trying to run the service on the cheap and this has led to a deterioration in the standard of service to those in need and of morale amongst the workers. If this is going to continue, there is little point in trying to plan a future NHS.

Next, I shall list a number of components required by a primary health care service which have been recommended from as far back as 1962, or even earlier. The majority of these have already been activated, either by statute or by forward-thinking doctors in various parts of the country. For the majority we have to thank the Porritt, the Gillie, the Peel and the Harvard–Davis committees, not forgetting the Fraser–France working party. Indeed, sheer repetition must have made the implementation of some recommendations inevitable. They include:

1 health centres and the building of primary health care teams
2 appointment systems and the attachment of health visitors to general practice
3 encouragement of trainee general practitioner schemes with measures to remedy possible abuse (Porritt) leading on to every entrant to general practice being specifically and vocationally trained for the work (Gillie)
4 trained secretarial staff
5 properly organised deputising services
6 direct and unrestricted access by GPs to consultants in charge of radiological and pathological departments
7 the continued employment of GPs in cottage hospitals in which they should maintain responsibility for their own cases, with consultant cover
8 GP maternity units sited as close to consultant staffed hospitals as possible
9 and an aim of the primary health care team to treat the patient in his own home throughout his illness.

A tenth, very major, recommendation might have been

implemented by now, but unfortunately it was stamped on by the Seebohm Committee:

10   close co-operation between GPs and skilled ancillary paramedical workers, including psychiatric social workers, probation and children's officers, mental welfare officers and various voluntary bodies. (Harvard-Davis included social workers and home helps as part of the group practice team.)

Mr Anthony (now Lord) Barber's seven suggestions for easing the burden of the GP's work (1964, chapter VI) have been largely implemented. The pool system has gone; doctors have been given financial encouragement to build group practice premises, to come together to work in partnerships and to employ what staff they need; local authority nurses, health visitors and midwives can now be attached to GPs' practices and new medical schools have been opened not only at Nottingham but also at Southampton and Leicester, together with a new clinical school at Cambridge.

So we have come a long way since the 1950s. At the beginning of the 1980s the remuneration of family doctors is, almost for the first time, not a matter of contention.

The introduction of approved deputising services has eased the burden of the doctor's work, but I am referring to work that extended over sixteen hours or more in twenty-four hours and involved regular tours of night duty. I am not referring to the introduction of a regular eight-hour day for doctors, or anything like it, but a lessening of what is, in effect, a heavy burden of work.

Whether it is ever going to be possible to decrease the number of unnecessary calls on the GP, I am doubtful. Although propaganda on television and by other means has helped there will always be a certain number of these calls, because some people are just not concerned about giving the doctor work to do – any more than they worry about the butcher or the baker. There will also be some who cannot judge whether a call is necessary or not and, the most important group of all, those who are in desperate need of help and advice and have no one other than a GP to turn to. These unnecessary calls, on paper, will always be a bone of contention, but a vocationally contented doctor should be able to take them in his stride.

There are two outstanding major worries. First, is the lack of uniformity of care throughout the country with an inability or disinclination in some areas by some doctors and local health authorities to implement the accepted criteria.

Inability may be for geographical or environmental reasons, including lack of adequate housing for the doctor and his family; a poor standard of practice premises which cannot be re-sited or rebuilt without help from the state; poor staffing through unwillingness by nurses, health visitors, receptionists and others to work in the area or on the premises; and an over-large, mixed and sometimes unruly list of patients.

There is inevitably a disinclination for doctors to maintain practice premises of a reasonable standard in areas where vandalism, petty theft and violence are rampant, and appointment systems are inoperable. Although these are special cases and must be urgently treated as such, there is little excuse for the remaining areas still to be without primary health care teams or trained non-medical staff. A doctor or group of doctors showing no inclination to progress towards the 1980s since the Porritt report was published could be said to be straining democracy too far.

The second matter for concern is the artificial division of care into two, with health and welfare working in separated compartments.

There is an increasing determination, especially at field level, to remedy the defect in care which government has created. This may mean local initiative being taken in some areas and not in others, so that again there will be an inequality of care from area to area. The hope must be that local efforts will eventually gather in force until they become irresistible (as happened with the building of primary health care teams, the institution of appointment systems and the training of receptionists and secretaries) and will reach a stage when government will be forced to make a national move to rectify the errors of its predecessor. Since any future scheme of care *must* presume unification of health and welfare, even though this may take a decade to re-create, one wonders why the Royal Commission narrowed its recommendation for encouragement of integration and further development merely to Northern Ireland. How, for example, can one talk of economies and yet at the same time recommend 'no radical change in the responsibilities for either the health or the personal social services'? The expense of separation applies not only to money but also to efficiency.

Making use of all this accumulated evidence I can now set down a plan for a primary health care service of the 1980s, starting with the premises in which the team will work.

It is impossible to be dogmatic about primary care premises, except to say that a reversal of policy from the encouragement of health centres to their condemnation is both illogical and unrealistic. The focus of primary care should be health centres or purpose-built group practice premises. Either could be doctor-owned or wholly or partly state financed (through Family Practitioner Committees). An allowance should be made to doctors to cover the use of their premises by members of allied professions working with the group and for their use by undergraduate and post-graduate students.

The term 'group practice premise' can be used even if the building only accommodates a single-handed practitioner, since he will be working in a group with colleagues from other caring professions.

Premises should be built to approved designs, making allowances for the demands of preventive care, under-graduate and post-graduate teaching, a common room and a study particularly designed for those in training, a possible future growth of the caring team (by the addition of welfare and other workers in the social services at present isolated from the health team), and technological advances in organ-isation and treatment. Premises should be designed and built with the maximum of co-operation and communication

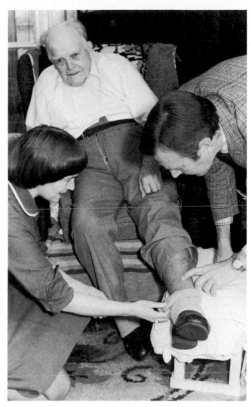

23 Caring for the old – and the young
(photographs by Dr John Woodward)

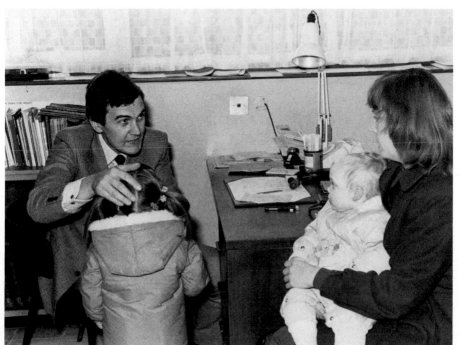

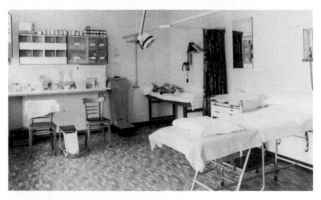

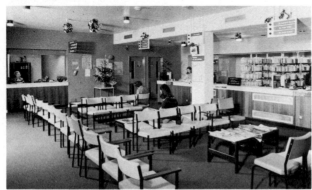

24 A modern surgery and waiting room *(Pulse)*

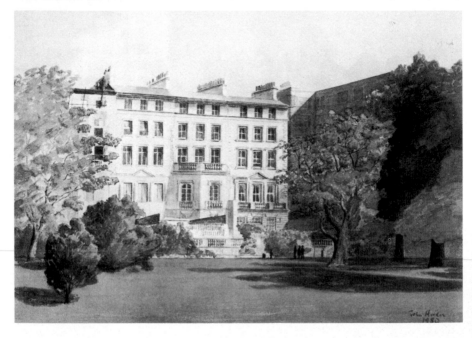

25 The Royal College of General Practitioners, painting by the President, Dr John Horder *(photograph by courtesy of Modern Medicine)*

between the Family Practitioner Committee, doctors, nurses and others who are to work in and operate from them. Once built, premises should be run with the minimum of interference by the state, i.e. FPCs or local health authorities, tenants being given overall control of administration, maintenance and repairs. Standard charges should be introduced, together with guaranteed security of tenure.

All those working in primary care should be trained personnel, including secretaries and receptionists, responsibility for whose training should be accepted by the government. Since they are the first and last members of the team to see the patient and have the responsibility of supervising his care when not in the doctors' or nurses' rooms, it is inequitable that they should be the only untrained members of the team. There should be an insistence on inter-professional training from the student years onwards.

Primary care premises should come under the aegis and custodianship of Family Practitioner Committees, which must never be abolished. These in turn should be part of a district health authority, area authorities being gently phased out. Districts, within agreed and acceptable levels, should grow steadily in importance and responsibility, it being understood that the best administration and service is required at or as near as possible to the grass roots.

No one should be allowed to administer local services who has not been intimately and actively involved in the day-to-day hurly-burly, agony and urgency of practice at primary care level. It is an insult to field workers to be directed from behind by staff officers who specialise in theory yet are tyros in practice.

There should be regional autonomy, with the absolute minimum of interference from the Department of Health and Social Security. Efficiency with economy should be rewarded and not stifled, thus accumulated savings should be retained by those who make them. A case can be made for the family doctor service to be provided through regional health boards, in the interests of functional and administrative unity, but only if the independent contractor status of the GP can be preserved and the primary care service guaranteed its fair share of the financial cake with, and not after, the demands of the hospital and other services.

Every effort should be made to ensure an equal standard of care between one section of the population and another. This is one of the most vexed problems to solve, for it includes the provision of purpose-built, properly sited and approved types of buildings with an acceptable range of equipment in all areas. This inevitably involves government help in rural and inner city areas where the particular needs of the people and of the caring professions, though recognised, have never been resolutely pursued. Priority should, therefore, be given to the building of health centres (even if of a temporary nature, and mobile!); to improvement grants for existing premises; to smaller lists without loss of income; and to an acknowledgement that many doctors in these areas, for various reasons, cannot live on or near their practice premises and so merit help in housing and travelling.

Every GP practising within the health service should have the right to part-time private practice without financial detriment and with an acknowledgement of the benefit that this can bring through competition and extra finance made available to the service.

There should be continuous ongoing research into future needs, particularly in relation to workload in general practice and to increasing involvement of family doctors and their colleagues in preventive medicine and teaching.

Help in reducing workload may come from development of computerisation and other technological aids to administration, research, teaching and care of the patient. Professor Wilkes (*Pulse*, 39, 2, 1979) considers that within the next twenty-five years, 40 per cent of practices will be computer-aided, yet it would be most unwise to budget for a lessening of the demands on a GP's time in the future. Science may produce new cures and change the face of medical care, but there will always be room in general practice for more time devoted to other primary care activities which cannot be adequately covered today.

The GP's daily round must be seen against a backcloth of decreasing hours being worked by the society within which he lives. He can never expect overtime payments; and even the present average forty-hour week has always been completely unrealistic for him. He will need to be helped in adjusting to a more leisured society in years to come.

In addition to computerisation, trained non-medical staff and increasing health education it may be possible to broaden the training of nurses and health visitors so that they can take more work from GPs, although they too work longer hours than the majority of the population. Moreover, nurses and health visitors working with doctors tend to increase the workload, for the positive and wholly acceptable reason that they uncover hitherto unknown, usually subacute or chronic, illnesses in patients – anaemia and chronic urinary disease or even malnutrition in the elderly. This is, of course, one of the objects of having a caring team and one of the methods of improving the standard of care.

'Feldshers' and 'barefoot doctors' must be mentioned in this context, if only to be dismissed, for this would involve training and paying for yet one more group of workers.

The health centre (care centre would be a better title) is, then, the focal point of primary care and members of the team should emerge from it to work within the community, the service giving them maximum encouragement to care for the patient at home.

As close a liaison as possible must be built up with the personal social services. Home care, and especially terminal care and care of the mentally and physically handicapped, implies home nursing, health visiting and provision for night care and although this need not necessarily be done by trained personnel, without whom home care would break down, it is the responsibility of the health service; while welfare workers, home helps and meals on wheels come under the social services. Locally, at any rate therefore, the concept of care must be seen to be united within itself, and not dangerously divided.

This factor alone underlines the need for available money in the primary care service to be concentrated on workers, not on offices, paper and administrators. There can be no excuse for an administrative module of something like 20 per cent of the total work force in the service.

Field workers must become used to working and learning together so that they can provide a total service as economically and effectively as possible, for the good of the patient/client and for their own professional satisfaction.

The community hospital programme ought to be regenerated. Family doctors, with their hospital and other colleagues, could meet together in these hospitals which should at best be sited in the grounds of the teams' health centres. Many patients now referred to district hospitals could then be cared for in their 'own' hospitals, once they have been fully assessed and investigated. If it be necessary in the first place to admit them to a district general hospital they could later be returned to the smaller one within their own community, closer to their families and under the care of doctors and nurses they know, and from there could go back home.

I wonder how much longer the state will be able to afford the 'hospital dumping' of patients who need never have been admitted in the first place if the primary care service had been properly organised, or who are retained in beds in large wards after the genuine need for hospital treatment is passed, simply because there is nowhere else for them to go? We know how expensive it is in patient satisfaction to keep district general hospital beds filled with those who could be adequately cared for in a community hospital or at home. Someone ought to start looking at the accounts again. With the growth of community hospital care, and with superspecialist units in the background, district general hospitals could be built more economically, with more effective use of building space, personnel, equipment and services.

Doctors working in general practice should be vocationally trained and ideally have higher degrees (the MRCP, DCH, for example) and/or an MRCGP. The Royal Commission accepts that experience alone does not guarantee good quality, nor, in my view, does the possession of higher qualifications. The essential is that those who are not, by personality or intention, potential GPs should be dissuaded as early as possible in their careers, and certainly during their vocational training. It is the duty of the teacher to divert them to an alternative and more appropriate discipline.

It is difficult to go along with the Royal Commission in its apparent belief that better standards will be achieved by supervised audit, by a greater involvement of Community Health Councils or by setting up panels of external assessors for each appointment of a principal, to ensure that standards are maintained. If ever there were recommendations calculated to destroy general practice as we know and value it, these are they.

Yet, in order to reduce criticism to a minimum and expand care to a maximum, GPs should be prepared to impose self-discipline, which includes self-audit. In addition, they should accept the need for continuing education throughout their practising years; admit to their discipline only those who have undergone vocational training and proved their worth; undertake an active role in uncovering the sick doctor and helping him, if necessary through the GMC's health committee; resolve to maintain up-to-date and forward-looking methods of practice; and use only supervised and acceptable deputising services. Even though no service can be perfect, it is in all the above particulars that doctors can be open to the charge that they have not themselves played a sufficiently active part in putting and keeping their own house in order.

If doctors fail in these responsibilities, then the state must intervene on behalf of the patient. This book has shown that most of the ingredients of an acceptable and worthwhile service are now there for the asking, on paper at any rate. They have been obtained through a great deal of toil and sweat extending over three decades, with or without the help of the state. It is, in my view, unwise for the profession to continue, in a paranoid way born of years of travail, to shift the blame for all the defects in the service onto someone else. The rational thing to do now is to put our own house in order first and thus be able to build future criticism on a more solid foundation. Just as doctors from time to time have had enough, some patients today feel the same way and it is no good our ignoring them.

I detest using such harsh words, but it is time someone from inside the profession used them. Bashing the doctor has become an acceptable game, played by a number of people for largely unacceptable reasons, but I hate the thought that others may join in because they are being deprived of a primary care service – which they may well have seen enjoyed by their friends in other areas – and because they feel that their doctors are, in some way or the other, letting them down.

In summary, if family doctors – oppressed and harassed as they have been, cynical and tired as many of them are after these past argumentative years – can show the loyalty to their patients that they have continuously received from the majority of the community to date, they will greatly help themselves and eliminate the need for outside interference. This may be unpalatable but I believe it to be true.

Community Health Councils, reconstituted to represent the community as a whole and not merely mouthpieces of local pressure groups, could be of immense value as friends of doctors as well as of patients. They are needed in the immense task of providing primary care, for GPs, like any other section of society, will respond to positive encouragement and to constructive criticism. Conversely, they will react adversely to constant nagging and negatively-oriented activity; and if Community Health Councils have open access to Family Practitioner Committees, as recommended by the Royal Commission, they will run the risk of attracting the suspicion and distrust of doctors and thus lose the unbiased image they need to create if they are to carry out their role effectively. It is much better they should get to know as many doctors as possible, individually or in their group practices, tackle them face to face about any defects or criticisms that have been uncovered and show a willingness to help in finding solutions with the doctors and not apart from them.

Thus patients with problems should be directed in the first place to the Family Practitioner Committee. With

Service (disciplinary) Committees, the General Medical Council, the Ethical Committee of the BMA and the civil courts there are already enough channels of complaint against GPs (more, in fact, than for any other section of society) without adding to them the lowering presence of a Community Health Council, especially if it is politically oriented.

The general public has long since recognised that in the family doctor service, despite its failings, they possess something valuable. Those who represent them should respect this opinion and encourage it. CHCs can guard the primary care service without taking on the role of policeman.

Three final items: money should never be allowed to come between a patient and the family doctor. A working party should research the possibility of introducing a limited list of free, essential and effective drugs, as currently prevailing in some other health services, with a charge on patients for drugs not listed. This in no way absolves the GP from his responsibility in careful and economical prescribing. Lastly, encouragement should be given to experimentation in different methods of delivering primary care, aimed at meeting the needs of the varied areas in the country for which it is responsible.

This completes my vision of a primary health care service which could work effectively within the NHS to the maximum advantage of the patient/client and the primary care team, in that order. It is built upon the evidence adduced in this book; inevitably it is also coloured by a firm belief in what is best for the caring professions if they are to get the most satisfaction from and fulfilment in their work. I hope, however, that this is fairly balanced by the acknowledgement throughout that everything done is primarily and essentially for the good of the patient.

It has also the advantage of consistency. For the past three decades many of us have believed in this type of service and have steadily worked towards its achievement against what have at times seemed overwhelming odds.

One other comment is imperative: any further improvements should be introduced quietly over the next decade or so, with resistance to any violent unheavals or changes of policy for political reasons. The health service deserves a period of peace and quiet.

I am only too well aware as I write this that the government and the profession will almost certainly be facing each other across the table to discuss interminably new government proposals or service needs, which may never more than marginally fit together. I fear, too, that levels of remuneration may be a paramount item on the agenda. Nothing, however, will alter my view that this chapter outlines a primary health care service which will bring maximum benefit to the patient and as much fulfilment in his work as any doctor should expect to obtain. It can also be run far more economically in terms of money than the service as it is exists today. I hope that an organisation like it will evolve with the least possible argument for all those involved in making it work.

Epilogue

The family doctor 1981

Have a good General Practitioner to whom you can talk and in whom you have faith. The best general practitioners realise their important function in protecting the patient from modern medicine (though they may not express it in those words), the worst will put you off with a pill and without an interview, or else send you at once to a specialist (who may be the wrong specialist) without taking time to evaluate your symptoms.

Don't let general practice die out. This would be a tragedy. The general practitioner is more necessary in the world of modern techniques and specialisation than ever before. His fate is in your hands; the hands of the discriminating public.

Lord Platt, MD
Private and Controversial

As we have seen, the general practitioner of the early twentieth century was a very different animal from the seventeenth-century apothecary. The Great Plague and the Great Fire of London, the oppression by physicians, the increasing needs of the poor and the emergent middle classes in the Industrial Revolution, the progress of preventive medicine and other social, economic and environmental factors, brought about his gradual metamorphosis, adding a bit here and chipping away a bit there to fit him into a society increasingly aware of the need for a primary physician – part doctor, part priest and part social worker – who would be available to the community at all hours of the day or night to *care for* the sick.

Because he had grown up in this way, from the apothecary's shop, he seemed in no need for any special education. There were not then, any more than there are now, any higher degrees in the innate qualities which were the major tools of his particular trade. Any other qualities needed for family doctoring he learnt as he went along. So much depended on the man himself, his flair for diagnosis and total devotion to his patients, fighting for their lives through the exhibition of sheer willpower combined with common sense.

The vital questions now are whether these basic qualities still exist; whether they are still as necessary as ever or whether they have been discarded (partly or wholly) to make room for others thought to be more relevant to the era of the welfare state? In the answer to these questions we shall find the family doctor of the 1980s.

A close analysis of the last thirty years distinguishes four closely linked elements contributing to the development of today's family doctor: the government, the patient, advances in diagnosis and treatment, and the doctor himself.

In preceding chapters, particularly chapter XII, I have described fully the activities of government since the inception of the NHS, the pressure by patients on the primary care services and the response of family doctors to organisational developments within the service over these years.

What surprises me is the extent of the advances in diagnosis and treatment and the impact these must have had on primary care, both in the nature of the doctor's work and in his ability to help his patient. Their influence on him is of far greater consequence than I imagined when I first set out to draw a picture of the family doctor as he exists today.

The first thing to understand is that these advances have not, as forecast by the architects of the Act, reduced the GP's workload. New, highly complex and sophisticated methods of diagnosis and treatment have involved the patient's own doctor and not just the hospital service. The consequence is that his work has become more rewarding, for he is now clearly seen as a doctor in his own right, working in an important part of the service. In other words, this element more than any other has served to change the pattern of his work and with it his image as a family doctor. Its progress, too, has been inexorable; sweeping aside on its journey, and taking precedence over, the adverse elements represented by recurrent arguments on levels of remuneration and the pressure of demand by patients.

This being so, I must spell out in more detail some of the work of the modern GP. First, enormous strides have been made in the diagnostic field, many of them provided by laboratory and X-ray departments of hospitals and available to GPs.

Then, coming on to treatment, whilst accepting that some techniques are so elaborate and complicated that they are only available to, or have to remain under the guidance of specialists (renal dialysis, organ transplantation and the chemical treatment of malignant disease are examples), many others are safe in the hands of GPs, working hand in hand with specialists. We have come a long way from the days when the range of effective drugs available to the GP were 'the alkalies in urinary infection, salicylates in acute rheumatism and digitalis in some forms of heart disease.'

The revolution started with the introduction of the drug Prontosil, proceeded to penicillin and other antibiotics, and has gone on to the deployment of an increasing variety of drugs for the treatment of depression and anxiety, diseases of the heart and circulatory system; those which correct hormone imbalance; and those which alleviate asthma, hay fever, rheumatoid arthritis and osteo-arthritis, to mention only some.

These have always been the cases most frequently seen in the GP's surgery, but nowadays most of them, even though some involve surgery or assessment by specialists, are capable of being diagnosed in the first place by GPs and given continuous care by them. The fact that many still cannot be cured, but merely held in check, adds to rather than subtracts from their work. A cure involves much less time.

The weekly programme of inoculations and vaccinations which GPs now undertake, together with the use of the antibiotics, has eliminated some diseases and the dangerous potentialities of others (progress which no one should belittle). Modern science has also brought within the GP's range the diagnosis and treatment of numerous diseases for which hitherto he could do little other than exhibit his compassion, sympathy and understanding, together with a tonic, sedative or analgesic dressed up as a pill or a rather unpalatable mixture.

The highly sophisticated modern drugs cannot be prescribed without care and time-consuming assessment. They frequently have unpleasant, undesirable and even dangerous side effects and it is hazardous for patients to stop taking them without medical advice. Consultations, therefore, have to be arranged so that the patient is not left without treatment. In these circumstances, but in no others, it is forgivable for doctors to issue duplicate prescriptions in moderate amounts or to allow their trained receptionists to prepare them for signature.

In short, although the diseases from which patients suffer may not have changed to any degree, the pattern of treatment certainly has. Today the GP has to deal with many important chronic patients who need to be seen regularly, require careful reassessment each time and their treatment frequently adjusted. Acute cases are now in the minority. When they are seen, they can often be accurately and immediately diagnosed and successfully treated. Few cases are now hopeless in that they are going to die tomorrow or the next day. They are going to live and to visit the doctor for years.

Thus GPs, willy nilly and not unhappily, have become a part of the scientific revolution.

Yet this is not all, for hospital radiological and pathological departments are now open to GPs and hospital doctors available for consultation in the patient's home. Moreover, the development of physical medicine and rehabilitation have provided the primary care service with a variety of ways to keep patients active and mobile. The state, via the health and personal social services, provides ambulances, nurses, health visitors, midwives, social workers, home helps, meals on wheels and various types of personal and domestic equipment, so that many patients – including the elderly, the mentally and physically handicapped and those suffering from incurable disease – can be nursed and treated in their own homes instead of having to be transferred to hospital or other chronic institutional care.

In addition, today's GP is expected to have some knowledge, if only a smattering, of the rarer conditions he is likely to meet, such as drug dependence, alcoholism, cot deaths, baby and wife battering; he should be *au fait* with such matters as the age of consent, of majority and criminal liability; with the rights and needs of women seeking to have their pregnancies terminated and in the use and misuse of 'the pill'. He has to be aware of the various social tragedies or misfortunes that have medical overtones.

The pace of change in medical techniques also means that the GP has continually to update his knowledge. He has to be a perpetual student – a further time-consuming necessity.

So the family doctor in the 1980s can no longer afford to know less and less about more and more. Added to this, he is working within a sophisticated and permissive society which is better informed and more litigious minded than in the past. The press and television have beset him with problems which his predecessors in the 1950s did not have to face. He is, in his work, competing with programmes on television describing and displaying for all to see the nature and treatment of disease and with groups of well-meaning but medically non-qualified people who offer treatment for this or that type of patient and even presume to advise him on what he should be prepared to tell patients about their illness and its prognosis.

He is at the receiving end of startling and controversial opinions on the prevention and possible hazards involved in the treatment of some diseases, like whooping cough, and has to be prepared at short notice to drop everything in favour of coping with an emergency (such as a massive programme of vaccination against smallpox).

Clearly, therefore, the family doctor today has to be a different man or woman from the one known to our grand-fathers and great grandfathers. His visits to the house and his accessibility to the patient may have decreased but the quality of his work and his skill and effectiveness have improved beyond question. There must be no further harking back to the good old days for time has proved that they were far from good in many respects.

Thus, the man or woman who enters general practice today faces the enormous responsibility of welding together the traditional concept of the family doctor, apothecary and friend of the 1950s and the 1980 version of a vocationally trained, well qualified general practitioner and sub-specialist. The degree of this responsibility can be gauged when we see that I have so far omitted from his work the most necessary and time-consuming item of all – the one for which he is needed more than ever today and which has been mainly accountable for the image of him built up over the centuries – his role as counsellor and friend.

It is surely no wonder that our image of the family doctor we feel we need and the flesh and blood doctor whom we now find in our homes and in his surgery, are two different people. Yet I do not believe this need be so.

I want to face the facts as they are and not as they seem to be: the young doctor today has discarded the three piece suit, the stethoscope curled inside his hat, the solid Humber or Rover and the spacious house with a drive and lawn. Instead, he may have long hair, jeans, an open shirt, a sweater or a sports jacket and a small car. He may live on a housing estate separated from his place of work. His wife may have been replaced by a receptionist and his seemingly endless hours of duty lessened by the employment of a deputy. But surely that does not deny him the right to call himself a family doctor, nor mean that Mrs Jones can no longer lean on his car and talk to him as she did in 1950 or that his patients are no longer able to tell him and his wife all their woes and secrets?

A glance at the other side of the coin should be reassuring, for this young doctor no longer feels alone all of a sudden when he leaves his hospital. Apart from the fact that he will probably join a group practice, he has undergone special training in family doctoring before being let loose on his patients; there has been a programmed transition from hospital to community and the primary health care team.

Today he has available to him at any time the immediate back up support from hospital consultants, including radiologists and pathologists.

In his own surgery he works closely as a team with nurses and health visitors; he may have his own portable electrocardiograph machine, a well-equipped treatment room (with an ample supply of sterile syringes, dressings and clothing) and a common room for informal conversation with others engaged in care, such as priests and chemists, or for clinical meetings with hospital colleagues.

Similarly in his maternity work, with the midwife he knows, he can look after the patient throughout her pregnancy and confinement. His antenatal care can be of such a quality that all but the most unexpected complications can be diagnosed early and their consequences avoided. Even when hospital confinement is chosen, he and the midwife can follow their patient into hospital and help to look after her. Moreover, early discharge back home can be arranged under such ideal circumstances.

He can run clinics for special groups of patients on his premises, which ideally are purpose-built. He has an appointment system for his patients whose notes are already on his desk waiting for him. He has a secretary on whom he can off load a good deal of his office work, including some of his telephone calls, and a typist to whom he can dictate his letters, if he does not put them on tape. He has receptionists and an appointments clerk (who may by now be specially trained for their jobs) who receive his patients for him and should also be able to relieve him of much of his administrative work.

He has special post-graduate courses available to him in a variety of medical centres; he may one day be selected as a teacher himself, be appointed to do sessions in his local district hospital or be fortunate enough to work in his own community (cottage) hospital. If that were not enough, he will soon have a computer on his desk.

Surely, we should not ask more of him than this. Yet I would be foolish if I did not share with others surprise and concern that these many desirable developments – adding up to almost exactly what the GPs of the 1950s thought must be achieved if family doctoring were going to be able to maintain its traditional role in society – seem to have *undermined* rather than reinforced the doctor-patient relationship of the 1980s.

Somehow, and somewhere in all this, the family doctor seems to have lost his identity. He has become just another doctor, a relatively unrecognisable member of a team working in a building resembling in appearance and function a small factory. We hear patients talking of going to 'that place along the road' ('No, not that one, the other one') and of seeing a doctor they cannot describe by name but only by appearance. We are told of areas in which patients do not even know the name of the doctor with whom they are registered and, worse still, live in fear of not being able to get a doctor at all when they are ill.

Patients have a feeling of being caught up in an impersonal state service where they are really rather a nuisance and considered as numbers rather than human beings.

The outstanding reasons for this must be, first, that in making room for all his new commitments within the NHS the family physician has had to neglect or even discard his role of being more than just a doctor to his patients, one who can be consulted by them for many other reasons than physical or mental illness; and, secondary but very pertinent to this, in improving his conditions of practice (for his patients' sake as well as his own) and becoming part of a primary health care team the doctor has become lost to his patients, sometimes to a degree of complete inaccessibility when he is most urgently needed; he has falsely believed that he can be replaced as an individual by any one of his team, or even by an approved deputy; and he has assumed that the passage of time has outdated and outmoded the concept of a one-to-one, family doctor-patient relationship.

His patients would emphatically deny all this. More than ever before they still need, and should have, a family doctor. So a preservation process is urgently necessary: to restore the old-fashioned doctor without at the same time losing his contemporary skills and sophisticated methods of practice.

This cannot be left to government, except in ensuring better communications within the service. It involves only the doctors and their patients. Patients must first concede that the new type of family doctor, whatever he looks like and wherever he lives, is every bit as good at his job and almost certainly better trained than his predecessor; then they must recognise the changed nature of his work and the range of his responsibilities, which now extends far beyond simple treatment in home or surgery; they must try to come to terms with receptionists and not regard them as dragons because they are too over-worked to smile and too busy trying to protect their doctor from unnecessary demands to be polite; they must learn to value the services of their doctor and not to misuse, or even abuse, them, and they must be prepared to take a more active part in helping to make the service work, particularly in the fields of community relations and community responsibility. Moreover, if they are not getting a satisfactory service they should have no qualms about saying so out loud. Passive submission merely encourages conditions to worsen.

Family doctors must first concede that they are still

needed as such by their patients. This may involve modifying the complicated machinery of modern health care in such a way that they can be as close to their patient today as were their predecessors yesterday.

In short, the need for up-to-date vocational training should not be allowed to eliminate the vital constituents of primary care identified during the course of this book. Practising from a health centre should not become synonymous with inaccessibility.

Let me give perhaps a trivial but symbolic example. In the old days, a patient was accustomed to queueing in order to see his doctor, and didn't usually complain about it. It was a recognised part of the consultation and enhanced the doctor's reputation – the bigger the queue the better the doctor must be.

So the appointment system, which was invented to eliminate the queue, is not necessarily a failure if patients still have to wait to see the doctor. But it *is* a failure if patients dread visiting an impersonal health centre where each patient seems part of a faceless crowd to the doctor and a natural enemy to his receptionist. And this can happen, I know, for at the last visit I made as a patient one receptionist was so busy bemoaning her lot that she ignored me completely – and the other one, who eventually attended to me, was eating an apple! The net result was that I felt I was in the way.

It is easy for the new type of premises in which family doctors work to appear impersonal and cold. But this difficulty would be largely overcome if everyone working in it would accept, as did the doctor and his wife in the 1950s, that their visitors are not there to buy a joint of meat or a pound of potatoes, but are sick and often apprehensive. The size of the building need make no difference at all; nor should the number of people working in it. The doctor who once had to be a whole team in himself can now be seen to be one member of a tightly knit and caring team. In fact, a team can actually help create an atmosphere of friendliness and willingness to help.

Patients accept being referred to a strange doctor if they

are told it is only for this once and given an explanation why their own doctor is absent. They understand a five minute allocation of their doctor's time if they know that this is only a preliminary assessment and that there will be a fuller examination later, if needed (and this can be made easier if the doctor sinks comfortably back in his chair rather than leaning forward with his elbows on the desk and a strained look on his face).

Doctors and their colleagues can help too if they can rid themselves of the paranoid belief that *all* the calls on their busy time are unnecessary, inconsiderate or contrived by insufferable malingerers. So far as primary care is concerned, in this respect the callers are sick. They may need no more than a smile and a few kind words; the modern family doctor and his team must be prepared to offer both.

As well as doctors and patients each contributing something in the journey back to family doctoring, teachers in hospitals and trainers in general practice need to ram home to students from the first moment they meet and go on dinning it in until they finally part, that the only person who *really* matters in primary care is the *patient*. Buildings, equipment and sophisticated treatment are there to create a better caring service for the patient and only secondarily to provide more comfort and better working conditions for the caring team.

Sadly, some students who are born family doctors lose their natural bedside manner after a term in a modern health centre or group practice and after listening to their seniors' conversations. Sadly, too, some patients revert to private treatment in a despairing effort to find care which, although no better than that available in the NHS, has a more personal feeling to it.

If today's GPs wish, deservedly, to regulate their professional lives to fit into a shorter working week I see no reason why they should feel ashamed or guilty, for they can retain the respect and confidence of their patients so long as they are still *family* doctors and fully paid up members of a general practitioner fraternity as it has been recognised over the centuries.

If, on the other hand, they are tempted to become purely mechanical purveyors of medicine to their patients, or form fillers, sieves for the hospital service or impersonal members of a large and fragmented network, shifting cases or chores they do not want onto someone else and operating petty or selfish restricted practices, they can do that too and no doubt spend happy days shooting, playing golf or sailing. But if, as a result, they lay the whole service open to justifiable criticism, the fault is theirs and not the state's or their patients' and they will lose the respect of society.

Having said all this, I know that I only have to take another journey to a village or a thinly populated part of the country to find the kind of family doctoring I know and have always wanted. I know, too, that in the more densely populated towns it is still possible to find areas of excellence and single-handed or groups of doctors maintaining a wonderful standard of service to their patients. No blame, either, should fall on doctors and nurses in those difficult areas where urgent help is awaited from the government to create some semblance of a service to patients at present deprived of it. Dedication and good intent are everywhere still to be found in plenty. It is a pity that some doctors, some patients and some governmental gaps in care are between them attracting too great a share of the limelight.

What is needed can be summed up to some extent by 'small is beautiful'. It is a readjustment to human scale so that our health service becomes equally attractive and rewarding to doctors and patients alike, making the most of the tremendous scientific and technological advances that have occurred since the NHS Act, but not forgetting that the sick need comfort and sympathy – the individual treatment offered by a family doctor.

References

PROLOGUE

Stevenson, R.L. 1912. *The Works of Robert Louis Stevenson*. Vol. 14: *Underwoods*, 63. London: Chatto & Windus.

Gibson, Sir Ronald. Introducing the Family Doctor (address to senior students at St Bartholomew's Hospital, London, 12 April 1955). *Lancet* 27 August 1955, 408–13.

Gibson, Sir Ronald. Letter to a Young Doctor (BBC talk). *Listener* 6 September 1956, **56**, 1432, 347–8.

CHAPTER 1: THE EARLY YEARS

1   Himsworth, Sir Harold. The Integration of Medicine (Linacre Lecture). *Brit Med J* 23 July 1955, 4933, 219.

2, 9, 10 Poynter, F. N. L. (ed) 1961. *The Influence of Government Legislation on Medical Practice in Britain*. London: Pitman Medical Press.

3, 4, 5, Macdonald, G. G. General Medical Practice in the Time of Thomas Vicary (Thomas Vicary Lecture). *Ann Roy Coll Surg Eng*, January–June 1967, **40**, 1–20.

6   Bryant, Sir Arthur 1966. *The Mediaeval Foundation*, 98. London: Collins.

7, 8   Whittet, T. D. From Apothecary to Pharmacist. *Chemist and Druggist* 18 July 1964, 63–4.

11   The Worshipful Society of Apothecaries of London 1978. *Handbook*.

12   Guildhall Mss. 8251, 8252, 8256.

13   Phayre, T. 1915. *The Boke of Chyldren*. London: Livingstone.

14   Debus, A. G. 1963. In *Chemistry in the Service of Medicine*, F. N. L. Poynter (ed). London: Pitman Medical Publishing.

15, 16   Whittet, T. D. Lecture to Bedfordshire and Hertfordshire Faculty, Royal College of General Practitioners, 18 May 1979.

17 Bayles, Howard. The Rose Case. *Chemist and Druggist* 1940, **132**, 473 and **133**, 8.

18 Good, J.M. 1796. *The History of Medicine so far as it Relates to the Apothecary*. 142–201. London: G. Dilley.

19 McConaghey, R. M. S. 1961. The History of Rural Medical Practice in *The Evolution of Medical Practice in Britain*, F. N. L. Poynter (ed). London: Pitman Medical Publishing.

20 Whittet, T. D. and Newbold, M. Some Eminent Cambridge Apothecaries. *Trans Brit Soc Hist Pharm*, 1977, **1**, 195–212.

21, 22 Stevens, Rosemary 1966. *Medical Practice in Modern England*. New Haven and London: Yale University Press.

23 Trevelyan, G. M. 1942. *English Social History*. 844. London: Longman.

CHAPTER 2: THE NINETEENTH CENTURY

1,21,24, McConaghey, R. M. S. Notes on the Evolution of
28 General Practice prior to 1858. *J. Coll Gen Practit*, **195**, 1, 267–78.

2 Turner, E. S. 1958. *Call a Doctor. A Social History of Medical Men*. London: Michael Joseph.

3 Whittet, T. D. From Apothecary to Pharmacist, 2. Apothecaries Take up Medicine. *Chem and Drug* 25 July 1964.

4, 6, 9 Bishop, W. J. Evolution of the GP in England. *Practitioner*, 1952, **168**, 171–9.

5 Cule, J. History of General Practice. General Practice and the Medical Act of 1858. *Update*, July 1973, 35.

7 *Lancet* 1830, **1**, 538.

8 *Lond Med Gaz* 1830, **6**, 619.

10,11,12 Henry, D. G. Nineteenth Century Anticipation –
25 Twentieth Century Realization. *J Coll Gen Practit*, 1966, **121**, 255–60.

13 Birkenhead, Lord Cohen of. Hastings and the G.M.C. *Brit Med J* 23 July 1966, 5507, 191–7.

14, 17 Alcock, T. Medical Review: Transactions of the Associated Apothecaries and Surgeon–Apothecaries of England and Wales. *Lancet* 1823, **1**.

References

15   Paget, Sir James 1902. *Memoirs and Letters*, 19–20.
        London: Longman.

16   Plowright, O. General Practice in England. *J Coll Gen
        Practit*, 1963, **6**, 542.

18   Horner, N. G. 1922. *The Growth of General Practice in
        England*. London: Bridge.

19   Rivington, W. 1879. *The Medical Profession*. Dublin:
        Fannin.

20   Allbut, Sir Clifford. The Universities in Medical
        Research and Practice (presidential address to BMA). *Brit
        Med J* 3 July 1920, 3105, 7.

22   De Styrap, J. 1890. *The Young Practitioner*. London: H. K.
        Lewis.

23   Percival, T. *Medical Ethics* (ed Chauncey Leake) 1927.
        Baltimore: Williams & Wilkins.

26   Cox, Alfred. General Practice Fifty Years Ago. *Brit Med J*
        7 January 1950, 77–8.

27   Grant, I. D. Status of the General Practitioner, Past,
        Present and Future. *Brit Med J* 1 November 1961, **1280**.

29   Nicholls, Lucius. My Grandfather's Practice. *Lancet* 24
        December 1966, 1413.

30   Pickles, William N. A Hundred Years in a Yorkshire
        Dale. *Practitioner* 1951, **167**, 322–9.

CHAPTER 3: 1900–1938

1   Stevens, Rosemary 1966. *Medical Practice in Modern
        England*, 33. New Haven and London: Yale University
        Press.

2   Horner, N. G. 1922. *The Growth of the General Practitioner
        of Medicine in England*. London: Bridge.

3, 8, 9 Hutchison, Sir Robert, Bt. Medicine Today and Yester-
        day. *Brit Med J* 7 January 1950, 72–3.

4   Grey-Turner, G. Surgery in 1900. *Brit Med J* 7 January
        1950, 73–4.

5   Marsh, Charles. *Early Medical Practice in Bath*. Bristol
        Medico-Chirurgical Journal 1964, **79**, 111–12.

6   Pickles, William. Trends in General Practice. 100 years in
        a Yorkshire Dale. *Practitioner* 1951, **167**, 326–7.

7, 13   Godber, Sir George. General Practice, Past and Present

199

(second Monckton Copeman Lecture). *J Roy Coll Gen Practit*, 1968, **16**, 179.

10   Cox, A. General Practice Fifty Years Ago. Some Reminiscences. *Brit Med J* 7 January 1950, 78.

11,12,16 Elder, H. H. A. Forty Years in General Practice. *J Roy Coll Gen Practit* 1964, **7**, 328–41.

14   Newholme, Sir Arthur. 1915. *Special Report on Maternity and Child Welfare*. Cmnd. 8085.

15, 21 Hughes, David. Twenty-five years in Country Practice (James Mackenzie Lecture). *J Coll Gen Practit* 1958, **1**, 5–13.

17   National Insurance Act 1911. London: HMSO.

18, 20 Wigg, J.W. and others. The Biography of a General Practice. *J Roy Coll Gen Practit* 1967, **14**, 85–7.

19   Vaughan, Paul 1959. *Doctors' Commons: A Short History of the British Medical Association*. 201-2. London: Heinemann.

CHAPTER 5: THE BIRTH OF THE NHS

1   Consultative Council on Medical and Allied Services 1920. *Interim Report on the Future Provision of Medical and Allied Services*. (Dawson Report). Cmnd. 693. London: HMSO.

2   Vaughan, Paul 1959. *Doctors' Commons*. 216–18. London: Heinemann.

3   Medical Planning Commission. Draft Interim Report. *Brit Med J* 1940, **1**, 743.

4   Ministry of Health 1942. *Social Insurance and Allied Services*. Cmnd. 6404. London: HMSO.

5   *A National Health Service* 1942. Cmnd. 6502. London: HMSO.

6   National Health Service Act 1946. Cmnd 6761. London: HMSO.

7   Interdepartmental Committee on the Remuneration of the General Practitioner. *Report* (Spens Report). 1946. Cmnd 6810. London: HMSO.

8   *General Practice and the Training of the General Practitioner* (Cohen Report). 1950. London: BMA.

9, 14   Medical Services Review Committee 1972. *A Review of the Medical Services in Great Britain* (Porritt Report). London: Social Assay.

References

10   *Brit Med J*, 1952, **1**, 113–30 (s).
11   *Brit Med J*, 1952, **2**, 282–6 (s).
12   College of General Practitioners 1952. *Memorandum and Articles of Association of the College of General Practitioners formed the 19th day of November 1952*. London: Linklaters and Paines.
13   Royal Commission on Doctors' and Dentists' Remuneration 1957–60, February 1960. *Report*. Cmnd 939. London: HMSO.

CHAPTER 6: 1960–1964

1   Royal Commission on Doctors' and Dentists' Remuneration 1957–60, February 1960. *Report*. Cmnd 939. London: HMSO.
2   *A Review of the Medical Services of Great Britain* (Porritt Report). 1962. London: Social Assay.
3   *Medical Staffing Structure in the Hospital Service* (Platt Report) 1961. London: HMSO.
4   Sub-Committee, Standing Medical Advisory Committee 1963. *The Field of Work of the Family Doctor* (Gillie Report). London: HMSO.
5   Fraser Working Party July 1964. *Interim Commentaries*. London: HMSO.

CHAPTER 7: 1964–1968

1   *Brit Med J* 4 April 1964, 3089, 115 (s).
2   *Brit Med J* 1964, 5387, **2**, 17–23 (s).
3   *Lines of Communication* (now *BMA News Review*) August 1964.
4   *Brit Med J* 1964, **3**, 103–5.
5   *The Times* 20 July 1964.
6   Debate on the Family Doctor Service. *Hansard* 27 July 1964, **699**, no. 151. London: HMSO.
7, 9 *Daily Telegraph* 12 February 1965.
8   *Daily Express*, 12 February 1965, 8.
10   *St Bartholomew's Hospital Journal* 1 March 1965, **69**, 3.
11   *Brit Med J* 1965, **1**, 61–70 (s).
12   A Charter for the Family Doctor Service. *Brit Med J*, 1965, **1**, 92–5.

13   GMS *Voice* 18 March 1965.

14   *Joint Report on Discussions with the Minister of Health upon the Charter for the Family Doctor Service* 2 June 1965. London: BMA.

15   Review Body on Doctors' and Dentists' Remuneration, May 1966. *Seventh Report*. Cmnd. 2992. London: HMSO.

16   Prince, John (Health Correspondent). NHS Winter Breakdown Warning. *Daily Telegraph* 23 September 1966.

17   *The Training and Employment of Non-Medical Auxiliaries in General Practice*. July 1963. London: BMA.

18   Trained Medical and Non-Medical Auxiliaries. *GP* January 1964, **1**, 3; 1, 2, 11, 12.

19   Royal Commission on Medical Education 1965–8, April 1968. *Report*. Cmnd. 3569. London: HMSO.

20   *Memorandum of Evidence to the Royal Commission on Medical Education* 1965. London: BMA.

21   BMA 1948. *The Training of a Doctor*. Butterworth Medical Publications.

22   Royal College of General Practitioners 1962. *Training for General Practice*. London.

CHAPTER 8: 1968–1970

1   Committee on Local Authority and Allied Personal Services, July 1968. *Report*. Cmnd 3717. London: HMSO.

2   Ministry of Health 1968. *The Administrative Structure of Medical and Related Services in England and Wales*. London: HMSO.

3   Working Party of the BMA Council on NHS Administration, June 1968. *Report*. London: BMA.

4   Brit. Med. J. 1969 **1**: 55–68 (s).

5   Royal Commission on the Reform of Local Government in England, February 1970. *Report*. Cmnd 4276. London: HMSO.

References

SECOND INTERLUDE

1   Gibson, Sir Ronald et al. Psychiatric Care in General Practice: an Experiment in Collaboration. *Brit Med J* 21 May 1966, **1**, 1287–9.
2   Gibson, Sir Ronald. The Middle Aged in General Practice Health. *Joint Symposium of the Society of Health and the Royal College of General Practitioners* 1964, **79**, 6, 306–10.
3   Gibson, Sir Ronald. The Satchel and the Shining Morning Face. *Brit Med J* 1971, **2**, 549–52.
4   Board of Science and Education, January 1971. *The Problem of Euthanasia*. London: BMA.
5   House of Lords, *Report*. 12 February 1976, **368**, 31, 196–226.
6   Gibson, Sir Ronald. The Management of the Hopeless Case. *Proc Roy Soc Med* (GP Section) 20 November 1957, **51**, 2, 111–16.
7   Gibson, Sir Ronald. Ethics and Management of Advanced Cancer. *Brit Med J* 13 October 1962, **2**, 977–80.
8   Gibson, Sir Ronald. Impact of Malignant Disease on the General Practitioner. *Brit Med J* 7 October 1964, **2**, 965–9.
9   Gibson, Sir Ronald. Home Care of Terminal Malignant Disease. *J Roy Coll Physcns* Jan 1971, **5**, 2, 135–9.
10   *Professional Conduct and Discipline* 1979. London: GMC.
11   *The Handbook of Medical Ethics* 1981. London: BMA.
12   World Medical Association. *International Code of Medical Ethics. Declaration of Geneva*. Sydney, 1968. *Brit Med J*, 1968, **3**, 493–4.
13   *Brit Med J* 1974, **2**, 313–23.

CHAPTER 9: 1970–1972

1   Report of Working Party on the Constitution of the GMC. *Brit Med J* 1971, **1**, 55 (s).
2   Review Body on Doctors' and Dentists' Remuneration 1970. *Twelfth Report*. Cmnd. 4352. London: HMSO.
3   Stevenson, Derek. Letter to members of the BMA. 1 June 1970.

4   Crossman, Richard 1977. *The Diaries of a Cabinet Minister*, Vol. 3. 925–6. London: Hamish Hamilton and Jonathan Cape.
5   Ibid, 928.
6   Ibid, 935.
7   Ibid, 941.
8   Ibid, 936.
9   Ibid, 942.
10   *Brit Med J* 4 July 1970, 37–40 (s).
11   *General Practitioner* 6 July 1973, 14–15.
12   DHSS 1978. *Collaboration in Community Care – a Discussion Document*. London: HMSO.
13   DHSS, Welsh Office 1974. *Community Hospitals. Their Role and Development in the National Health Service*. HSC (15) 75. Cardiff: HMSO.
14   DHSS 1971. *NHS Reorganisation: Consultative Document*. London: HMSO.
15   DHSS 1972. *National Health Service Reorganisation: England*. Cmnd. 5055. London: HMSO.
16   *National Health Service Reorganisation Act 1973*. London: HMSO.

CHAPTER 10: 1972–1976

1   *Industrial Relations Bill* (Bill 60) 45/1, 1 December 1970. London: HMSO.
2   DHSS 1971. *The Organisation of General Practice*. Report of a sub-committee of the Standing Medical Advisory Committee (Harvard–Davis Report). London: HMSO.
3   DHSS 1970. *Domiciliary Midwifery and Maternity Bed Needs*. Report of a committee of the Standing Maternity and Midwifery Advisory Committee. London: HMSO.
4   BMA Board of Science and Education, January 1971. *Report on Euthanasia*. London BMA. *See also* Prince, John (Health Correspondent) 99% of Doctors Are Against Mercy Killing. *Daily Telegraph* 22 January 1971.
5   Gibson, Sir Ronald. The Management of the Hopeless Case. *Proc Roy Soc Med* 20 November 1957, **51**, 2, 111–16. *See also* Home Care of Terminal Malignant Disease. *J Roy Coll Physns* January 1971, **5**, 2, 135–9.

References

6 BMA. Working of the Abortion Act. *Annual Report of Council 1970–71,* Appendix 5, 52. (Memorandum by a Special Panel of the Board of Education and Science, February 1971.) *See also Report of the Committee on the Working of the Abortion Act,* Vol. 2, April 1974, Cmnd. 5579–1. London: HMSO.

7 BMA. *Annual Report of Council, 1973–74,* 5–6.

8 *Brit Med J* 1966, **2,** 170 (s).

9 Turner, R. D., Jones, R. V. H. and Streeter, Jacqueline. (DHSS Primary Care Sub-Committee of NHS Computer Research and Development Committee.) Computers in Primary Care: Where Next? *Brit Med J* 1980, 6246, 281, 1020–1 (s).

10 The final report of CURB was *confidentially* submitted to the Advisory Council on the Misuse of Drugs; only a summary was made public. January 1977.

11 *Sunday Times Weekly Review.* 14 September 1980, 33–5.

12 Stevenson, John. How I Averted a Health War – Barbara. *Pulse* 27 September 1980, **40,** 39, 4.

13 Castle, Barbara 1980. *The Castle Diaries.* London: Weidenfeld.

14 DHSS 1975. *The Separation of Private Practice from National Health Service Hospitals: a Consultative Document.* London: DHSS.

15 BMA. *Annual Report of Council, 1975–76.* 3–4.

16 DHSS, April 1975. *Report of the Committee of Inquiry into the Regulation of the Medical Profession* (Merrison Report). Cmnd. 1018. London: HMSO.

CHAPTER 11: 1976–1979

1 Review Body on Doctors' and Dentists' Remuneration, May 1977. *Seventh Report.* Cmnd. 6800. London: HMSO.

2 BMA. *Annual Report of Council 1977–78.* 3–4. London: BMA.

3 *Pulse* 1977, **35,** 2, 1.

4 Committee on Child Health Services 1976. *Fit for the Future.* Vols. 1 and 2. London: HMSO.

5 *Link* April 1975, 12, 18.

6   BMA. *Annual Report of Council, 1978–79*. 7. London: BMA.

7   General Practice Charter Working Group. Report. *Brit Med J* 1979, **1**, 564–72. *See also General Practitioner* 16 February 1979, 6–13.

8   *Pulse* 23 June 1979.

9   *Brit Med J* 1979, **2**, 215; 1979, **2**, 1377; 1980, 280, 575; 1980, 280, 872. (Report stage, not concluded.)

10   *BMA News Review* December 1979, **5**, 12.

11   Royal Commission on the National Health Service, July 1979. *Report*. Cmnd. 7165. London: HMSO. *See also* BMA, April 1977. *Evidence to the Royal Commission on the National Health Service*. London: BMA.

12   DHSS, December 1979. *Patients First*. London: HMSO. *See also* circular on reorganisation (HC(80)8).

13   Review Body on Doctors' and Dentists' remuneration, May 1978. *Eighth Report*. Cmnd 7176 *and* June 1979, *Ninth Report*. Cmnd. 7574. London: HMSO.

14   Review Body on Doctors' and Dentists' Remuneration, May 1980. *Tenth Report*. Cmnd. 7903. London: HMSO.

15   Royal Commission on Doctors' and Dentists' Remuneration, 1957–60, February 1960. *Report*. Cmnd. 939. London, HMSO.

CHAPTER 12: HEALTH CARE IN THE 1980s

1   GPs' ploy to raise earnings. The *Guardian*, 27 January 1981.

EPILOGUE: THE FAMILY DOCTOR 1981

Platt, Lord 1972. *Private and Controversial*, p. 59. London: Cassell.

Health and Prevention in Primary Care, 1981. London: R. Coll of Gen. Practit.

DHSS, 1980, *Health Service development: structure and management*. HC(80)8. London.

Primary Health Care in Inner London, report of a study group commissioned by the London Health Planning Consortium, May 1981.

Toxteth GPs' surgeries wrecked in riots *General Practitioner,* 10 July 1981.

Index

The Family Doctor

Callaghan, J., Prime Minister 162
Cambridge Clinical School 174
Cameron, Dr (now Sir) James 142
capitation method of payments to GPs 78
care, equal standards necessary 178
care of the dying, management of 124-6
care of the poor 22
Carlill, Adam de 18
Carr, Mr (now Lord) 150
cassiodorus and herbal medicine 16
Castle, Barbara 136, 157, 159, 160
fights for NHS 158
and pay beds 157-8
Central Committee for Hospital Medical Services ballot of consultants 158
central pool system of NHS payments 77, 86-7, 89
certificates, care in issuing 133
cervical cytology and general practice 112
Chamberlain Act (1930) 49
chaperones during examinations 132
Charing Cross Hospital pay beds 157
Charter of General Practice 99
Charter Working Party (1979) objectives welcomed 164-5
chemists and druggists supplant apothecaries 21
chronic sick 117
Church, the, and medicine 16
class status of patients 123
clinical freedom in NHS, fight for 148-9
clinics; for chronic sick, value of 117
for special groups of patients 191
club doctor, functions of 38
new, 116
Cohen, Lord, report of 76
College of General Practitioners 79, 85
faculties 79-80
College of Physicians (1518) 19
Colleges of Physicians and Surgeons, diplomas 30, 32
Committee of Inquiry into the Regulations of the Medical Profession 160
Commonwealth Medical Association ethical code 131
communications 44
Community Health Councils 166, 181, 182, 183

community hospitals 148, 166
programme, need for 180
complaints against GPs, channels for 183
compulsory retirement of GPs 166
computer aids for GPs 65, 66, 164, 178, 179
confrontation with government 101, 124-42
consultants: reliance on GP 10
and specialists, confrontation over pay beds 157-9
consultants and Specialists Committee 142
continuing education for GPs 164
contraceptive service, fees 168
list 155
supplying 155
contract practice abuses 38-9, 48
Corrie, John, MP, amendment to Abortion Act 165
cot deaths 189
cottage hospitals 112
employment of GPs in 173
system 46
transferred to state 73
Court, Professor Donald, report of 162-3
Cox, Dr Alfred and sickness clubs 38
Crossman, R., Secretary of State for Social Security 109, 110, 136, 138, 141, 167
and abortions 155
on Seebohm report 144-5

Danckwerts, Mr Justice and GPs remuneration 78
dangerous drugs, overprescribing 156-7
Dawson of Penn, Lord, health service committee of 72, 73
death, easy, doctor's responsibility for 125
Declaration of Geneva (1947) amended (1968) 131
declining urban areas, need for doctors 166, 172
dentists under NHS 81
Department of Health and Social Security (DHSS) 109, 177
depression (1930) maximum relief in 49
deputising services 67, 155, 173, 174, 181
diagnosis: methods of 41
science of 36

208

Index

210

Index

211

Index

In this new book, Richard D'Aveni identifies the rise of strategic capitalism as the fundamental threat to America's future and national security and provides a four-pronged strategy for preserving the American Dream.

—Clyde Prestowitz
Author of *The Betrayal of American Prosperity*
and President of the Economic Strategy Institute

The economic warfare China is engaging in through communist capitalism is extraordinarily seductive, and poses great risks to U.S. firms and the U.S. economy. But democratic capitalism works to its fullest potential when nimble and motivated capital markets and investors build upon consistent strategic federal investments in basic research, in a tax environment with internationally competitive corporate tax rates.

—Gregory T. Lucier
Chairman and Chief Executive Officer, Life Technologies, Inc.

The rise of China as a global economic power is one of the single greatest events in our lifetime. . . . We can't [adopt] a defensive position. We must hold our place as the greatest economic power in the world; we must set the example and trust in the power of capitalism.

—Michael T. Dan
Recently Retired Chairman, President,
and CEO of The Brink's Company

As competition around the globe continues to intensify, the United States can no longer take the approach that "countries don't compete" and must create an innovation policy agenda that will advance their position on the global playing field.

—Bill Nuti
Chairman and Chief Executive Officer, NCR Corporation

It's not too late for America to be the architect of [a] new economic order and create a more strategic form of capitalism. . . . The first step for American corporations in addressing China's emerging economic strength is to understand the global playing fields and their new rules. America's CEOs must learn firsthand what is driving this change and its long-term implications.

—Dinesh C. Paliwal
Chairman, President, and Chief Executive Officer
Harman International Industries, Inc.

If we hope to mirror China's success, America needs a wider application of public-private linkages that advance technology development . . .

—Michael Morris
Chairman and Former Chief Executive Officer
American Electric Power

While our nation has demonstrated a unique capacity to unite in times of crisis, we have also shown a tendency to undermine this attribute when under the strain of an impending crisis—highlighting our differences, rather than celebrating the potential for them to disappear. In these moments . . . we must be strong as a nation to resist behaviors which give fanaticism a voice . . . forcefully reject partisan behavior which demands blind adherence to orthodoxy, and . . . recognize that the politics of blame discourages bold risk taking and innovation which will be critical to generating economic growth and creating jobs.

—George S. Barrett
Chairman and Chief Executive Officer, Cardinal Health, Inc.

Only through the design and execution of a successful national growth strategy will we find solutions to our challenges. . . . If the President and Congress do not show the courage and the political will to do what must be done, our continuing trajectory toward second-class status in the world is assured.

—Peter Nicholas
Cofounder and Chairman, Boston Scientific Corporation

As free trade agreements multiply across the globe, a significant number of these arrangements outside the United States are falling short of WTO standards, discriminating against U.S. interests, and diverting trade. To prevent U.S. exports from being compromised by the growing "spaghetti bowl" of illegal trade preferences, the United States will need to insist that these illegitimate fair trade agreements be reformed.

—Fernando Aguirre
Chairman and Chief Executive Officer
Chiquita Brands International

The solution to the emerging global economic threats is clear. Great leadership, the courage to lead and think differently, an audacious roadmap, and a partnership of government, people, and business can reverse the U.S. decline and position the country once again for growth and greatness.

—Salvatore D. Fazzolari
Former Chairman, President, and
Chief Executive Officer, Harsco Corporation

We have many strengths in the U.S., but we also need to recognize that other countries are evolving to become more competitive. This new global competitiveness is a good phenomenon for us and the world.

—David M. Cote
Chairman and Chief Executive Officer, Honeywell Corporation

China is simply too large to ignore. . . . Clearly, U.S. multinational corporations have proven to be nimble and adaptable in determining what they need to do to win in China and other emerging economies around the world. The U.S. government must also do its part to help American corporations get access to and fair treatment in all of the emerging markets.

—Steve Angel
Chairman, President, and Chief Executive Officer, Praxair, Inc.

America needs a better economy. To achieve it, the United States must increase the quality of its labor pool, create greater efficiencies in the manufacturing environment—and direct its strengthened capabilities to a cause that the country can rally behind.

—Patrick M. Prevost
President and Chief Executive Officer, Cabot Corporation

America's position as the leader in innovation isn't just threatened; we've relinquished it. . . . I implore policy makers to make [advanced K–12 education] programs a top priority, [especially in science, technology, engineering, and math]. They are critical to keeping America not just as the leader in analytics, but the global leader in technology and innovation.

—Jim Goodnight
Chief Executive Officer, SAS Institute

For a free e-book featuring insights from CEOs about a strategy for America, please visit www.radstrat.com.

STRATEGIC
CAPITALISM

THE NEW ECONOMIC STRATEGY
FOR WINNING THE CAPITALIST COLD WAR

RICHARD A. D'AVENI

New York   Chicago   San Francisco   Lisbon   London   Madrid   Mexico City
Milan   New Delhi   San Juan   Seoul   Singapore   Sydney   Toronto

The *McGraw·Hill* Companies

1 2 3 4 5 6 7 8 9 0   QFR/QFR   1 8 7 6 5 4 3 2 1

ISBN   978-0-07-178116-9
MHID   0-07-178116-1

e-ISBN   978-0-07-178117-6
e-MHID   0-07-178117-X

McGraw-Hill books are available at special quantity discounts to use as premiums and sales promotions or for use in corporate training programs. To contact a representative, please e-mail us at bulksales@mcgraw-hill.com.

This book is printed on acid-free paper.

Library of Congress Cataloging-in-Publication Data

D'Aveni, Richard A.
  Strategic capitalism : the new economic strategy for winning the capitalist cold war / by Richard D'Aveni.
    p. cm.
  ISBN-13: 978-0-07-178116-9 (alk. paper)
  ISBN-10: 0-07-178116-1 (alk. paper)
  1. Capitalism--History--21st century. 2. Capitalism--Political aspects--United States. I. Title.
  HB501.D36 2013
  330.12'2--dc23

                                                            2012025363

To my mother, Marion E. D'Aveni:
Thank you for giving me, by deed or genetics, the love,
intelligence, logic, drive, mental discipline, organization,
inquisitiveness, and counterintuitive insight that so greatly
contributed to this book, and that have made me what I am.

Contents

Foreword

We Are Already in a Trade War with China and We Are Losing, Badly

To remain economically competitive with other countries, particularly China, we need to deal with reality.

First, our leaders must realize that we are already in a trade war with China and we are losing, badly. Failing to address China's unfair and protectionist trade practices has cost us millions of manufacturing jobs and devastated our middle class. We need to vigorously enforce our trade laws. This does not require a new program. We simply need to enforce the rules of existing trade agreements.

Critics will argue that this is protectionist, but there is nothing protectionist about holding other countries to their agreements. President Reagan understood this when he said, "To make the international trading system work, all must abide by the rules." And if nations do not abide by the rules, we need to act with greater resolve.

Second, America needs a national industrial strategy. Our economic competitors have one. We must correct the mistake we made in believing that a service-based economy could replace a manufacturing-based one as the country's wealth creation engine. Manufacturing used to account for over 30 percent of our GDP [gross domestic product]; today it has dropped to 9.9 percent. We need a strategy to get manufacturing back to 20 percent of GDP.

Finally, we must invest in our nation's infrastructure. Investments the United States made during and after World War II fueled our economic growth in the second half of the twentieth century. Much of that infrastructure is reaching the end of its useful life and new investments are required.

A creative way to fund these investments would be to allow companies to repatriate overseas earnings, estimated at over $1 trillion, tax-free by putting that money into infrastructure bonds. Each $1 billion spent on infrastructure creates 35,000 jobs. Then, over time, multinationals would be able to draw that money back.

Remaining economically competitive requires focusing on three basic fundamentals: fighting unfair trade practices, boosting manufacturing, and improving infrastructure. These are among the many initiatives advocated by Richard D'Aveni in this thought-provoking—and controversial—book. Even if you don't agree with Professor D'Aveni's wide-ranging agenda for remaking American capitalism, you would do well to examine his no-holds-barred ideas. He grasps the new global reality like few other thinkers, and his passion for his subject is sure to stimulate needed debate over a fresh approach to assuring another century of prosperity for America.

Daniel R. DiMicco
Chairman and Chief Executive Officer
Nucor Corporation

As Chairman and CEO of North Carolina-based Nucor Corporation, Dan DiMicco runs a $15.8 billion Fortune 200 steel company. Mr. DiMicco is a member of the board of directors of Duke Energy, the American Iron & Steel Institute, and the World Steel Association. Mr. DiMicco also served for several years on the United States Manufacturing Council. In 2010, the *Harvard Business Review* named Mr. DiMicco as one of its 100 Best Performing CEOs in the World.

Nucor is North America's largest steel manufacturer and largest recycler; it recycles one ton of steel every two seconds. It operates over 200 facilities primarily in the United States and Canada. Through the David J. Joseph Company, Nucor is also one of the leading scrap companies in the United States. Nucor is best known for its breakthrough technological firsts in mini-mill steel production, electric arc furnaces, thin slab casting for flat rolled steel, and thin strip casting for coiled steel.

Preface

In the 1990s, my research revealed that companies were competing with one another in a radically different way. Rather than competing to create enduring advantages or to form oligopolies that would reduce rivalry and increase profits, companies were using sequences of bold, aggressive, surprisingly temporary advantages to achieve dominance over their rivals. They were not suing for peaceful coexistence among oligopolists. They were competing to create disruptive advantages that constantly undermined, neutralized, or made obsolete the key advantages of industry leaders. They had harsh new strategic tools that broke earlier rules of the game.

Once heresy, in my view—that competitive advantage is much less sustainable given fierce and escalating competition—is now commonly held. Indeed, what I labeled *hypercompetition* has now moved up a level—from competition among corporations to competition among nations.

With the rise of the new economic powerhouses, especially China, we are witnessing a new form of capitalism in which states compete against other states—or, more accurately, in which the various states' forms of capitalism compete with one another for economic success.

Joseph Schumpeter argued that the forces of creative destruction are integral to the efficient working of a capitalist system. Schumpeter's ideas are widely accepted. I am arguing that those same forces work upon the system itself, so that a better-adapted form of capitalism will eventually destroy or displace the incumbent system. This dynamic process is at work around the world.

No capitalist system that succeeds in the global economy lasts for long in the same form. China has shunted aside the notion of continuity over millennia, as dynasties disintegrated and new ones eventually replaced them. To gain an advantage, competitors have to disrupt the disruptor. And creating disruptive competitive advantage is what the national agenda must be about. What are we the best in the world at? The competitive advantages of nations determine how, and how much, wealth is distributed.

The United States in particular has still not adapted to this new world, insisting that corporations should compete with one another without excessive help from their governments. Meanwhile, China in particular has coordinated the efforts of its business entities for state purposes and introduced a slew of new competitive weapons.

The United States is facing a China that has marched onto the global playing field aiming to win by changing the rules of competition in a way that breaks the United States' most basic rules of capitalism. What we are witnessing are the first moves in what I call the capitalist cold war. This book is my response to that threat. In it, I set out my analysis and conclusions and offer some (deliberately radical and provocative) solutions. I do this not out of some misguided notion that I have all the answers, but out of a deeply held conviction that the United States is in danger of sleepwalking off the edge of a cliff.

My argument is simple: that the traditional view of capitalism as practiced in America and most of the West is outdated and inadequate to explain the situation we find ourselves in. It is only by challenging long-held assumptions and considering radical alternative policies that we can hope to understand and respond to the new world order.

I have spent the last five years collecting facts, doing strategic analyses, and coming up with implications and strategies that are being used in this competition among different types of capitalism. This book is the result.

It comes to four important conclusions. First, the countries that compete most effectively have adopted elements of *managed capitalism*. This approach, my research makes plain, need not be the sole preserve of emerging markets. Second, the country that sets the standard of success at managed capitalism is China. Third, China is playing to win—to become the world hegemon. That is, it aims to displace the United States as the world's economic leader by becoming the global rule maker and privilege taker. My fourth conclusion—perhaps the most obvious, but also the most worrying—is that the United States and its allies in the free world have a lot to lose in terms of prosperity, economic freedom, geopolitical power, national security, and even democratic values if China becomes the world leader.

Strategy, Not Ideology

I approach the subject of the different types of capitalism as a strategist. I don't argue for one pet ideological approach or another, as if I were in a theoretical or imaginary world. I also do not argue that one solution—one type of capitalism—works better than others in all places or in all circumstances. I argue for what works in an imperfect world, a world in which many countries are vying for the biggest share of the global economic pie.

Because of my pragmatic approach, I know this book will be controversial. I challenge the widespread belief in the importance and efficacy of free markets, open trade, stockholder-oriented corporate governance, social programs, wealth transfers, and the stimulation of artificial demand through massive government borrowing and easy credit. I believe that national leaders, like many professors in the classroom, have limited the debate needed on capitalism by sticking to politically correct discussions. They have tied their hands and closed their minds.

Whether or not leaders say so in public, the reality is that China and the United States are fighting with different forms of capitalism, and they are vying to shape a new world economic order. This means that national leaders who are concerned about the nation's competitive strength should think about how to modify their versions of capitalism to provide companies with the best backing possible. National leaders cannot force their economies to fit their ideological ideas of what's supposedly "best." Instead, they have to take the time to understand the transformation of capitalism that is underway and then devise pragmatic ways to manage the transformation in their favor.

A lot is at stake. The leaders of the United States have to win if they are to preserve our fragile democracy. That means not just raising the return on capital, but creating a strategy to raise the fortunes of the population as a whole. From the perspective of the nation, it makes no sense to have a capitalist system that maximizes stockholder wealth by transferring capital to foreign markets where the growth and costs are better, while leaving the vast majority of the nation's people without jobs and unable to pay their mortgages. Stockholder-oriented corporate governance has become a formula for the milking of a mature nation (the cash cow) to invest in emerging nations (the stars). If there are no limits on the milking, the cow ultimately is milked dry and dies.

The evidence shows that the nation with the strongest capitalist model will lead the world. China today has seized the initiative from the United States. But this is not an issue for America alone. National leaders of countries throughout the world face the challenge of using a smart capitalist strategy to take back control over the next version of capitalism employed in the world economy. Where will the new rules of capitalism come from? Will they come from the United States, or from China? Will a mix occur? Where will other nations fit in?

Strategic Capitalism outlines a specific plan for how the United States can restore itself to economic greatness. If acted upon, the plan would not trigger global recession, as some might fear or suggest. Instead, it would accelerate the process of change so that China focuses more on production for its internal markets than on exporting, and we in the West reallocate and better focus our own efforts, resources, and budgets. The book also provides a logical framework, strategy analysis tools, and strategy proposals for use by other countries seeking to establish their capitalist strategies. I believe that the issue of making our brand of capitalism more strategic should dominate the debate in future U.S. presidential elections and will dominate the debate in the halls of Congress and the White House for the next two decades. The struggle for world economic leadership will continue, and nations must prepare for the competition—and clash—of capitalisms that is already in progress. In many ways, the survival of the democratic world depends on it.

Richard D'Aveni
Bakala Professor of Strategy
Tuck School of Business at Dartmouth College
Hanover, New Hampshire, USA
August 2012

Introduction

A Turning Point in History

Today, we face a turning point in American history—a time requiring reinvention. Even as the job market picks up temporarily, we are warned of a "new normal," an economy in which good jobs are disappearing overseas and average wages are depressed by foreign competition. We are warned about tepid growth, unstable careers, fewer opportunities, and dependence on foreign imports for survival, and even the loss of America's position as leader of the global economy is foretold.

Underlying the new normal are two central players: the United States and China. Today we face a crisis in our ability to compete, particularly with China. China has emerged from a meager capitalist adolescence to vibrant adulthood. It has mastered manufacturing so quickly that even companies as American as Apple now make almost everything they sell in Chinese plants. China has acted so aggressively to build its manufacturing enterprises that it has taken more than two million American jobs in the last decade. It has grown at such speed that, if its current growth rates continue, its economy will surpass that of the United States before

2030. Meanwhile, the United States has spent a decade sitting idle, distracted by wars and terrorism.

There are alternative explanations for America's current ills. Some commentators point to an aging population, for example, or technological unemployment—the tendency for information and communications technology and other technologies to replace human labor. But my focus is on the impact of China's system of capitalism on U.S. competitiveness. My research indicates that this is a major contributing factor.

China is what one might call a *hypercompetitor*. It has a new system of capitalism that is disrupting America's system—some would even say undermining it. In industry after industry, it has many countries on the run, often with hard-boiled business practices that most developed countries would not accept if China were not so large.

But China is also what a sporting person might call a "worthy competitor." It challenges all comers to raise their game. As for the United States, I believe that China is doing the American people a favor. It is delivering a timely economic kick in the pants. The big controversy rests on whether the United States will be able to get up after it is kicked in ways that are much more severe than ever before.

Strategic Capitalism—The Way Back to Greatness

So, what are we to do? Now is not the time to rely on ideological or theory-based ideas that encapsulate what *used* to work. Most ideologies and theories are not appropriate anymore. They freeze a nation's thinking, paralyze its ability to adjust, and doom the nation to continued decline. Only a fool continues doing the same thing and expects different results. Now is the time to devise new mechanisms and systemic innovations.

That is the subject of this book: how to fix America's capitalist system so that it can win in a much more competitive world—how to restore the nation's finances, reinvent the nation's economic system, reseize the initiative from rivals, and remake the global economic world order for economic gain. I call this *strategic capitalism*.

The pages ahead amount to a guidebook to strategic capitalism. They urge leaders to look at the future strategically, and to craft a strategy for winning over the long term. Unlike many books, this one does not promote an ideology, whether from the left, right, or center. It promotes pragmatic thinking that comes from anyone with good ideas. It champions the need for new conversations about our competitors. It urges leaders to step over the party lines and do what is necessary and what works.

The need for a new capitalist strategy would not be so great if the United States and other developed countries didn't face such a crisis. But a grave economic threat has enveloped us, and the nature of it is hard to dismiss: at this moment in time, China's version of capitalism is allowing it to grow much faster than the United States, albeit from a much lower base. Of course, it is an oversimplification to say that China does capitalism better than the United States. The wealth of the United States and other Western nations was built on a highly effective form of capitalism. It is the desire to replicate that sort of wealth creation that is driving China's current dynamism. But it is also clear that the form of capitalism that China is pursuing is very different from the one that brought the United States its success in the twentieth century.

The writing is on the wall. While the United States once ruled global trade, as of 2011, China exported to the United States $295 billion more in goods than the United States exported to China. Meanwhile, China has become the top trading partner with seven of the G-20 countries.[1] Modern China plays capitalist hardball better than the United States does. Its momentum is palpable.

At the start of this century, Western economists argued that China's economic miracle would not last. China would adopt Western-style democracy and free markets, or it would not be able to handle the stresses and strains of the country's growing pains. But the economists were wrong. What's more, China has not just become a manufacturing hub for low-tech goods that poor peasants can make. It has leaped to the top rungs of manufacturing sophistication. In many cases, China makes things that the United States no longer can—laptops and lithium-ion batteries, for instance. The U.S. Department of Defense estimates that China's technology lags that of the United States by only five years.

The era of hypercompetition has highlighted another fact of life among competing nations: few national leaders are playing by win-win rules. They are playing by win-lose rules. When Chinese negotiators get together with their U.S. counterparts, they invariably issue press releases that gush about "mutual benefit." Both countries reap big returns from economic interchange, the thinking goes. But the negotiators always try to get more for their nation. The benefit is mutual for some industries, but it is unequal for nations as a whole. China's goliath trade surpluses are testimony to that fact. The truth is, the United States has dawdled in showing that it is up to the task of competing with China. The trade deficit with China in 2011 was the biggest ever, up 8 percent from the year before.[2] Alarm bells have sounded in Washington, but no cogent strategy has emerged.

Deadlock—Disaster or Decision?

Several things have impeded action. One is that the United States is short of cash. Indeed, the United States and Europe are effectively bankrupt. The twin Ds, deficits and debt, have put tight financial handcuffs on the United States. With no money, there's no action. And the situation is worsening. The Congressional Budget Office estimates that by 2020, U.S. debt payments will consume so much of the government budget that the only things the country will be able to pay for are defense and interest on borrowing. No money will remain for healthcare, welfare, education, safety, environmental protection, or entitlement programs, assuming a balanced budget. Worse than the lack of money is that the debate over taxes completely distracts politicians from looking past the next budget battle to the global economic battle that is brewing.

Another impediment to action is that U.S. leaders appear to be irrevocably smitten by the theory of free markets, competitiveness, and the practice of laissez-faire capitalism. (They are not alone—some economists retain their belief in the efficiency of markets no matter what.) Many U.S. leaders are equally committed to large social programs. The modus operandi today is simple: let companies pursue completely open trade, give Wall Street a completely free hand in allocating U.S. capital, force corporate executives to maximize stockholder wealth only, and let the government redistribute some of the wealth to those who have been left out. This approach powered U.S. success during most of the last century. Few people questioned it (including me). But taking this approach today often enriches companies and channels money to the poor, while impoverishing nations and the middle class. So long as the United States remains stuck with its free-market, social-program infatuation, action to challenge China will remain limited.

The third set of handcuffs is the focus on the short term. Executives try to please shareholders who demand short-term returns. Leaders appeal to voters who demand quick-fix solutions and entitlements. The executives make investments in China—fueling China's competitive ability—because they see dollar signs in the Chinese consumer market of the future. Government leaders fail to make adequate investments in the United States—investments that could launch new, job-creating industries—because they don't see votes in doing so. The short-termism of both kills long-term strategy making.

Perhaps the most disappointing factor impeding action is simple denial of the facts. Few Americans can believe that the United States has lost its edge to such a degree. Many people see this when the economy is in trouble, but with any slight upturn in the economy, people start to think that everything is fine again. Few recognize the 40-year decline in inflation-adjusted income that we have endured, and even fewer believe that we need to change our system of capitalism in order to compete.[3] True, in a 2011 Pew Institute poll, Americans counted China as the United States' greatest threat.[4] But the evidence is that most Americans don't actually want to make any sacrifices for the good of the nation. No one wants to give up his entitlements. No one wants to compromise her ideological positions by admitting that those positions have failed. Many people act as if Europe's and America's debt crisis is not serious and assume that it will fix itself. It is, and it won't.

Adding to the Americans who don't believe in the threat are those who won't talk about it. Most corporate CEOs—and I've talked to hundreds of them—simply will not go on record criticizing China. They tell me regularly that they don't know what to do—they are damned if they enter China, because of the risk and their fear of becoming controlled by the Chinese government, and they are damned if they don't, because of the size and growth of Chinese markets and their potential to create shareholder wealth. But they wouldn't dream of starting a public conversation about the bind they are in, because that would threaten shareholder value or trigger Chinese retaliation. The subject is taboo.

But the time has come for real leadership. An honest debate about the situation can help the United States break out of its rigid stance. It may make everyone uncomfortable—but it will make the United States economically stronger, and it will make future profits, jobs, wages, and living standards better for our children and grandchildren.

Facing the Hard Facts with Courage

Any strategist will tell you that the first step in building a great strategy is facing the hard facts. Let me emphasize four such facts. Each should shake American beliefs to their core:

- *America has an uncompetitive form of capitalism.* Economic growth and trade numbers show that China's version of managed capitalism works better in certain ways. Therefore, America will need some form of industrial policy to compete with China's managed capitalist system.

- *Maximizing shareholder wealth at the corporate level does not maximize the wealth of the nation now that the world is global.* Jobs move to low-cost countries, and investment moves to large, high-growth markets like China. Therefore, the government must break this cycle.

- *The power of Wall Street and financial markets to determine which industries get liquidated or expanded is becoming a weakness.* The United States is abandoning strategic industries and industries that provide jobs for the working and middle classes. Therefore, the government will have to reduce the power of Wall Street if we wish to save industries that are useful to society, even if they are less profitable.

- *China is taking advantage of the United States because we are sticking to free-trade ideals when the rest of the world isn't.* The United States is currently caught in a dilemma: we can't disengage from trading with China without hurting our economy, but continuing to consume too much from China will impoverish the United States, strengthen China, and create even larger trade deficits unless China becomes more cooperative.

To face these hard facts, we must face an overarching and divisive issue: the role of government is about to expand. This is a radioactive issue that we can no longer avoid. China has brought it to the fore. Compared to the United States, China has a strong and coordinated leadership that is able to pursue a single-minded economic strategy. That said, Beijing is having some trouble keeping the regional party bosses in line, with some of those bosses freelancing and getting rich in the process. And China is alienating middle-class professionals who are crucial to innovation. Corruption at regional and national levels have had a negative effect, but China's policies have been effective overall. The United States will be required to match China if America is to have a chance.

In response, naysayers will undoubtedly repeat the line, "The government shouldn't be in the business of picking winners and losers." That's unfortunate, because the U.S. government will have to do even more than that to balance the scales with China.

The reality is that free markets alone cannot beat good strategists. Many people in the West will argue, of course, that central planning and industrial strategy is a broken concept. They will point to the failings of the former Soviet Union, among others, as proof. But the last Cold War was a different situation. It was a contest between capitalism and communism—and capitalism won. What we are seeing now is a contest between two very different forms of capitalism. To win this capitalist cold war, the U.S. government will have to throw its weight behind U.S. industry and business.

This is not the leap in the dark that some suggest. The inability of the U.S. government to manage economic strategy is vastly overstated. The U.S. government has created or aided many industries that are global winners, including agriculture, aerospace, biotechnology, advanced materials, pharmaceuticals, and software. The big problem today is that most economic decisions (regulations, industrial policies, protectionism, and so on) are made behind closed doors in Congress—a place where campaign contributions and lobbying sway decisions without close scrutiny. Often hidden in bills that are so long that no member of Congress can read them before voting on them, economic decisions are made by professional politicians who have no expertise in the industries they regulate, and they are made in so many committees that compromises, conflicts, inconsistencies, and holes abound.

The real problem is that U.S. industrial policies are scattershot because policy makers aren't thinking strategically or coherently enough. They haven't been daring enough to educate voters on the need for a more coordinated approach. The upshot is that no one is looking at the big picture. For example: Are we making so many laws that we make corporate change impossibly slow? Do the laws work at cross-purposes? Do we have a strategy and a unified purpose behind all these laws?

So the problem is not that government can't do strategy. It is that it is not set up to do strategy for the nation. President Obama's

2011 proposal to create a single organization that would be responsible for the economy is a first step toward the kind of agency we need if we are to develop a national capitalist strategy. He suggested that the Commerce Department, the U.S. Trade Representative, the Export-Import Bank, the Overseas Private Investment Corp., the Trade and Development Agency, and the Small Business Administration be consolidated into one department.

Some fear that this would give the president too much power, or that such a department would promote corruption and central planning on such a scale that free markets would be destroyed. However, these are issues that can be resolved. Just think back to the days when the Federal Reserve System was created to regulate the banking industry. Political influence was reduced by giving the Fed autonomy, and corruption was reduced by several laws coupled with strict enforcement. Removing Congress from the equation would speed decision making, break deadlocks, and reduce the influence of campaign contributions. Rather than using the logic of ideology or ineffectual theory, the goal should be to use the power of systematic strategic thinking and problem solving.

Perhaps the greatest challenge for U.S. leaders will come from dealing with global politics. Negotiations with China will require strongly coordinated U.S. economic policies. The tools of tariffs, regulations, incentives, and investment in U.S. industries will all become important. It appears that China will not compromise on trade and other economic issues based on U.S. complaints alone.

So the challenge for U.S. leaders will be to put teeth behind their complaints. The United States will need a strong government if it is to deal with China. It has to be prepared to call China's bluff. Moreover, because global political relations often support economic affairs, the United States has to play the negotiating game more aggressively.

If it comes down to it, and China does not budge, there may be an intense economic cold war between capitalist systems. This would not be the optimal scenario. Hopefully, China will recognize its interdependence with the United States and will blink before a capitalist cold war gets out of hand.

This book sets the goal of preparing for the worst, while hoping for the best. The goal is not to have a capitalist cold war that destroys the economies of both nations. It is to prevent one. However, if it comes down to it, the United States must be able to win a capitalist cold war. This would be better than simply giving up, as we have done so far. It is better to stop the gradual decline of America while we still can than to end up like the proverbial boiled frog.

The Power of Systematic Strategic Thinking and a Problem-Solving Mentality

For companies and countries, success will increasingly come from strategy. What has changed is the units of analysis—we are moving from competitive strategies for large corporations to competitive strategies for entire nations and their networks of economic allies.

The tasks required to create such a strategy are straightforward, and are set out in the rest of this book. But that's not to say that the steps of strategy making are easy. And implementation is even more difficult. This type of strategic thinking will involve many systemic innovations that will take people beyond their comfort zones. And it will take courage to champion these innovations. The notion of crafting a national economic strategy will itself strike many people as heresy. Received wisdom says that economies run by planners always fall short of those that are left to operate on their own. The market, we are told, has hidden intelligence; left alone, it ensures an efficiency of operation among businesses that government planners cannot match.

But there is a curious lack of consistency in this thinking. The executives who lead the companies that drive the economy don't operate with a distaste for strategy at all. In fact, they would laugh if their colleagues in other companies said: "We don't have a strategy, and we don't need one because the market will take care of us."

To be sure, developing a strategy doesn't always lead to success. Many people are bad at it. As in any decision-making process, the conclusions from hard analysis and planning cannot foresee all future turns of events. But not planning is simply not an option. The British businessman Sir John Harvey Jones once quipped: "Planning is an unnatural process; it is much more fun to do something. The nicest thing about not planning is that failure comes as a complete surprise, rather than being preceded by a period of worry and depression."

The role of national leaders is to prevent complete surprise. My aim is help them in that task.

The choices are stark. First, the United States can allow the current trends to continue and capitulate to China's economic advances. Second, it can fight back by improving the competitiveness of its current system so that the United States can remain dominant. Third, it can be more proactive about promoting free markets and hope to convert China to its free-market ways. Fourth, it can retreat from the concept of global free markets and open trade with enemies and friends alike. Instead, it can build a new trade bloc in which it can set new rules of capitalism for loyal allies and trading partners and be able to build the prosperity of the entire bloc, while China builds its prosperity at the expense of the rest of its bloc.

If you follow the reasoning in this book, you will conclude that none of the first three alternatives remains available. Either the United States won't accept them or China won't. Neither country will cede future wealth to the other. Neither will cede future control of global capitalism to the other. Each will vie for dominance. That is the nature of great powers over the millennia. The United States and China will remain locked in a relationship of "frenemies," dividing the economic wealth of the planet, but not sharing economic systems, values, or allies.

As Alexis de Tocqueville noted in 1835, "The greatness of America lies not in its being more enlightened than any other nation, but rather in her ability to repair her faults." This is still true today. The United States has allowed its economy to evolve to a point where it no longer controls the rules of the game. But in the following pages, I describe how to retake the lead—how to define the problem, how to perform the unnatural process of planning expertly, and how to restore the United States to greatness.

Capitalism in a Nutshell

Generic Capitalisms. There are four generic or pure forms of capitalism: laissez-faire capitalism, social-market capitalism, managed capitalism, and philanthropic capitalism. Capitalist systems are made up of different mixtures of the generic capitalisms. When the mixture of generic capitalisms is chosen to enable a system to outperform, beat, neutralize, make obsolete, or undermine rival capitalist systems, it known as *strategic capitalism*.

Laissez-Faire Capitalism. The first generic form of capitalism, laissez-faire capitalism, is an economic system based on private ownership of the means of production, distribution, and exchange, and characterized by the unfettered freedom of capitalists to operate or manage their property for profit in competitive, free markets. The goal is to maximize the efficient use of capital.

Social-Market Capitalism. The second generic type of capitalism is social-market capitalism, an economic system designed to redistribute wealth and, through regulation, protect the public and working people from exploitation. It aims to create a healthy society by countering the concentration of wealth that results from laissez-faire capitalism. It is intended to strengthen a nation's social backbone by building prosperous middle and working classes with ample consumer buying power, while providing a social safety net for those who are perceived to be unable to help themselves, including the poor, oppressed minorities, and the elderly.

Managed Capitalism. The third generic form of capitalism is managed capitalism, an economic system in which government technocrats or committees coordinate state and private entities to build a strong economy with healthy employment and reliable growth. Through long-term planning, they invest in long-term research and development (R&D), nurture new industries, protect industries from the bankrupting rigors of global competition, build national corporations with global economies of scale, create other long-term competitive advantages, and sustain strategic industries that are critical to economic and military security. The goal is not to maximize the efficient use of capital or labor, but to accumulate national wealth so that the state can create economic or military power vis-à-vis foreign nations and their corporations.

Philanthropic Capitalism. The fourth generic type of capitalism is philanthropic capitalism, a system to build the creative and scientific base of a country in areas that would otherwise receive little or no funding from corporations or the government. National leaders set philanthropic policy by using the tax code to tighten or relax restrictions on giving, restricting or allowing deductions for gifts to universities, foundations, hospitals, scientific and medical research centers, the arts, and other endeavors. The goal is to create national competitive advantages over decades through developing endowments that finance a distinctive national culture, style, knowledge, and other intangibles.

A Capitalist System. A capitalist system is a mixed economy made up of a blend of the four generic forms of capitalism— typically, one in which laissez-faire capitalism is modified to achieve goals beyond profit maximization for the private owners of wealth, including (1) the welfare of the needy (social-market capitalism), (2) the nation's goals for military or geopolitical power, economic power or position, and national security (state or managed capitalism), and (3) a variety of other societal, cultural, religious, personal, or nonmaterialistic needs (philanthropic capitalism).

Strategic Capitalism. Strategic capitalism is a capitalist system designed through the proactive, nonideological guidance of the government to manage the competition between capitalist systems to a prosperous outcome for its people and for the nation as a whole. The overall goal is to intentionally outpace, outperform, or disrupt rival capitalist systems that present a major threat to the nation's prosperity and power; to intentionally guide the nation's economy toward a better long-run competitive position; and to intentionally shape a world (economic) order that benefits the nation and its allies.

Capitalist Cold War. A capitalist cold war is a contest (that stops short of full-scale war) between two or more capitalist systems to see who is the rule maker and who are the rule takers. The intended outcome of a capitalist cold war is that the winner sets rules for the global system of finance, trade, international regulation, intellectual property markets, and other economic activities, which favor the growth and prosperity of the rule maker and its people.

Part 1

Analyzing Capitalist Systems and How They Act
The Four Cs of Capitalism

Part 1 covers the four Cs of capitalist dynamics:

- Competing
- Combining
- Controlling
- Capturing

Capitalism is dynamic. Excluding exogenous events, such as natural disasters and military conflict, capitalism changes because of the four Cs. The four Cs emphasize four processes that cause continuous change. Opposing capitalist systems *compete* by disrupting one another. In the course of this competition, countries *combine* different generic types of capitalism to form unique capitalist systems. Governments use different techniques to *control* capitalist behavior at home and abroad. Governments work to *capture* other nations within their sphere of economic influence in order to spread their form of capitalism around the world. And strategic capitalists attempt to guide the way their capitalist system competes with rivals, combines types of capitalism to form a unique capitalist system, controls capitalist behavior at home and abroad, and captures other nations in its capitalist system.

1

Competing Capitalisms

Hypercompetition and the Disruption of Superpowers

Let me make a prediction right off: history is going to repeat itself. The United States went through a period after World War II in which capitalism struggled to overtake communism; later, American capitalism was challenged by an emerging economic power, Japan. The Japanese version of capitalism easily stunned the smug and complacent United States. Over time, the United States righted itself, recalculated how to compete, and came back with new moves to secure its role as the world economic leader.

That was the 1980s. Japan had huge trade imbalances with America. The U.S. capitalist system had grown vulnerable. American businesspeople felt entitled. Companies enjoyed lofty profits, even though they had high labor costs and underutilized assets. The Japanese undercut the United States with lower costs and better quality. U.S. manufacturers somehow didn't see Japan's economic advances coming. It was as if an upstart boxer walked right up to the veteran and pulled the proud fighter's shorts down. A chill then ran through all of U.S. industry.

This comeuppance ended the complacency of the giant global industrial power. The United States reinvented the way it

3

conducted capitalism and rallied back. American oligopolies were reorganized, ineffective top management teams were removed, and stockholders and boards of directors were given more power. Wall Street played an active role in this switch, using hostile takeovers, forced divestitures, and friendly mergers and acquisitions.

And now another challenger has come along: China. Like Japan, China feels neither complacent nor unprepared. In a painful sense of déjà vu, the American veteran has his boxing shorts around his ankles, and industry is feeling another chill. We are now facing the questions of the decade: Will history really repeat itself? And will the United States again emerge as the champion?

My prediction—and my conviction—is that, yes, it will. The veteran boxer will right itself, recalculate how to compete, and come back with new moves that will give it the momentum to control the flow of punches and counterpunches in the economic ring. America will secure the heavyweight title for decades more.

But that leaves other questions: How will the old fighter do it this time? What approach will it use?

That's where I have another prediction. The United States will come up with an innovative round of economic moves and countermoves, and it will outsmart, outmaneuver, and outbox China. As part of the comeback, U.S. national leaders will rebuild the country's fiscal physique, rework its capitalist system, create a strategy for a succession of competitive actions, and reclaim the center of the global boxing ring. But America will not be able to use the same methods that it used to best the USSR and Japan. China is a much bigger and very different contender, and hypercompetition is now the global reality.

History Is Hypercompetition

What is hypercompetition between nations? It comprises a series of actions by rivals who are seeking to tilt the playing field to their advantage—in effect, to set the rules of competition. It also comprises moves and countermoves to disrupt or undermine the form of capitalism used by rivals. Hypercompetition is rough-and-tumble competition with the intent of diminishing rivals' advantages while creating surprising new competitive advantages for one's nation. It is a concept that characterizes the aggressive nature of global competition today.

The lineage of hypercompetition and the strategies it demands can be traced back to Sun Tzu. More than 2,500 years ago, the Chinese military leader advocated the power of surprise to disrupt and eventually destroy competitors. However, while they may be timeless and universal, the clever and swift actions championed by Sun Tzu sometimes are not decisive enough and take too long. This is when strategists look to the principles outlined by Carl von Clausewitz, the Prussian soldier and military theorist. Clausewitz advocated unleashing massive, overwhelming force with relentless extreme superiority at a given moment and a specific place.

From my two-decade study of hypercompetition, I have found that when nations (or corporations) engage in hypercompetition, they create competitive advantage by doing the following:

- Go on the offense for a decisive victory.
- Disrupt rivals before rivals do the same to them.
- Change the rules of competition often.
- Escalate competition before rivals do.
- Force others to play catch-up.
- Surprise rivals by making current advantages obsolete.
- Learn strategy from business, military science, and diplomacy.
- Prepare a strategy of future moves and countermoves.
- Execute the strategy faster than rivals can react.

Consider how Japan took advantage of the United States by disrupting and destroying national oligopolies and uncompetitive manufacturing industries—especially in autos, electronics, machine tools, and steel. To some extent, it is a moot point whether Japan intended to do economic harm to the United States. It can be argued that Japan was simply trying to rebuild its economy after World War II, but the effect was the same: it harmed U.S. economic power. (Of course, much the same could be said of China. But whether it is consciously setting out to overturn American economic superiority or not misses the point: the effect is the same.)

Japan developed a form of managed capitalism that featured domestic industry groups called *keiretsu*[1] and informal *zaibatsu*[2] (which were formally outlawed after World War II). They did not seek to maximize corporate profits in the short run. They sought to maximize employment in Japan and reinvestment in the long-term growth of the groups. The Japanese Ministry of International Trade and Industry (MITI), which championed a national strategy for economic growth, intervened in markets to make this happen. As part of its industrial policy, it favored one or two companies in each industry as "national champions." It also protected domestic markets and created export incentives to maximize the growth of the Japanese economy.

As it spread its influence in the 1970s and 1980s, Japan, Inc., also brought new management methods to the fore. These included *kanban* and *hourensou*. The two concepts facilitated collaboration and information flows, and they enabled just-in-time inventory systems, supply chain management, and speedy management decision making. Meanwhile, a new form of quality management transformed cheap Japanese goods into premium ones. "Made in Japan" went from an emblem that evoked contempt to one that inspired awe. With its newly developed prowess, Japan pushed Western companies out of automobiles, home appliances, cameras, copy machines, steel, consumer electronics, memory chips, televisions, and other industries. Manufacturing cities in Japan earned lustrous reputations. Manufacturing centers in the United States earned the moniker "Rust Belt."

In Japan's version of capitalism, government and industry develop a cozy relationship. Arm's-length relationships are considered unrealistic. Officials in regulatory agencies work hand in hand with businesspeople to improve each industry's global competitiveness and achieve the nation's goals. In the United States, arm's-length relationships between the government and corporations are the rule—or should I say the myth. Government regulators attempt to keep their distance to avoid corruption and bias. Even corporations avoid cooperation with one another for fear of being accused of collusion and other antitrust violations.

The United States Gets Blindsided

The United States became a sitting duck for the sharp aim of Japanese industrial groups and MITI. After the war, the United States had settled into a model of capitalism that emphasized oligopolies—a limited group of firms in each industry that influenced the total supply, capacity, prices, and quality of goods. The oligopolies were referred to by the names of the cities in which many of the firms were located: Pittsburgh meant steel; Hollywood, movies; Detroit, automobiles; Boston, defense and space electronics; Hartford and Boston, insurance. Oligopolies developed in airlines, aluminum, beer, carbonated beverages, chemicals, cigarettes, gypsum, industrial gases, synthetic fibers, tires, and mainframe computers.

Business strategist Michael Porter described America's capitalism in 1980 in his seminal book *Competitive Strategy*. He showed that five forces allowed oligopolies to thrive: high barriers to entering their markets, limited power of buyers, limited power of suppliers, few substitute products, and limited rivalry among the players. By following the principles that Porter highlighted, big companies could set premium prices, make good money, pay people handsomely, and support a growing American middle class, without getting caught in collusion or predation. Of course, this wasn't always good for the consumer. To keep up the good times, for example, Detroit used strategies like "planned obsolescence" to force consumers to buy a new car every five years and to keep the repairs and parts businesses flowing.

At the time, the United States didn't operate free markets in many industries. Archaic regulations affected airlines, alcohol distributors, automobiles, banking, bus transportation, chemicals, healthcare, insurance, railroads, securities, trucking, utilities, and many other industries. Regulations guaranteed airlines, defense contractors, and utilities a "fair rate of return" on assets or cost-plus pricing. Some regulations hindered new firms' entry into markets like pharmaceuticals. Others punished aggressive firms for "predation." All told, while many people thought that these regulations were protecting the public from oligopolistic practices, many others realized that the regulations helped to protect existing companies. It gave industry veterans "sustainable" advantages. In essence, the government maximized the welfare of producers at the expense of consumers. And the Japanese took advantage of this mistake by undermining the oligopolies through better quality, lower prices, and better service.

Before 1970, many U.S. companies enjoyed a honeymoon from fierce competition. That explains why U.S. manufacturers reaped the highest return on assets of the century in the 1950s and 1960s. Their results came easily in the wake of the destruction of global capacity during the war. Consumers around the world thirsted for new products, and the United States, largely alone, had the capacity to make them. The high point of the period came from early 1961 to mid-1969. U.S. gross domestic product (GDP) grew by 53 percent, or 5.1 percent a year. The United States was literally reaping the spoils of war.

The good times set the United States up for a fall. It learned to operate with a capitalist system that, in hindsight, made it weak. U.S. oligopolists let their free-market competitive muscles atrophy. The Japanese not only muscled up but came out fighting in a new way. For one thing, the Japanese started treating customers well, aiming to please them with better quality and lower prices. For another, they treated their suppliers well, aiming to develop partnerships that would create efficient supply chains in which everyone shared the savings. They supported their approach by refining their manufacturing skills to such an extent that the United States could not quickly match their speed or quality. As U.S. customers flocked to buy goods from Japan, U.S. companies collapsed.

At first, the United States reacted like a stunned boxer. It wobbled and followed a tortuous, uncoordinated path. The government presented no strategy. Policy makers didn't even agree that they should have a strategy—and they didn't. As businesses sought to compete, they often ran a ragged race until the Japanese firms outran them. Many of them sold out or liquidated. High-wage jobs disappeared. They reappeared in the same industries in Japan.

The United States was at a turning point. The industries that plunged into crisis included machine tools, autos, steel, small home appliances, consumer electronics, and memory chips. Political pressure from the United States helped to establish voluntary import goals for U.S products, limit exports of certain goods, and set goals to balance U.S.-Japanese trade. Some deals stuck—import limits on steel and autos, telecom procurement agreements, and semiconductor import agreements. But others came too late, or were too laxly enforced, to help save U.S. industries.

Once-prosperous cities, in turn, tipped into decline: Detroit, Buffalo, Rochester, Cleveland, Pittsburgh, Flint, Syracuse, Erie, Utica, Toledo, Youngstown, Lansing, Saginaw, Gary, South Bend, Elkhart, Milwaukee, Indianapolis, and Chicago. To this day, except for Chicago and Pittsburgh, most of these cities are still languishing. This is an important point: although the United States recovered its economic poise, it did so at a great cost. That cost was the hollowing out of America's manufacturing base.

In the years that followed, as we shall see, the United States moved to become a knowledge-based economy. However, it never rebuilt its manufacturing core. Something was permanently lost—America's manufacturing self-reliance. This is one of the reasons why the United States has proved so vulnerable to competition from China.

The Reagan Revolution

When Ronald Reagan came to power in 1980, he responded with an ideological conviction that would leave a lasting legacy: laissez-faire capitalism would unleash the country's latent economic power. Reagan believed that free markets would spur better decision making than was possible in government. They would allocate capital to its highest and best use more efficiently. And, in turn, they would encourage the wealthy to invest more cash to create more jobs, with the accumulated wealth "trickling down" from the rich to the poor.

Among the highlights of Reagan-era thinking were the following: Deregulation (initially begun under President Carter with airlines in 1978 and railroads in 1979) would spur lower costs, better service, and more business start-ups. Quashing union power would create more flexible labor markets. Open international trade based on free-trade rules would create more wealth for all. Privatizing government functions would make services cheaper and better. Moving R&D efforts out of government and into private companies would make R&D more productive. Getting the government out of industrial policy would allow the fittest industries to flourish.

Along with the Reagan revolution came many benefits: Cheap imports gave consumers more choices of affordable products. Low down payments and government support encouraged homeownership. Tax cuts for individuals and business left more money for people to save, spend, and invest according to their own wishes. Hostile takeovers forced companies to maximize wealth for shareholders. Perhaps most important, new corporate strategies emerged that whipped U.S. firms into trimmer, more agile, and more imaginative fighting shape.

By the end of the 1980s, the laissez-faire capitalism championed by President Reagan had captured the hearts and minds of politicians in both parties. One of them was President Clinton, who in the 1990s did not reverse the Reagan model, but instead supported open trade, notably the North American Free Trade Agreement (NAFTA). Clinton worked diligently to open several industries in Japan to U.S. exports. When needed, he raised the specter of a trade war to force Japan to open its doors.

This new brand of laissez-faire capitalism, reprising some of the methods used in the United States prior to 1900, disrupted the surge in Japanese strength. Two periods of sustained GDP growth in the United States ensued: the Reagan boom from late 1982 to mid-1990, at 37 percent (4 percent a year), and the Clinton boom from early 1991 to late 2000, at 43 percent (3.8 percent a year). Shareholder wealth skyrocketed.[3] Observers credited laissez-faire capitalism with creating 16.3 million jobs under Reagan, from January 1981 to December 1988, and 22.8 million under Clinton, from January 1993 to December 2000.

Laissez-faire capitalism worked to counteract Japan, Inc. Indeed, it grew in stature and came to be regarded as the savior of American business. People widely believed in the new formula for success: deregulation, an orientation toward stockholder wealth, a powerful Wall Street monitoring firms and CEOs, outsourcing and offshoring to cut costs, using nonunion workers for flexible and less expensive labor, product lines favoring higher-value-added products and services, and efficiency and quality as the guiding stars of manufacturing success. Laissez-faire capitalism gave the United States everything it needed to take on the world: lean, hypercompetitive firms that were ready to fight companies based in low-cost nations.

Japanese Stagnation

The new U.S. approach to capitalism stalled Japan. We matched its costs, improved our quality, became more proactive, disrupted Japanese strategies, and undermined Japanese competitive advantages. Japanese firms persisted with their strategy, in particular seeking to compete with greater efficiency and higher quality. But the United States and other global manufacturers caught up. As the gap between Japanese and U.S. quality narrowed, consumers noted the diminishing returns on buying Japanese goods. Meanwhile, Japanese consensus-based decision making constrained innovation and change. The Japanese didn't have the bold moves to outdo the Americans the way they once did.

The United States also forced changes on Japan that made the country less competitive. For example, before the 1980s, a six-day workweek was common, but the United States complained, using the Organization for Economic Co-operation and Development (OECD) and the International Labour Organization (ILO) to pressure Japan to make five-day workweeks the standard. While workers enjoyed more freedom, productivity fell. Japan's educational system faced the same pressure to move to a five-day week, and the country began the phase-in of this in 1992. In the eyes of many Japanese, this reduced the drive, work ethic, stamina, and intellectual capabilities of schoolchildren, which in the long run would undermine Japanese corporate productivity.

The United States also forced Japan to join the world financial market. This, more than anything else, sapped the power of the Japanese economic engine. Japan's financial swoon happened this way: the Bank of Japan kept interest rates low to supply Japanese firms with inexpensive capital (among other reasons). Japan also lowered its interest rates to help the United States during the temporary but severe Black Monday stock market crash in 1987. The rock-bottom interest rates led real estate buyers to bid up prices in Japan. In turn, banks lent billions to buyers who were eager to get in on the action. However, the Bank of Japan was ultimately forced to raise interest rates to enter the global system. Real estate prices softened. The Ministry of Finance stiffened rules on real estate transaction volume. The Bank of Japan then raised interest rates to 6 percent. Real estate prices and the stock market collapsed.

Japan's banking sector, mired in a credit crisis, could no longer fuel the country's economic engine. Japanese companies lacked access to capital as banks rushed to shore up firms that were thought to be too big to fail. Little money was left for long-term investment in R&D and modernization. Many firms struggled with high debt loads and low growth. Mergers of weak firms arranged by the government often simply created larger losers.

This extended the crisis. American processes such as bankruptcy, hostile takeovers, or liquidation would have returned money to the system for productive investment more quickly, but these were almost taboo in Japan. Many industries in Japan lost the ability to compete vigorously.

Japan has gotten deeper into financial trouble over the years. Its public debt has grown to more than double that of any other developed country, reaching 230 percent of GDP in 2011. Though massive, the debt has not triggered a crisis, as the Japanese people hold most of it. But Japan continues to suffer from the debt burden. Government deficits have constrained recovery. Among other things, they have ensured that Japan, Inc., has not come up with a second capitalist act. From the point of view of a laissez-faire capitalist, Japan has not matched the United States in efficient capital allocation, raw GDP growth, or creation of shareholder value.

However, economists have no reason to believe that Japan has failed on all dimensions. Japan's handling of its capitalist system has much to recommend it. By some economic and quality-of-life measures, it has advanced in an impressive way.[4] It has kept unemployment low (4.2 percent), increased life expectancy by 4.2 years since 1989, and to this day generates a $50 billion trade surplus with the United States. To be sure, the Japanese stock market has languished, as has GDP growth, but Japan retained a good standard of living and it remains a strong (number 3) player in the ongoing contest of capitalist hypercompetition.

The contest between the United States' and Japan's form of capitalism is instructive. Japan's form of capitalism differed sharply from that in the United States prior to the 1980s. Moreover, the United States had embraced the values of Presidents Franklin Roosevelt and Lyndon Johnson. These men had molded capitalism around unionism, labor protections, public reliance on government, regulation of big business and banking, progressive income tax rates, and massive wealth-transfer programs to the elderly and poor. Government in that era aimed to reduce poverty, protect people from greedy bankers and companies, and build the backbone of a stable capitalist democracy—a large working and middle class.

This earlier capitalism, with its oligopolies, was not up to Japan's challenge. To be sure, it helped the United States rule the world economically for nearly three decades. But Japanese capitalism disrupted it. In turn, Reagan-era laissez-faire capitalism, a new form of capitalism that also differed sharply from that in Japan, disrupted Japanese capitalism. The striking conclusion: each version of capitalism undermined or disrupted the previous version. This is hypercompetition between nations.

China's Turn

While Japan has sought to regroup in the game of capitalist hypercompetition, another country now has the United States on the ropes, namely China.

Interestingly, the approach that the United States used to beat back the economic threat from Japan—primarily laissez-faire policies along with a few aggressive managed-market actions—will not work against China. This is precisely my point: strategic capitalism does not advocate one form of capitalism as the only solution. Rather, it takes a pragmatic approach, using whatever blend of capitalist policies is necessary to counteract the threat.

The fact is that China can't be pushed around the way the United States handled Japan, so we need a different approach.

On the surface, China favors a capitalist strategy similar to that of Japan in the 1980s. Key elements include protection of home markets, government subsidies for domestic industries, close ties between business and government, dependence on exports, theft of intellectual property, and lean social programs. It also includes artificially low interest rates, an artificially undervalued currency, high savings and investment rates, firms working for national growth rather than profit maximization, long-term financial horizons, and government-controlled industrial policy.

But for all the similarities, the resemblance is in some ways superficial. Behind the scenes, China uses state-owned banks to allocate funds among firms. It encourages big state-owned enterprises to compete against one another. This contrasts with Japan's use of MITI and *amakudari*[5] to exert control over private-sector *zaibatsu* and *keiretsu*. It also has a long history of entrepreneurial traditions developed earlier in China, which contrasts with the samurai traditions of loyalty and military-style obedience in Japan.

Another difference is that China does not look to America for military protection, as Japan did. This has given China more autonomy in resisting American influence. In contrast, China actively seeks leverage over the U.S. government by financing U.S. budget deficits. China has thus been able to resist American efforts to force China's banking system into the world financial markets and to revalue the yuan to market levels.

Yet another difference is that China's population is much larger than Japan's. This has given China more leverage over foreign countries, investors, and corporations. It has also given China options that Japan didn't have. For example, as Japan became more successful, it lost its low-labor-cost advantage. China still has almost a billion peasants that it can deploy in low-value-added manufacturing. Meanwhile, China can still upgrade manufacturing in the coastal areas, where wage rates and standards of living are rising quickly.

The Chinese are also building a mercantilist system. Chinese state-owned enterprises are buying up raw materials in Africa and Latin America. China's growing network of suppliers will feed its manufacturing processes and in turn fill its export pipeline to the United States and Europe. China's appetite for imported iron ore, oil, copper, aluminum, cobalt, niobium (tantalum), and other minerals has been growing at more than 21 percent yearly. For many of these materials, it is estimated that at least 60 to 80 percent of China's needs must come from imports. China's size gives it a huge amount of leverage over supplier nations.

China is taking ownership of supplier corporations either through state-owned enterprises or directly though its ministries. This gives the Chinese government the option of using its acquired resources as instruments of state policy. It can influence the foreign policies of other nations or undermine free trade in commodities the way the Organization of Petroleum Exporting Countries (OPEC) does. Among China's targets is Latin America.[6] The reality is that many nations are gradually falling into China's economic sphere of influence. Of course, commentators will argue that the United States acquires far more assets abroad than China does. This is true, but U.S. acquisitions are driven by corporate strategic objectives rather than by national strategic aims. Again, my argument is that China is acquiring foreign assets in a state-directed and strategic way in a deliberate attempt to increase Chinese economic power.

In Africa, China is locking up assets through mercantilist relationships. It has invested in the copper industry in Zambia and the Democratic Republic of the Congo. It is buying forest products in Cameroon, Gabon, Mozambique, Equatorial Guinea, and Liberia. It has spent billions of dollars securing drilling rights in Angola, Nigeria, and Sudan. And it has cut exploration or extraction deals with Chad, the Democratic Republic of the Congo, Ethiopia, Equatorial Guinea, Gabon, Kenya, and Mauritania.

At first glance, China's interest in Africa appears little different from that of the United States or the European Union. Its trade with central Africa, for example, is only 0.15 percent of its total trade volume, comparable to that of the European Union and the United States. But here the comparison ends. Across Africa, Chinese firms have muscled out other companies, winning contracts to pave highways, build hydroelectric dams, upgrade ports, lay railway tracks, and build pipelines. To gain access, China offers soft loans designed to encourage Chinese-built infrastructure. The loans offer below-market interest rates and concessions like long repayment periods or interest holidays.[7]

China's activities have become so aggressive and extensive that some Africans have become suspicious. Many worry that China is trying to re-create colonialism as it elbows out foreign competition and moves in Chinese migrants. Chinese expatriates in Africa number 400,000, including 100,000 in Zambia and 120,000 in Nigeria. China is using its economic relationships to court

African votes in the United Nations (UN) to isolate Taiwan. Rene N'Guetta Kouassi, the head of the African Union's economic affairs department, has warned, "Africa must not jump blindly from one type of neo-colonialism into Chinese-style neo-colonialism."[8]

China is also attempting to monopolize certain raw materials. It domestically mines 95 to 97 percent of the world's 17 rare earth elements. Dysprosium, gadolinium, praseodymium, and other rare earths have useful electrical, optical, and thermal properties. They are used to make smaller, more powerful magnets for cars, computer disk drives, motors, generators—and missile guidance systems. Others are used to improve heat resistance in jet-engine turbine blades and brighten images in night-vision goggles. They are essential to green-energy technologies, including solar cells, wind turbines, and electric and hybrid car motors.

The future of many technologies depends upon access to rare earth elements, and China has recently restricted supply by setting export limits. The Chinese government imposed an unannounced embargo on shipments of raw rare earths to Japan during a disagreement over disputed islands. China has also imposed export quotas and raised taxes from 15 to 25 percent on crucial alloys. U.S. rare earth mining companies, such as Molycorp Minerals, plan to expand U.S. production, but developing new mines will take five to eight years.

In short, China is throwing its considerable economic weight around in a way that has not been seen since the United States introduced the Marshall Plan after World War II. My point isn't that such actions are inherently wrong. Far from it. Rather, my argument is that the United States isn't as good at doing it as it once was. And my other point is that if a nation is going to throw its weight around, it is better that it is a democratic nation like the United States, with checks and balances on its power, than an authoritarian, one-party state with none.

Some people will argue that in an increasingly multipolar world, the likelihood of a single dominant hegemon is receding. It is true that the world is becoming more and more connected via technology and trading relationships. But the fact remains that the United States is currently the only viable counterweight to Chinese power—the only guarantee of a bipolar, let alone a multipolar, world. It is therefore in the interests not just of Americans but of people all over the world that the United States remain economically strong. Most great empires, from the Roman Empire to the British Empire, have declined not because of a single military defeat, but because their economies were unable to sustain themselves over time. In order to maintain its military and political influence, the United States must safeguard its economic power.

It is unrealistic to suggest that the United States will regain its economic leadership over the entire world. The center of gravity is likely to shift toward Asia, which now accounts for 60 percent of the world's population. My argument is that the United States must retain its economic leadership over a smaller capitalist ecosystem (a capitalist bloc) or sphere of influence. This U.S.-led bloc or sphere will then be in a stronger position to negotiate with the Chinese sphere.

It can be argued, too, that China is simply seeking to assert its rightful place in the world. Lacking the political assets that the United States has acquired in more than a century of diplomacy, China is using economic policy to serve political ends because it cannot gain influence by military or cultural means. This argument says that it is not necessarily about economic domination, but simply about China's attempt to gain the influence to match its size, which is perfectly natural. Unfortunately, the same argument could have been used to explain Germany's economic buildup just before World War II. I am not suggesting that the Chinese agenda is the same, but economic appeasement is not in the best interests of either the United States or the free world.

China's Disruption of U.S. Capitalism

With managed capitalism, China has taken the same approach as Japan. But it has added the weight of its larger population, state control of financing, the mercantilist approach, and its willingness to play tough with foreign suppliers and buyers. That has brought the United States into a growing economic confrontation. We are witnessing the opening round of hypercompetition between China and the United States. Some may argue that China's actions are simply the result of its desire to raise its own economic game, rather than a deliberate policy to undermine the performance of the United States. I do not share that view, but even if that were the case, the intention is less important than the effect on U.S. interests. The ways in which China has disrupted America's rules of capitalism can be seen from the following observations.

During 2010, the United States spent $365 billon on goods from China. China spent just $92 billion on goods from the United States. The U.S. trade deficit with China has grown by 27 times since 1990. The United States has lost leadership in many global markets. China is now the largest exporter of high-tech products.[9] In 1998, the United States had 25 percent of the world's high-tech export market, and China had just 10 percent. Ten years later, the United States has less than 15 percent, and China has 20 percent.

The United States has become dependent on China. China is now the United States' biggest supplier of components critical to the operation of U.S. defense systems, including U.S. missiles, supercomputers, and other military equipment. Chinese producers have grown so large that they can determine world prices in industries as different as steel and antibiotics. In steel, China produces 11 times as much as the United States. This allows the Chinese government to influence global steel prices. It also raises the possibility that China can put the few remaining American steelmakers out of business.

Of course, China has not entered the global fray without creating some dependencies of its own. Above all, it depends on Americans' voracious appetite for consumer goods. If China weakens the U.S. economy too much by reducing U.S. manufacturing jobs, it will actually undercut itself. A vicious cycle would ensue as successive expansions of Chinese exports undercut the demand for products from the very plants that make the exported products.

China also depends on the stability of the U.S. dollar. The Chinese central bank holds more than $3 trillion in foreign currency reserves, mostly U.S. dollars. It has lent so much money to the U.S. government that it has become a creditor held hostage by the goodwill of its debtor. If the United States defaults, China will suffer a loss of more than $1 trillion. If China stops lending to reduce its reliance on the United States, China can hurt America—by lowering the U.S. debt rating and in turn raising interest rates—but it could easily hurt itself more.

As Philip Coggan argues in his book *Paper Promises: Money, Debt and the New World Order*, a new world order will emerge from the current economic and financial crisis, and it will be governed by the creditor nation of the future, China.

Coggan points out that China's priorities are very different from those of America and Britain, who pioneered the last two world monetary systems. He warns that many promises have been made both to creditors and to citizens in the form of future benefits. Those promises cannot all be kept, so there will be winners and losers.[10] For Coggan, the big question is the imbalance between China and America and whether China will continue to stockpile dollars. The answer is no. China will reach a point— probably in the next five to ten years—at which doing so is no longer worth it. If America hasn't ended its dependency on borrowing from other countries by then, there will be a crisis.

The exact depth and form of that crisis is not yet clear. It may be a crisis for the United States alone, or it may be one that affects China and the other developing economies around the world. Let's be clear: China still has many hurdles to cross before it becomes the dominant economic power in the world. Its role as hegemon is not certain. Remember, it once seemed certain that the Japanese economy would surpass that of the United States, but those predictions did not come true. Similarly, China's future is not preordained. As with Japan, the United States has it within its power to influence the outcome. But whereas America was able to rely on its political and military influence to persuade Japan to accept many of our rules of capitalism, China is a different proposition.

The reality is that China's size and population mean that it is less susceptible to this sort of soft American power. The fact remains, though, that the United States is still the master of its own destiny—but only if we act soon. Of course, China itself may also suffer a setback or become the victim of its own growing pains. This could take a number of forms. The Asian currency crisis of 1997 is an example of what can befall even the most dynamic emerging economy, although, for the time being, China's currency exposure is hedged through its large holdings of U.S. dollars. There are other crises that could affect China's development, including potential public unrest if the Chinese people become sufficiently frustrated that the country's newfound wealth is not being distributed to the wider population fast enough. This is one potential bear trap that the Chinese leadership could fall into.

That said, the size of the country and its dispersed population makes it easier for the Chinese authorities to crack down on dissent using divide-and-rule tactics.

Those who believe there is no intent on China's part to undermine America's economic position—and therefore no evidence that China is a hypercompetitive rival to the United States—should consider what that huge shift has meant for the general Chinese population. If China were simply intent on making its own people wealthier, it could easily have distributed more of the wealth that it created. There is no doubt that Chinese consumers have suffered so that the country can subsidize people elsewhere in an attempt to get into markets—from the United States to Africa. That is a strategic decision.

A recent report by the Brookings Institution makes the point that the Chinese leaders believe they are heading ever more surely into a zero-sum future: for every economic step gained by China, another country must accept a step back. U.S. intelligence analysts' interceptions of Chinese officials' communications indicate that

Chinese policy makers increasingly assume a zero-sum approach in relations with the United States, and they see a future in which China comes out the long-term winner.[11]

China's decision to act as a creditor to the West is also a strategic choice that one must consider when determining China's strategic intent. This strategic choice is not consistent with a desire to improve the way of life for the mass of the Chinese people in the short term. China has pursued a strategy based on deferred consumption at home in order to create access to foreign markets (and dependence upon Chinese products in those markets). The question is how long the Chinese leadership can continue to pursue that policy at the expense of keeping a large proportion of its people poor. That is a calculated gamble, aimed at disrupting the West— and insulating China from possible future shocks.

Remember, this is only the opening round. Yet it is already clear that China is disrupting the West's rules of capitalism in areas such as ignoring intellectual property rights, deferring home consumption, and manipulating its currency. China has taken advantage of the United States' modern form of capitalism.

Japan earlier took advantage of the United States' postwar form of capitalism by destroying oligopolies and noncompetitive manufacturing industries through strategies that took advantage of oligopolistic strategy. The United States watched helplessly (or smugly) as Japan hollowed out the U.S. manufacturing base and pushed jobs into service industries. Now China has taken advantage of the United States' near blind faith in laissez-faire capitalism. Its push toward global mercantilism and economic nationalism has such power that it has neutralized the United States' power to set the global rules for competition and trade. The United States does not have the leverage to force China to change, as it did with the Japanese. It must find a new way.

Three Challenges

Put in the historical context of our economic battles with Japan and now China, hypercompetition between forms of capitalism presents three very important challenges to those who would plan our economic strategy:

- *No form of capitalism works forever.* When one form of capitalism is competing with another form of capitalism, the rules of capitalism must adjust to the punches that are being thrown. Thus, one cannot rely on any ideological or theoretical approach that says that one approach fits all times and all situations. Capitalism evolves and competes with different versions of capitalism.
- *The world is currently engaged in a win-lose game.* China is playing to win at the expense of America's form of capitalism, and China is ignoring the theory of free trade that insists that open trade maximizes the total growth of the world economy. China has no incentive to change its approach because it also wins when the United States loses.
- *Superpowers are actively and aggressively disrupting one another to create an uneven playing field with new rules of capitalism.* Therefore, strategists cannot base an economic strategy on theories that predict that the world will reach a long-run equilibrium. Constant disruption will not allow a long-run equilibrium to develop.

A strategy based on an ideology or economic theory can create competitive advantage, but it depends on the game the rival is playing, and it works for only a short period before the rules of capitalism get changed. Competitors probe for weaknesses and then exploit them. Truly great competitors find ways to undermine, make moot, neutralize, or make obsolete the competitive advantages of their rivals' capitalist systems.

The unbridled call by some U.S. policy makers for doubling down on our commitment to laissez-faire capitalism and social programs mistakes the challenge of the present for the challenges of the past. Promoting more free trade and open markets seems to have worked against Japan in the 1980s and 1990s, but it was not a strategy for the permanent economic salvation of America, and it is not working against China. China has different competitive advantages from those that Japan had, and hence different tactics will be required to overwhelm those advantages. This, in turn, will require new competitive advantages in America, as well as the abandonment of old advantages that are no longer relevant to the current economic situation.

In a sense, the United States is suffering now from arrested capitalistic development. It has developed powerful motor and thinking skills based on thinking that was suitable for the last two centuries, but it has not yet taken its thinking to the twenty-first century.

This is the juncture where my prediction comes in. U.S. leaders, though in their painfully querulous way, are grasping the new reality. They are noticing that we are tangled up in our boxing shorts. For a while they will trip over those shorts. But eventually, they will pick themselves up and learn a new way to compete.

The United States is on the cusp of recognizing that just as businesses go through phases of creative destruction, capitalist systems do as well. The time is now for the United States to launch a post-Reagan revolution to take the battle to our competitors with a fresh approach, a hypercompetitive strategy fit for the twenty-first century.

2

Combining Capitalisms

Comparative Advantage and Capitalist Systems

Imagine the exhilaration that was in the air as the founding fathers of the United States sat down in 1786 to draft the Constitution. Working from the ideals of Montesquieu, Jean-Jacques Rousseau, John Locke, and Edward Coke, they sought to design a more perfect nation, incorporating democratic principles into a new republic. They had a wealth of emerging thought about government and freedom to inform them. They combined and recombined their ideas until they had created a republic that would fit the circumstances of the new country and its place in the world.

They knew that they were undertaking the biggest social experiment of all time: creating a government that relied on the people to rule themselves. The founding fathers feared rule by tyrants, but they feared rule by an uneducated, unruly mob even more. At the time, they did not know what combination would work. So they combined checks and balances, the electoral college, a bicameral legislature, a strong presidency, flat taxes, and a great deal more to see how it worked. The founding fathers also recognized that this new form of government would need continual refinement. And they were right: over time, the original republic that they created has been modified to become a universal democracy, adding "one person, one vote" as one of its core principles.

If we listen to many U.S. leaders today, they are telling us that we don't need to innovate the way the founding fathers did when it comes to our capitalist system. Instead, they have presented us with either/or choices:

- For or against free markets?
- For or against managed capitalism?
- For or against social programs?

The choices are framed as false dichotomies, and they are often asked as if the answers don't depend on global circumstances, our current financial condition, or the actions of rivals that are trying to disrupt our system of capitalism.

But, like the founding fathers, we have more than either/or decisions. We can build a more perfect capitalist system that uses elements of different types of capitalism, or we can even apply different types of capitalism to different industries as needed. Different types of capitalism can be combined in many novel ways to create entirely new versions of capitalism.

My argument is that we have failed to see the nuances of the different forms of capitalism that nations choose over time. Legacy programs from one era carry over to another. Changes made are often layered on top of old capitalist ideas and institutions. Through our failure to see how different types of capitalism can be mixed, which mixtures work, what different mixtures achieve, and how other countries mix their capitalisms differently, our economic thinking has become too rigid, and our vision of capitalism has become blurred.

The good news is that we are positioned to lead again. As we grasp the realities of hypercompetition, our capitalist system needs reinvention and rebuilding. We have smart people in industry, academia, and government who can do so. We just need to let them out of the intellectual straitjackets that constrain their thinking.

American democracy has evolved from the republic conceived by the founding fathers to a universal democracy. The nation's health and success demanded changes in democracy. In the same way, our form of capitalism has, and can again, evolve to promote further economic success.

Four Generic Types of Capitalism

Let us examine some of the nuances of capitalism. We oversimplify the world when we identify a country as a laissez-faire capitalist (e.g., the United States), a social-market capitalist (e.g., Sweden), or a managed capitalist (e.g., China). In truth, every nation has some mixture of four generic types of capitalism: laissez-faire, social-market, managed, and philanthropic capitalism. The reality is that the different types of capitalism exist as pure types more in theory than in practice. Although the struggle of competing capitalisms rages among nations, as discussed in the last chapter, the struggle among different types of capitalism also rages within nations.

Each generic type trades off two key goals: economic freedom (free markets) and income equality, as shown in Figure 2-1. At one end of the freedom spectrum, governments use central planning, and people have no property rights. At the other end, governments exert zero control and allow totally free markets and unlimited private property rights. At one end of the income-equality spectrum, governments assiduously redistribute income to reduce economic class differences. At the other, they provide no income redistribution and allow individuals to accumulate wealth as the reward for taking risks with their investment capital.

Figure 2-1 illustrates that each of the four types of capitalism aims at different goals, operates with different competitive rules, and stimulates different capitalist behavior. Our muddled thinking about goals, rules, and behavior has led to unproductive debates about the best strategy for the future.

To show that we have more options than we think, let's first look at each form of capitalism to clarify our terms.

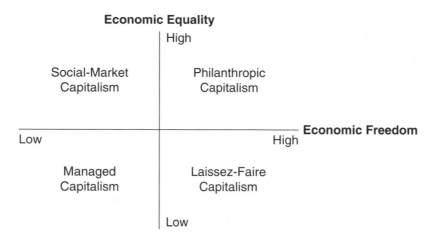

FIGURE 2.1 Four Generic Capitalist Strategies

Laissez-Faire Capitalism

In theory, laissez-faire capitalism is an economic system in which the production, distribution, and exchange of goods and services depend on private citizens investing capital and making profits. People operate within freely evolving, transparent, and efficient domestic product and financial markets, as well as within open international trade systems. Government interference is minimal or nonexistent. The word *laissez-faire* is French for "let it be."

Laissez-faire capitalism promises people that they will live in a society with unfettered competition, free of regulation, with the chance for upward social mobility. Its supporters believe that laissez-faire capitalism allows workers, investors, and consumers to create a better life through the efficient use of capital and incentives for working hard and taking risks that offer the opportunity for greater rewards. Consumers are believed to receive lower prices, better quality, and greater variety. In theory, the economy grows faster than without a free market.

Pure laissez-faire capitalism rarely exists. Economists largely agree that the pure form would be impossible in complex, modern economies because anarchy would result. Voters in democracies instead want their governments to intervene to smooth economic cycles and create jobs, so some regulation is required. Still, laissez-faire advocates argue for limited government. And laissez-faire thinking and limited government have remained a core tenet of conservative economic thinking in the United States since the presidency of Ronald Reagan.

However, many people believe that laissez-faire capitalism allows the rich to gain at the expense of everyone else. The top 1 percent of Americans, for example, controls 93 percent of the wealth. The capitalist class of investors, asset managers, investment bankers, and traders has control of the money and thus of investment priorities. As a result, wealthy investors may direct investment to dubious social purposes—for example, treating male baldness in the developed world receives more investment than curing malaria in the developing world. Companies also have little incentive to pay for their "externalities," such as pollution, social costs due to offshoring, product liability, and collapsed banking systems. In other words, free markets do not always self-regulate in the interest of society.

Managed Capitalism

Managed capitalism is an economic system in which mostly private enterprises compete in markets that are nominally free but are subject to comprehensive government control. The state intervenes in the economy to protect specific businesses or industries. It also directs private firms to achieve state goals. The state, large firms, and labor unions coordinate their efforts to ensure multiple national goals: economic growth, low unemployment, positive trade imbalances, restrained imports, access to raw materials, energy availability, food production, industrial development, and the support of foreign policy or military goals.

Managed capitalism differs markedly from communism. In managed capitalism, the state allows ownership of private property, affirms the right to make a profit, prohibits monopolies, and permits income-class distinctions to develop. Managed capitalism does not, by itself, address social goals, such as progressive income taxes or wealth-transfer programs from the rich to the poor. Instead, it relies on a "rising tide to raise all ships," and encourages high savings rates as the only way for people to take self-responsibility for retirement, healthcare, unemployment, advanced education, and catastrophic events.

Managed economies theoretically combine the power and resources of the entire state to achieve unified national goals. Technocrats, not politicians, conduct planning and lead implementation. They work toward clearly stated national goals, and they hold hearings and planning sessions to gather input on national direction. They sidestep coordination with lobbyists and politicians to minimize parochial or politically driven decision making.

In the United States, President Richard Nixon championed a form of managed capitalism in building the Cold War military-industrial complex. Perhaps more than any leader before or after, he pressed for a tight linkage between government and private defense contractors. Technocrats managed the defense industry to ensure that advanced tanks, communication systems, missile systems, and other strategic military equipment came on line quickly. He even decided where the defense industry should be located, moving many contracts to universities and firms far away from Route 128 near Boston. Nixon also announced the War on Cancer. The National Institutes of Health (NIH) took the same managed approach. The Defense Advanced Research Projects Agency, or DARPA, was held up as a model approach to forward-thinking R&D. Nixon also used wage and price controls to control markets directly during times of oil shortages and stagflation.

Managed capitalism has its downsides. Planners may miscalculate prices and supply and demand. Market inefficiencies may develop, and technocrats may cover them up, leading to failed management. Technocrats may also make poor choices, leading to political scuffles over direction. In the United States, managed efforts have yielded many successes. Industries that have benefited include aerospace, agriculture, computers, communications, defense, telecommunications (the Internet), pharmaceuticals, medical equipment, and software. Products and technologies that founded industries have emerged from work at NASA, the Department of Defense, the National Institutes of Health, the National Science Foundation (NSF), and the Department of Agriculture.

Truly managed-capitalist governments control their economies through many intrusive actions: state ownership of private firms, wage controls, price controls, capacity controls, production limits, licensing procedures to prevent or encourage market entry, industry cartelization, creation and support of national champions, trade protection, government subsidies, and state-sponsored R&D to advance specific businesses or industries. Some regulations or controls improve profits, and others reduce them for the public good. Note that managed-capitalist intrusion stops well short of communist central planning, which assigns personnel to state-supervised activities, plans the budgets of state-owned monopolies, and sets all output requirements.

At the extreme, managed capitalism is "state capitalism." Through corporatized state agencies, a controlling share of stock in publicly listed firms, and other means of control, the state acts like a giant corporation. Corporate losses become public, and everyone essentially shares them with the state. If subsidies persist too long, poorly performing enterprises may be propped up beyond their useful life, eating up a lot of government money. Worse, managers may lose their incentive to fix inefficiencies, reduce labor costs, and stay competitive with foreign firms. However, state capitalism does not have to be implemented through Soviet-style central planning that determines every aspect of production, consumption, investment, and savings by the government and public.

Social-Market Capitalism

Social-market capitalism is an economic system in which the state provides social security, unemployment, health, welfare, education, and other benefits for the poor, needy, elderly, and working class. The government encourages private ownership of businesses and competitive markets. It avoids price setting. It regulates markets and protects labor rights through national collective bargaining laws. It also regulates markets to constrain investors from exploiting markets for personal gain at the expense of stability—the way Wall Street bankers profited at the expense of U.S. financial stability in 2008. Some of the biggest social market programs in the United States were created by Presidents Franklin Roosevelt and Lyndon Johnson.

Social-market capitalism redistributes money from wealthy and middle-class people to the poor. Besides reducing income inequality, it encourages widespread consumption by those who receive government benefits. It also cuts poverty and, in theory, crime. Government aims to aid the poor and their children in finding jobs, thus spurring economic growth and contributing to society's well-being. Without such aid, children in high-poverty areas often receive less education and are essentially removed from the productive economy as adults, becoming economic liabilities. But as people move up, they pay rent, buy cars and homes, invest their savings, and, in turn, build GDP. This can be a virtuous cycle, as reducing poverty also cuts other expenses associated with it—for example, healthcare costs related to emergency room visits by the uninsured.

Social-market capitalism has its downsides. Critics argue that government money isn't always used for its intended purpose as a result of bureaucracy, fraud, poorly designed programs, and so on. Critics also say that wealth transfers drain both investment capital from the wealthy and funds that the government might spend for economic purposes. This diversion of funds may reduce programs that create long-term advantages for the nation, including industrial development, research, military hardware, infrastructure, communication systems, and energy and water projects—all of which may create more jobs than the social-market wealth transfers that displace them.

Wealth transfers also take investment and spending money out of the hands of the rich. The wealthy may decrease their consumer expenditures and, if taxes are high enough, feel a reduced incentive to work, build businesses, and hire people. In turn, the transfers may also reduce the incentive for the wealthy to invest in the United States and it may reduce the incentive to work by recipients of the largesse. In the United States, the top 10 percent of earners pay almost three-quarters of all federal income taxes. The bottom 40 percent pay nothing. In fact, many people in the bottom 40 percent receive payments from the government because their tax credits exceed their liabilities. The risk, on balance, is that taxation may shrink the overall incentive to work and the amount of capital available for investment and growth.

Philanthropic Capitalism

Philanthropic capitalism is an economic system in which privately owned enterprises compete in laissez-faire markets that run on profit motives, self-interest, and greed. However, the owners of capital make voluntary gifts to the poor, the needy, and charities for religious, educational, scientific, or other altruistic reasons. These charitable gifts can support institutions and causes that are critical to economic growth: universities, research centers, libraries, research hospitals, and so on. In effect, the philanthropists recycle back into the country the wealth the country helped them produce.

The notion of philanthropic capitalism was perhaps best embodied in the thinking of U.S. steel baron Andrew Carnegie in the late 1800s. Carnegie believed that business and philanthropy were separate endeavors. However, he asserted that the wealthy had the obligation to use their money to benefit society. And he was true to his word. He spent billions (in 2012 dollars) to promote the spread of literacy, culture, and higher education. Other early industrialists, including J. P. Morgan and John D. Rockefeller, did the same. Their example continues to set the standard for philanthropists like Bill Gates and Warren Buffett.

The United States has become the world's best example of a country using the principles of philanthropic capitalism to its advantage. Despite the Great Recession, 60 percent of Americans give to charity. Individuals give 10 times as much of their income as people in France do, for example. Charitable gifts have built the endowments of hundreds of major universities, research hospitals, technology and research centers, and medical research foundations for more than 300 years. This transfer of wealth has created many of the crown jewels in the United States' treasure of innovative institutions, leading to new technology, industries, health benefits, and wealth for millions of people.

The American leader who is best known for promoting a form of philanthropic capitalism as policy in recent decades is President George H. W. Bush. Bush called for a "thousand points of light" to do charitable works. The thousand points never materialized to replace government social programs. But when his son, George W. Bush, rose to the presidency, his April 2002 statements reinforced the essential approach: "Government cannot solve every problem, but it can encourage people and communities to help themselves and to help one another. . . . I call my philosophy and approach compassionate conservatism." In essence, the Bushes wanted charitable giving to replace some of the need for social-market capitalism.

Philanthropy can come from two places: people and businesses. In a twist, many CEOs and strategists today argue that Andrew Carnegie was wrong in saying that philanthropy and business should stay separate. For example, John Mackey, CEO of Whole Foods, urges business leaders to integrate philanthropy into their business goals. He says that businesses also have obligations to customers, employees, and the broader communities in which they reside. Even the well-known strategist Michael Porter called for businesses to focus more on helping society in his 2011 *Harvard Business Review* article titled "Fixing Capitalism." In contrast to some of his earlier theories, he called for corporations to create "shared value" for the stockholders and society—a return to what was once called the "multiple stakeholder approach" in the pre-Reagan era.

The debate over whether businesses should divert funds to philanthropy has a long history. Economist Milton Friedman has argued that the only obligation of businesses is to maximize share-holder wealth. This viewpoint prevails in many corporate circles. But people like Gates and Mackey, while embracing the arguments for free markets in Adam Smith's *The Wealth of Nations*, also cite Smith's earlier work, *The Theory of Moral Sentiments*, which focuses on people's desire to help their fellows. Mackey argues that the desire to help others can be a powerful motivator for business success. Capitalism based on philanthropy remains a utopian ideal, yet it plays a key role in national wealth.

No system of capitalism works for all seasons. Success depends on tuning the mix for the times and the country. In other words, a capitalist system that works well in one country may not work the same way in another because of many factors, including the culture, norms, institutions, corruption, religion, geopolitical circumstances and rivalries, and financial condition of the nation.

Capitalist Systems in Different Countries

We can learn a great deal about various capitalist systems by looking at the choices that other countries have made. Policy makers do not throw their weight behind just one generic type of capitalism, as some politicians would have us believe. In reality, the choice isn't between one generic type versus another. It is a choice of what mix to use and how much weight (comparative advantage) to give to each of the generic capitalisms within the mix.

Figure 2-2 illustrates the mixes of generic capitalisms and the comparative emphasis assigned to each generic capitalism in 15 countries.[1]

Note that the white, gray, and black dots denote light, medium, or heavy comparative advantage assigned to each type of generic capitalism. One caution when interpreting Figure 2-2: the dots do not indicate which countries have the best of each kind of capitalism. They only indicate the relative weights within each country. In other words, the table does not report competitive advantage, nor does it compare one country to the next. Still, the table is instructive for understanding capitalist systems because the mixture

Generic Capitalism	USA	China	France	UK	Germany	Italy and Spain	Sweden	Brazil	Japan	South Korea	Taiwan	India	Singapore and Indonesia
Laissez-Faire Capitalism	●	◐	○	●	◐	◐	◐	◐	○	◐	◐	○	●
Social-Market Capitalism	●	○	●	●	◐	●	●	◐	◐	◐	◐	○	○
Philanthropic Capitalism	◐	○	○	◐	◐	○	◐	○	○	◐	○	◐	○
Managed Capitalism	◐	●	●	○	◐	●	◐	◐	●	●	●	●	●

Circle Color = Level of Comparative Advantage: Black = High Importance, Grey = Moderate Importance, White = Low Importance

FIGURE 2.2 Capitalist Systems in 15 Countries

and the weights assigned to each generic type of capitalism reflect each nation's comparative advantages and thus its implicit goals related to economic freedom and economic equality.

Let's look at some specific capitalist systems more closely: those of France, the United Kingdom, Singapore, Japan, Germany, and the United States. Each offers a different way of seeking economic success. We did not find any country that executed only one of the generic types of capitalism. Some have done well by executing certain mixes, but not all mixes work well. The questions are: What (intentional or inadvertent) capitalist strategies are nations using to ensure that their capitalist systems meet their goals? And what choices should other nations make in order to stay competitive?

France's Mixture of Social-Market and Managed Capitalism

France has committed itself largely to social-market and managed capitalism.[2] In France's case, the country has traded off the workforce flexibility and cost efficiency of laissez-faire capitalism for the job protections and employment security that come with strong unions and heavy social benefits. It has also traded off the strong private-enterprise incentives of laissez-faire capitalism for the support of large "national champions" enabled by managed capitalism. National champions include global enterprises such as France Télécom, Renault, and Air France-KLM.

France, like a host of other European nations, earns the ridicule of laissez-faire advocates. Workers in France have a 35-hour workweek. The country's companies enjoy protection from foreign competition. They also get periodic bailouts, showing that they have not stayed fit to compete globally. French workers receive generous pensions and the retirement age is 62, and this partly explains why the nation faces a huge pension-funding shortfall. Taken as a whole, the evidence is that France has made choices that will limit its growth. GDP in 2010 rose only 1.6 percent, and France did not make its growth projection of 2 percent in 2011.

One can argue that France has succeeded in its aim to create a strong social support system. Though it scorns totally free markets, it nonetheless has established a portfolio of global companies. More French firms (39) occupy the ranks of the Fortune 500 than do German ones. In fact, France leads 10 out of 50 industries analyzed by *Fortune* magazine.[3] This is in spite of some spectacular failures, such as efforts in the 1980s to create national champions in the electronics industry using Thomson and Honeywell Bull.

To the extent that France has succeeded, it has done so because of its strong institutional support for managed capitalism: an elite corps of civil servants, chosen and educated at taxpayers' expense at the École Nationale d'Administration, guides the economy in choosing national champions and in choosing R&D investment targets. France does not strongly support entrepreneurship. In a world in which companies like Google rise from nothing to a global empire in a matter of years, France does not provide incentives for start-ups to flourish.

Being stretched beyond its means (like many countries), France has not done well recently. The French budget, burdened with social spending, exceeds that of Germany, even through Germany's GDP is one-third larger. If France is to remain competitive, whether within Europe or with China, the evidence suggests that it will have to reduce its commitment to social-market capitalism and experiment with new ways to execute managed capitalism. However, the May 2012 election indicates that the French people may not have the will for an austerity program, as suggested by the election of a socialist president.

The United Kingdom's Mixture of Laissez-Faire and Social-Market Capitalism

The United Kingdom has committed itself largely to laissez-faire and social-market capitalism.[4] With the reforms of Margaret Thatcher in the 1980s, the United Kingdom embraced laissez-faire capitalism. Although post–World War II lawmakers turned the United Kingdom into a managed economy, the pendulum swung under Thatcher. Moreover, financial losses in the 2008 panic prompted leaders like David Cameron to reduce social-market capitalism even more, cutting benefits and relying on more philanthropy (1.1 percent of GDP) to play a bigger role.

Thatcher also moved the country away from a long focus on managed capitalism, especially by privatizing companies. The British treasury had been drained for years by costly government-supported firms, leaving the British with little appetite for keeping up with industrial policy. In this case, Cameron's government proposed a small turnabout, establishing 21 enterprise zones, or industrial parks, to encourage innovative industries. This move recognized the United Kingdom's lagging position in innovation. For example, 5,672 patents were filed from the United Kingdom in 2009, compared to 16,311 from Germany. The United Kingdom had cut funds for R&D. It spends less on R&D as a percentage of GDP (1.8 percent) than France (2.0 percent), Germany (2.5 percent), or the United States (2.7 percent).

The recent choices of the U.K. government show that the country has decided to trade off the societal supports of social-market capitalism for the efficient capital and labor efficiency encouraged by laissez-faire capitalism. It has also decided to favor laissez-faire efficiencies over the long-term business development supposedly enabled by managed capitalism. Though the United Kingdom utterly turned its back on managed capitalism under Thatcher, policy makers have recognized that maybe they went too far, letting China gut the country's manufacturing sector.

The United Kingdom has built up some vibrant businesses in the last two decades, notably in the financial sector. Until the 2008 financial panic, the shift to laissez-faire served the country well. However, the free-market thrust in financial markets ran amok, just as it did in the United States. Meanwhile, social-market expenses became a heavy burden: more than half of government spending goes to pensions, healthcare, education, and welfare. That is why the United Kingdom is now focusing on rebuilding the fundamentals of its capitalist system, slashing budgets by an average of 19 percent, the deepest cuts since World War II.

The recent approach in both the United Kingdom and the United States—free-market capitalism constrained by ad hoc managed capitalism and burdened with social-market capitalism—has yielded similar economic results: large deficits and high national debt. Burdened by social costs, and faced with a decline in manufacturing and stalled advances in knowledge industries, both economies have grown uncompetitive with China. As of May 2012, the voters in the United Kingdom, unlike those in the United States, seem to have accepted the near-term pain of cuts in a turnaround economy, and have elected a conservative government to undertake the surgery.

Singapore's Mixture of Managed and Laissez-Faire Capitalism

Singapore has committed itself to a unique mix of managed and laissez-faire capitalism.[5] Since the 1970s, the country has guided the growth of pillar industries, nurturing oil refining, chemicals, electronics manufacturing, and biotechnology. To attract foreign direct investment, it has invested in modern infrastructure and rigorous, globally competitive school systems. It also offers a low

17 percent corporate tax rate. Its approach allows it both to build a native manufacturing sector and to attract many global companies, including Philips, Shell, and Intel.

Singapore has traded off the social support of social-market capitalism for growth under both laissez-faire and managed capitalism. The country has no minimum wage, offers no unemployment insurance, and requires all citizens to pay for their own retirement, healthcare, and education. To ensure that people have the money they need, it requires that everyone save 20 percent of his earnings, matched by up to 16 percent by employers. All savings go into accounts that are invested in government bonds, providing a pool of money that civil servants can use to fund the works of managed capitalism at low interest rates.

The country essentially relies on dovetailing its two kinds of capitalism. Charitable giving and social support are both minimal compared to other developed countries. Singapore's approach, understandably not the product of a democratic regime, gives it a huge advantage in winning foreign investment. Companies are drawn to the country's free-trade policies, educated workforce, top-tier infrastructure, favorable tax rates, efficient civil service, and business-friendly regulatory regime. Singapore is rated number one, ahead of the United States (number four), in the World Bank's ease-of-doing-business ranking.[6]

Singapore shows how laissez-faire and managed capitalism can complement each other, but it also shows how much execution matters. The record of managed capitalism has proved to be mixed. The electronics sector, launched in the 1980s and 1990s, became unsustainable as Chinese manufacturing ramped up. One factor that probably hurts Singapore is that the government spends little on R&D, preferring to tap multinationals for their know-how and technology. The lack of homegrown research weakens innovation and entrepreneurship. As China hollows out even more Singaporean factory employment, Singapore will need to modify its strategy if it is to succeed, as one of seven jobs in Singapore is in the declining manufacturing sector.

Japan's Mixture of Managed Capitalism and a Touch of Social-Market Capitalism

Japan has leaned heavily on managed capitalism, using industrial policy to strengthen and protect a string of industries, starting with heavy and chemical industries in the 1960s and autos and electronics in the 1970s.[7] The country chose favored companies to lead each industry, urging mergers to achieve economies of scale. It also pressured or cajoled companies into dividing up product markets to limit competition and avoid duplication. Though frowned on by technocrats, some companies—in particular, Honda and Sony—flouted the wishes of government planners and engaged in free-market competition.

In choosing mainly managed capitalism, Japan traded off the potential for innovation under laissez-faire policies for a coordinated effort to create jobs and wealth that would raise all Japanese people into the middle class. Though many Japanese view laissez-faire principles favorably, to this day the government pursues managed capitalism with a heavy hand, choosing target industries and supporting their growth.

Early on, Japan emphasized wealth redistribution and social-market capitalism because World War II had left many Japanese impoverished. In the 1960s and 1970s, Japan created a social safety net that includes unemployment benefits, national health insurance, a national pension benefit, and a low-income benefit. However, the country did not spend lavishly on such programs. Instead, it focused on creating as close to 100 percent employment as possible by rebuilding its large and established pre–World War II businesses.

Japan had a well-functioning managed capitalist system by the 1980s. Helped by banks that supplied low-cost capital from Japanese savers, the country gained a clear competitive advantage in some industries, as mentioned in the previous chapter. The ministry that guided the economy appeared to be on track to help manufacturers trounce their U.S. competitors—and it would have gotten much farther along that path had it not been for a U.S.

political backlash that forced Japan to back off. Japan then agreed to export quotas and ended up building plants in the United States and cutting deals to open up its markets to U.S. goods.

Japan then stalled, as outlined in Chapter 1. Its banks lent corporations too much money at below-market interest rates. This lending created too much capacity, inflated real estate prices, and triggered a stock market collapse. The country has not recovered in the ensuing years, as Japan's managed capitalism has failed in several industries. What seemed like economic omnipotence turned into economic incompetence. And the government's resistance to writing off bad loans and liquidating poorly performing firms contributed to long-term malaise. But that's only part of the story. Japan also didn't adapt as well as it could have. Its planners didn't change to unlock the dynamism of free enterprise, preferring instead to support the traditional, slow-moving *zaibatsu* and *keiretsu* industry structures.

Japanese planners today are targeting new industries in which to create new global competitors. The industries include those making products for the environment, renewable energy, and healthcare for the elderly. Japan continues to offer subsidies, tax benefits, and support for industrial groups. The country also spends more on R&D as a percentage of GDP than any other nation. Will the renewed commitment to a fresh set of industries pay off? The answer is not yet clear.

Given current evidence, Japan may be making the wrong trade-offs. In an effort to dominate new markets and create large, stable target industries that generate full employment, it continues to trade away the free-market incentives of laissez-faire capitalism for the benefits of managed capitalism. It also persists with a measure of protectionism, with a weighted-average tariff of 4.9 percent, the thirteenth highest among developed nations.[8] Many other trade barriers are informal, such as complicated distribution channels, exclusive business relationships, legal barriers to market entry, and informal restrictions of foreign direct investment.

Japan was good at managed capitalism, but it faces a challenge for the future. One of the reasons appears to be execution. The biggest barrier: ministries have conflicting goals and don't coordinate. Technocrats in the trade ministry would like to lower the corporate income tax to attract corporate headquarters, as the Singaporeans do. (The rate in Tokyo is 40.69 percent, whereas that in Singapore is 17 percent.) But the finance ministry has control of taxes, and no entity coordinates policies across government. This, in turn, hinders Japan's ability to compete with better-coordinated competitors like China.

Germany's Mixture of All Four Capitalisms

Germany manages its economy with a relatively even mix of the four generic capitalisms.[9] It has shaken up its mix in recent years in order to stay competitive. Though many Americans hold up Germany as an example of going too far with both social-market and managed capitalism, Germany has changed this. It has crafted a strategy that draws on the strengths of each generic type of capitalism. While most Western countries grew weakly coming out of the 2008 financial panic, Germany grew 3.6 percent in 2010.[10] By 2011, unemployment had fallen to 5.5 percent.

Germany uses some managed capitalism that both supports basic R&D and channels money directly to industries of the future. In the mid-2000s, it launched an official "High-Tech Strategy." It renewed that strategy in 2010. This strategy includes a slate of programs that speed up investment in energy, health, transportation, security, and communication technologies.[11] It has a specific aim: to remain a leader in high-skill, high-value manufacturing, enabled by a well-paid high-end workforce. Essentially, the Germans want to sell premium and niche products that are available nowhere else in the world.

In one program, Germany funds high-tech start-ups for two years. Companies can use the money for R&D and for taking products through to prototype or even market entry. The program started with €272 million.[12] Another program gives grants twice yearly to companies with under 250 employees. The money speeds growth in six fields of R&D that are deemed critical: biotechnology, nanotechnology, information and communication technology, manufacturing technology, energy, and optical technology.[13] The country aims to launch its businesses into "lead markets" by getting science and industry to work closely together.

The core of the German economy is the *Mittelstand,* or the numerous medium-size, family-run German businesses. Among the ways in which Germany supports this core is a rigorous education system that requires long stints in vocational school. Apprenticeships in 342 trades create a highly skilled workforce. Heavy investments in infrastructure provide excellent roads, railways, and other services. The German government, using tax benefits, transfer payments, and subsidies, steers investment to emerging *Mittelstand* industries. One example of the latter is feed-in tariffs that transfer money from old industries to new ones. A tariff paid by consumers who use fossil fuels goes straight to renewable-energy firms. All firms in the industry get their share. The more successful they are, the more they get.

Along with a devotion to managed capitalism, Germany remains dedicated to offering a full slate of unemployment, health, and pension benefits. For many years, it traded off the work incentives of laissez-faire capitalism for the safety net of social-market capitalism—and up to a decade ago, it earned criticism for its largesse and its disincentives to work. That approach was reflected in the country's economic results. In the early 2000s, growth slowed to just 1.0 percent, and unemployment hit 11.4 percent. The country's treasury labored to fund as many as 180 social programs.[14] Germany was limping, and critics called it "the sick man of Europe."

But the criticism dissipated when, unlike most developed countries, Germany rapidly got back on its feet after the recent downturn. That's because in the early 2000s the country's conservatives, fearing the worst during the slump of that era, slashed unemployment benefits, raised the retirement age (from 65 to 67), and upped healthcare copayments. The unemployment reforms were most drastic. They cut benefits to 12 months from 36 or more. They curtailed benefits if people didn't take a job that was offered to them. And for those who stayed on the dole for the long term, they required means testing, in which the jobless had to prove that they deserved benefits.

Stated simply, in just a few years, Germany remixed its capitalisms, reducing the emphasis on social-market capitalism. The economic picture then brightened. By 2007, GDP growth hit 4.4 percent, and unemployment fell to 8.2 percent. Poverty rates rose, to be sure. So did street protests across Germany. And the country couldn't shield itself from the recent downturn. Its growth tanked along with that of Sweden, the United Kingdom, the United States, France, and everyone else that was stung by the panic. GDP fell 3.5 percent in 2009. But by 2010, Germany was up and running again, rivaled in Europe only by Sweden, which had undertaken its own reforms in the 1990s.

Germany today has found a way for each form of capitalism to complement the others. The elements of managed capitalism provide for healthy industry through training, R&D funding, and a strategy to spur private initiative in future industries by offering tax benefits, transfer payments, and subsidies. The elements of laissez-faire capitalism, in which the government acts as coach rather than boss, allow plenty of room for private-sector growth. The *Mittelstand* is the bastion of laissez-faire capitalism in Germany. The social-market system redistributes wealth so that people have the cash to buy goods and enjoy a middle-class standard of living without draining the country's coffers. With that combination, Germany can win against China, with which it enjoys a trade surplus.

Assessing America's Mixture of the Four Capitalisms

So where does the United States stand? The United States has committed to a heavy focus on laissez-faire and social-market capitalism. America's mix of capitalisms resembles the United Kingdom's, but with one striking difference: the greater use of philanthropic capitalism. No other country has encouraged charitable donations that build institutions dedicated to science, medicine, education, and other knowledge as much as the United States has over the last two centuries.

An Underutilized Capitalist Tool—Philanthropic Capitalism

When Andrew Carnegie wrote *The Gospel of Wealth* in 1889, the steel tycoon argued against the notion that wealthy businesspeople should give their money away to their families. They should, he said, "administer it as a public trust during life."

Carnegie set the example, giving away more than $8.5 billion (in today's dollars), much of it for education. In one unprecedented move, he paid to build 2,500 public libraries in 1,400 U.S. communities. His philanthropy rapidly expanded a public institution that has formed the basis for a learned society in America. And he did this out of personal philosophy, not motivated by tax relief, as income taxes didn't exist until near the time of his death.

At about that time, the United States decided to increase its emphasis on philanthropy aimed at institutions and initiatives that support a humane, civil, and productive society. Since 1917, the deductions in the U.S. tax code have encouraged Americans to give away trillions of dollars, donating at a rate of roughly $300 billion each year. Today, roughly $12 billion of public and private funding for R&D is done in universities and colleges,[15] many of them built by philanthropy.

Out of U.S. institutions came many inventions. From Rutgers University came streptomycin (curing tuberculosis) in 1943. From Harvard University came the first program-controlled computer in 1944. From the University of Minnesota came the pacemaker in 1958. From Dartmouth College came the BASIC computer language. From the University of Pittsburgh came the combined PET/CAT scanner in 2000. These inventions, and countless others, all emerged from science labs and scientists who had been given a leg up by philanthropic capitalism.

To be sure, the funds coming from philanthropy remain small compared to federal and corporate dollars. But where does the government turn when it wants to do R&D? It turns to the endowed research institutions created by philanthropy. Philanthropic capitalism helps institutions ranging from schools to hospitals to research centers work at the earliest stages of inquiry and invention, stages of research that companies do not fund. It also supports a unique American strength, the endowment. Creative work funded by the storehouse of capital in U.S. endowments ranges from writing and filmmaking that feed Hollywood to biology and chemistry that feed the legal drug industry.

A Hidden Capitalist Tool—Managed Capitalism

The United States has generally forgone the benefits of long-term economic planning by downplaying managed capitalism. However, the United States has used some ad hoc managed capitalism as a result of erratic funding that comes from uncoordinated policy making and politics. Managed capitalism has led to many new products and industries based on the technologies spun off from R&D sponsored by NASA, DARPA, the NSF, and the NIH, among others. Agriculture, pharmaceuticals, utilities, banking, and the nuclear industry have all been protected and closely supervised or subsidized at one time or another. Many of America's managed industries have done well as a result of government funding, including the defense, agriculture, pharmaceutical, software, computer chip, and aerospace industries.

Despite the common belief, America already has an industrial policy. But this policy has stemmed from politics and historical events. The United States lacks any institution that can craft a coordinated, rational strategy. While the president and Congress are supposed to weigh trade-offs, find complementarities, and resolve the contradictions of managed capitalism, neither has. Both the executive and legislative branches suffer from dividing the tasks of managed capitalism among numerous legislative committees or executive departments. So coordination is nearly impossible.

An Expensive Capitalist Tool—Social-Market Capitalism

The United States' commitment to social-market capitalism in recent years shows that wealth transfers can put the nation at risk. Reviewing the federal budget, 58.6 percent goes to social programs, including social security, Medicare, Medicaid, low-income assistance, unemployment, health, low-income housing, and other social services. Only 23.3 percent of the budget is spent on the military and veterans' affairs. Gross interest on public debt is 12 percent. Investments in the economy and America's long-term competitive advantage are minimal: 9.1 percent for services such as workplace safety, education, law enforcement, transportation, and environmental protection—basic standards for the functioning of our economy. Technology has not been invested in. For example, space and science receive only 0.7 percent, energy only 0.4 percent, and telecommunications only 0.3 percent. Meanwhile, trade and economic development receive only 0.3 percent of the budget.[16] In sum, while most people mistakenly think that military expenditures are draining the United States' coffers, the truth is that social programs have crowded out investments in the long-term economic health of the nation.

Expenditures on entitlements and wealth transfers are most responsible for the budget deficits over the last few years. These deficits have created such high debt levels that the U.S. government risks defaulting on its loans. As public debt keeps growing, U.S. credit ratings will fall, and interest payments will grow. The Congressional Budget Office predicts that by 2020, U.S. interest payments will reach about $1 trillion per year. Military expenses aside, interest payments on the national debt will then eat up most of the government's budget, leaving little for domestic programs, such as health, housing, education, environmental regulation, and research.

Another major part of social-market capitalism is government efforts to save jobs and stimulate consumption in order to artificially keep the economy going. Only history will tell whether the American Recovery and Reinvestment Act of 2009—a.k.a. the stimulus package—had an effect on the economy, either preventing the economy from spiraling further down or actually starting a growth spurt in the long run. But many debate the effectiveness of the act.

It is also important to keep in mind that we have not yet paid for the stimulus package. At the time of its passage, the cost was estimated at $787 billion, but the final bill is not yet known. In addition, this sum did not include other recovery costs or profits from bailing out banks and auto companies. Many people doubt whether the act did anything more than fix some short-term problems. Few of the expenditures created a long-term national competitive advantage. Even the infrastructure repair work did not create an advantage. It contributed to road-surface repair, but it did not do much to reduce traffic congestion in the cities, make transportation more efficient and speedy, or reduce the usage of fuel. In fact, the entire act did little to reform America's capitalist system in any significant way. By and large, the act just flooded more money through an already faltering system.

Even if the stimulus package saved the country from a possible depression in 2008, it diverted attention from the root causes of our capitalist system's weaknesses. It stimulated U.S. consumption with tax cuts, and it created economic recovery projects that kept police, teachers, and other public employees working. However, other than some investment in renewable energy projects, it mostly amounted to short-term expenditures rather than investments in the future. That is, the money is here today, gone tomorrow.

Just as unfortunate, stimulating consumption perpetuated a consumption mentality that promises to hurt our economic power for years. As politicians spur people to consume more at lower prices, they seek cheap imports made in countries that threaten U.S. jobs. In other words, government stimulus leads to more consumption, leading to more imports and more jobs lost. This, in turn, leads to more debt, and the debt creates another threat, namely, raising borrowing charges—which are just more money poured on the debt fire, which only gets bigger.

Overall, the stimulus efforts increased the national debt from $10.6 trillion when President Obama took office to $15.3 trillion by February 15, 2012, an increase of approximately $4.7 trillion in less than three years in office. (This compares with the increase of $4.9 trillion during President George W. Bush's eight years in office.) The current national debt means that every man, woman, and child alive in America today owes $50,540. And there is no plan for how we will pay this back.

An Overestimated Capitalist Tool—Laissez-Faire Capitalism

Most people attributed the boom years during the Reagan and Clinton administrations to laissez-faire capitalism. However, this conclusion may be based on faulty reasoning. Cause and effect may be confused because of the timing of policy actions and policy outcomes. The boom years could have stemmed from the heyday of government R&D in electronics 10 and 20 years before. All of the boom industries of the 1980s—cell phones, computer chips, microcomputers, operating systems, and graphical user interfaces—stemmed from government-supported research done years earlier.

The same goes for the 1990s' boom, which included growth from the Internet, web backbones, fiber optics, portals, browsers, e-commerce, and Internet applications and software. Again, these industries got massive R&D support in their early days 20 years before, and came to fruition in the 1990s. One could conclude that the much-maligned policies of "government intervention" and "industrial policy" caused the booms. Laissez-faire capitalism, meanwhile, freed the business community to commercialize these technologies as they became ripe. A mix of "government-managed" and laissez-faire capitalism could have been the magic elixir in this case—along with a foundation of research infrastructure created through centuries of philanthropic capitalism that built the endowments of major research institutions. So perhaps U.S. managed capitalism may be a much more important reason for these booms than laissez-faire radicals would have us believe.

We may also be confused because times have changed. Theories that assumed creation of the wealth of a nation are, in practice, now creating wealth for just a few or even for other nations. Laissez-faire capitalism suggests that individual greed magically turns out to be good for the nation. The markets will create wealth for all by creating jobs. Thus, many people argue that if the corporations are profitable, workers do well. In February 2012, the stock market was flirting with a Dow Jones Industrial Average of 13,000. Yet unemployment was still more than 8 percent, and this number would be much higher (some analysts say even double) if the figure included all the people who have given up looking for jobs and those who are underemployed.

How can there be such a disconnect between the Dow Jones average and the economy? Probably the most important answer is that corporations have benefited by operating and selling overseas, while American workers have not fared as well. During the period of globalization, American workers have not benefited as companies have grown more efficient through outsourcing and offshoring. Consider the following fact: 90 percent of American workers have had stagnant wages for the last 20 years. Thus, people who are dependent on their jobs for most of their wealth have lost more than they have gained.

Often we ignore the failures of laissez-faire capitalism. Consider the massive failure of trying to transport laissez-faire capitalism to Russia in the early 1990s, where the nation's lack of religion made it difficult for so-called capitalists to differentiate between business and criminal activity.

Consider also the deregulation of the financial industry in the United States. Banks were allowed to compete freely, and what happened? The industry took on too much risk by maximizing its profits with risky subprime loans and derivatives. The banks nearly collapsed the country's entire economy. Over the last decade, free markets have led to three bubbles created by overexuberance: the Internet bubble, the real estate bubble, and the credit crisis. While some people dismiss these as "mere corrections," it is hard to explain why corrections are occurring so frequently in the last decade. And it is even harder to explain how free and efficient markets could have misvalued Internet, real estate, and banking assets by such wide margins.

Often we just assume that laissez-faire capitalism leads to a better economy. But let's examine the recent relationship between economic prosperity and the Economic Freedom Index (based on 10 elements of economic freedom that make up laissez-faire capitalism).[17] During the first decade of the twenty-first century, countries stressing managed capitalism have generated high GDP growth and created large trade imbalances by exporting to the more social-market and laissez-faire capitalist countries. They have also amassed resources from these countries, including jobs, intellectual property, foreign investment, global trade, raw materials, and oil.

One of the reasons that managed capitalism is doing well is that economic freedom no longer appears to provide the single key that will unlock national prosperity. I examined this hypothesis by analyzing a sample of countries that included the G-20 plus two of the most economically free nations according to the Heritage Foundation's Economic Freedom Index.[18] I found that in the first decade of the 2000s, the economic freedom index and prosperity (GDP per capita),[19] as expected by laissez-faire thinking, are very significantly correlated: approximately 0.70 (out of a perfect 1.0). But if one controls for a nation's geographic advantages and resources, such as climate, natural disasters, seacoast advantages, arable land, metals, minerals, clean water, oil, natural gas, precious metals, forestry, and food, the correlation between economic freedom and prosperity almost disappears. These results suggest that economic freedom by itself is less associated with prosperity than we originally thought.[20] Though these data provide just a spot check of economic history, they provide a counterpoint to economists who believe that economic freedom always begets wealth.

I also examined economic freedom relative to growth (in GDP per capita) at three points during the early 2000s. The nations with the least economic freedom grew faster than the United States and Europe. By 2009, the relationship between economic growth and economic freedom showed a *negative* statistical correlation.

Again, these results cast doubt on the idea that laissez-faire thinking is the single miracle elixir for economic growth. To be sure, countries with managed capitalism do not offer economic freedom to spur growth. Yet managed capitalists appear to have initiated a major game changer that will yield significant prosperity in the future. In contrast, economic freedom seems to create growth only in small city-states like Hong Kong and Singapore.

The United States developed its mix of capitalisms over time to suit its needs at given moments: philanthropic capitalism to deal with the illegitimacy of the industrialists in the early 1900s, social-market capitalism to deal with the poor during the Depression, managed capitalism to deal with World War II, and laissez-faire capitalism to deal with the new capacity that was coming on line as nations recovered from World War II. This evolution worked to create a very prosperous nation. But today, America's mix doesn't produce growth or employment results superior to those from China's mixture of capitalisms.

From Muddled Mixture to Miracle

What this all adds up to is a simple fact: America's mixture of generic capitalisms is now a muddle. We spend too much on some of the capitalisms, and too little on others. We rely too heavily on capitalisms that worked in the past but are dysfunctional in the present. We ignore the emerging formulations of capitalism that are necessary for the future. Meanwhile, we rely too little on the capitalisms needed to compete with the Chinese capitalist system in the present.

To be absolutely clear, what I am saying is that the U.S. approach to capitalism—which is based on the accumulation of a lot of old policies that do not fit the current circumstances or help to win against China—is nonstrategic.

Why has this occurred? No one is steering the ship. No one is designing our capitalist system and managing our portfolio of industries. The U.S. government is not set up to do it, and many U.S. leaders are opposed to the idea. Many others lack the vision to create such a big-picture strategy. Even though it seems logical to build a national economic strategy, many politicians fear placing so much power in one place. More important, many of them fear giving up their power over their current fiefdoms. This is a threatening situation for the United States and other nonstrategic countries that are facing China, which has perhaps the sharpest strategists since the ancient Romans.

While the United States has been averse to excessive managed capitalism, the crisis of the present opens a big opportunity to choose a fresh path to the future. Like the founding fathers, leaders today have the chance to reinvent our system of capitalism. Companies need the help of the U.S. government, and the American system of capitalism must include more managed capitalism. Germany, Sweden, South Korea, and China all practice different mixes of capitalism that include more managed capitalism than in the United States, and their recent economic performance has exceeded that of the United States in several ways.

We can decide to choose a new mix of capitalisms that will create an economic miracle for the United States and its people. We can take the best of each country's systems, resolve inconsistencies among the different capitalisms where we find them, execute our strategies with freer markets, create a nonpolitical national strategy-making process, and make something better. But we need a commitment to adopt a capitalist strategy—to becoming strategic capitalists.

As Yogi Berra once said: "If you don't know where you are going, you might wind up someplace else." Economists have long argued that the invisible hand of the market would direct us to where we should be going. We didn't have to know how to get there ourselves, and we didn't have to fear ending up "someplace else." That thinking was perfect for the era of incompetent managed capitalists. But today we face hypercompetition from very smart strategists. Our leaders will have to step up their game, paint a vision, and execute that vision to transcend the politics of division that is keeping the country from developing a unified strategy to rebuild a powerful new capitalist system for the future.

3

Controlling Capitalist Systems

At Home and Abroad

When Zhang Huamei filed for a business license in 1979, the 19-year-old became the first official capitalist in China.[1] A native of Wenzhou, China, she sold buttons and watch straps from a table in front of her home. Ms. Zhang had actually set up shop 18 months earlier. Now she had been issued a certificate to carry on legally. She went on years later to earn praise from the Chinese Communist Party. In 2005, she was celebrated in Beijing.

When Ms. Zhang first got going, the going was tough, even though her father encouraged her. "At that time, working for yourself was very shameful," she said in an interview later.[2] "My classmates were ashamed of me for starting my own business. They would turn their heads away when passing my house and pretend not to know me."[3] Mao Zedong's Cultural Revolution had ended just a few years earlier, and people continued to view capitalists as profiteers, quick-buck swindlers, and illicit speculators who were taking advantage of unsuspecting or unknowledgeable people. For years, the state had controlled all capitalist behavior.

But Zhang got started in business at an auspicious time. In 1978, two years after the death of Mao, Deng Xiaoping emerged, launching the "Reform and Opening" economic program and reversing the anticapitalist thinking that Mao had railed against during a 10-year purge. Out went slavish compliance with central planning. In came a reliance on market forces. Out went communes and in came townships. Out went tightly controlled state commerce, and in came more autonomous state-owned companies. Out went lifetime bureaucratic sinecures and lifetime employment, and in came jobs in which people were rewarded and promoted for productivity.

And out went contempt for businesspeople like Ms. Zhang, and in came official encouragement. In southern China, the government even set up special economic zones. In Shenzhen, the vibrancy of free-market capitalism came to rival that in Hong Kong. China began to create a new form of managed capitalism. It combined quasi-free markets with strong government guidance. It applied industrial policy supported by trade protection. It solicited foreign investment and encouraged competition with and among foreign firms.

Thirty-five years later, Ms. Zhang had expanded beyond her streetside table. Selling buttons globally, she became one of China's 960,000 millionaires, according to the 2011 *Hurun Wealth Report*. (The report defines people as millionaires if their net wealth exceeds ¥10 million, roughly €1.1 million or U.S.$1.47 million.) Now featured in press interviews, she represents the millions of people who pushed the frontier of private wealth creation in China.

Thanks to Deng, China now has an enormous middle class, larger than the entire U.S. population. The China State Information Center estimates that the middle class makes up a quarter of the Chinese population (as of 2010), based on earnings of ¥50,000 ($6,227) per year. And its numbers are growing fast. While estimates vary, roughly half of China's projected urban population will be middle class in 2025, making the Chinese middle class twice the size of that in the United States. It looks as if one part of the

American Dream—middle-class prosperity—is arriving in China at meteoric speeds.

"From poverty to prosperity, we owe that to the guidance and support of the Reform and Opening Policy,"[4] Ms. Zhang said in a 2011 interview.

Indeed, she owes it to a form of managed capitalism that other countries are having increasing trouble beating. It features China as the world's manufacturing hub, a preferred destination for businesspeople relocating factories of all kinds. It features more than 700,000 foreign-invested companies (as of 2011). It includes an economy that has absorbed more than $1 trillion in foreign direct investment.[5] And it features a populace earning wealth that would have been unimaginable a decade ago. The country now has more billionaires than any other country in the world besides the United States.

Ms. Zhang's and her countrymen's gains, however, have often come at the expense of other countries. The net growth in American jobs during the first decade of the 2000s was close to zero.

China has given the West a comeuppance. The Chinese people can and should be proud of their country's economic success. Not only has China taken manufacturing business from the West, but it has shown that it can build up its own manufacturing business faster than any other country. In 2007, it ran up against a shortage and soaring prices of polycrystalline silicon, the main material for solar panels. Foreign companies dominated production. A Chinese entrepreneur spent just 15 months raising $1 billion in capital and building a plant to supply roughly one-quarter of global production.[6] China went from a polycrystalline-silicon nobody to a giant in the blink of an industry's eye.

State Control of Chinese Business Enterprises

The gains in China stem from a simple fact: it has learned to operate as an expert managed capitalist. Part of those gains stems from harnessing market forces by private parties like Ms. Zhang. China has done much not only to encourage start-ups but also to privatize state firms, and with good reason: the productivity of private firms is double that of state-run firms.[7] Because of the growth of market-run firms, the private sector now makes up 50 percent of the economy. Free-market Westerners applaud this change.

But the private gains make up only half of the story, and the less revealing half. Central to China's success in implementing managed capitalism is its command and control of its other businesses, fully or partly state-owned enterprises, or SOEs. The Communist leaders in Beijing no longer set all budgets, control supply and demand, and micromanage every enterprise. But they and their subordinates do intervene at all levels. In other words, the state controls the vital organs of wealth creation, even if those organs harness once-heretical market forces to boost productivity, profits, and growth.

SOEs, in which the government owns all or the vast majority of the shares, produce 40 percent of China's GDP. Another 10 percent of GDP comes from firms in which the government holds a less-than-majority ownership. Together, there are 20,000 of these companies in all industries, a formidable force that is under the control of the Communist Party of China.[8] When Communist leaders express a new economic vision for the country—as they have recently in the twelfth Five-Year Plan—they have a massive organizational apparatus to put it into reality.

We can infer that one reason for China's ongoing success is cultural. The country's leaders have taken advantage of historical traditions of cooperation and technocratic government. Since the days of Confucius, Chinese culture has stressed collective and coordinated actions by administrators promoted for their technocratic expertise. (Only Mao and colonial times interrupted these Confusian traditions.) Unlike cultural norms in many countries in the West, the norms in China dictate that coordinated projects take precedence over those that are individualistic and uncoordinated. The Chinese people have largely accepted coordinated economic policies as a national project, in spite of repression of a variety of freedoms.[9] The Chinese believe in taking the long view toward accomplishing something big together. Despite preaching about teamwork in the United States, Americans appear to be at a distinct disadvantage when progress requires nationwide coordination.

The Chinese have appeared to embrace the rough-and-tumble free-market world, where every firm struggles on a level playing field with other global companies. But the truth is that the Chinese government retains a tight grip even on publicly traded firms. Firms competing overseas with other multinationals do not operate independently. A number of firms raise capital in the United States, but they still take their marching orders from Beijing. Aluminum Corporation of China (Chalco) is 42 percent owned by the state; China Petroleum and Chemical Corporation (Sinopec), 76 percent; and China Telecom, 71 percent.[10] China owns a controlling share in 70 percent of all listed Chinese firms,[11] and it uses that control to the state's advantage.

Although China insists on the inclusion of capitalist principles in SOE goals—a demand for profits, for example—these principles often take second place to state goals. The SOEs get plenty in return. China readily gives out favorable tax breaks, trade protection, and administrative support. Overseas, it helps them through export credits, soft loans, foreign aid, and diplomatic support. Even military assistance and training remain available for China's elite SOEs. Instead of letting foreign giants savage domestic companies, China's leaders have made sure that they have given Chinese firms everything that they need to do the reverse.

Chinese leaders use their SOEs to build the country's position in nationally important industries. So-called strategic industries include defense, electric power and the grid, petroleum and petrochemicals, telecommunications, coal, civil aviation, and shipping. The state mandates that it will retain absolute control of these industries. SOEs still dominate the so-called pillar industries including equipment manufacturing, autos, information technology, construction, iron and steel, nonferrous metals, chemicals, and surveying and design, even though China permits foreign competition. The pillar industries employ a lot of people and support infrastructure development. The state mandates that it will retain strong control over each of these industries.[12]

Chinese leaders, who directly control 120 SOEs from Beijing,[13] are also aiming to create an elite corps of "national champions," large, vertically integrated business groups serving entire industries. The current Five-Year Plan singles out for national champions companies in the auto, steel, cement, machinery, aluminum, rare earth, pharmaceutical, electronic information, shipbuilding, petrochemical, and textile industries.[14] According to *The Economist,* the government has decided that 30 to 50 of its best SOEs will be converted into "globally competitive multinationals."[15]

Provincial and city governments control many businesses as well. And over the last couple of years it has been official government policy to reduce the influence of the private sector while favoring improvement of the efficiency of the government-owned enterprises.

To ensure that the SOEs serve the state, Chinese leaders operate the levers of power at every level. Government-controlled central or regional investment funds, or holding companies, are staffed with government officials who guide the SOEs' investments and operations. In addition to controlling SOE shares, these funds can also choose and approve all top management personnel. For the 50 biggest SOEs, the Communist Party appoints people to at least the top three positions. The State-Owned Assets Supervision and Administration Commission (SASAC), the agency that acts as a holding company for central SOEs, appoints people to other top jobs as well.[16] A network of other state-controlled entities, including 300 provincial and municipal SASACs, controls job appointments at many other state-owned entities.

The SASAC may sound like a big Western investment fund, where managers aim for top returns for shareholders. However, it is part of the State Council, China's chief administrative organ. It has the authority to manage SOEs using "supervisory panels" for each SOE. Although not all SOEs sell shares to the public, when they do, they place those shares not on Wall Street or in London, but in Hong Kong. As a result, SOEs typically have a dual corporate structure. The main part of the enterprise remains legally controlled by the state, while a division may be more or less privatized via joint ventures or initial public offerings.

Chinese officials do not hide the fact that SOEs, even if they obtain capital from foreign investors, operate at the behest of the state. In the United States, SOEs must file Form 20-F annually. In the 20-F of China Southern Airlines, the following statement appears: "The Company is indirectly majority owned by the Chinese government, which may exert influence in a manner that may conflict with the interests of holders of ADRs, H Shares and A Shares."[17] The inference investors can draw is this: even if it would save the company money to buy planes from Boeing or Airbus, it may well buy them from the China Commercial Aircraft Company (COMAC), an SOE founded in 2008. China's commitment to fulfilling the state's goal of developing a domestic aircraft company comes first.

The state further gives SOEs and associated firms an advantage by controlling their purse. It provides financial support for exports (e.g., export credits and soft loans to foreign buyers of Chinese goods and services) through the Export-Import Bank of China (Exim Bank), the world's third largest export credit agency. In the same way, the government-owned China Construction Bank can provide money to control China's SOEs in the mining and infrastructure development industries. Diplomacy, sales and gifts of military equipment, training, and foreign aid are also used to secure business deals.

For these reasons and more, the 2011 report by the U.S.-China Economic and Security Review Commission concluded the following: "When it joined the WTO in 2001, China promised that the government would not influence, directly or indirectly, the commercial decisions of SOEs. China does not appear to be keeping this commitment. . . . If anything, China is doubling down and giving SOEs a more prominent role in achieving the state's most important economic goals."[18] China has figured out how to exercise enough control through a national decision-making hierarchy that it can formulate and execute its form of capitalism like no other country can.

State Coordination of the Overall Capitalist System

Along with its array of control structures, the Chinese Communist Party (CCP) has managed to coordinate government policies across its ministries to put the nation and its business enterprises squarely behind the goals and methods of the CCP. Though the regime remains notorious for corruption and infighting, it nonetheless ends up appearing to have a level of coordination that is not currently possible in most democracies. (See Figure 3-1.) This coordination helps China amplify, if not multiply, its competitive power to outperform the United States and other Western countries.

Jiang Zemin, Hu Jintao, and other Chinese leaders who built on Deng Xiaoping's legacy have aligned new commercial, economic, and social policies to a remarkable extent. China has a grip on both strategy and execution in ways that other countries seem unable to match. Whether this comes from the command-and-control structure or a shared desire to advance China's economic power is hard to say.

State Coordination of Trade and Commercial Policies

China's trade policy puts the United States in a particular bind. In a sense, the policy allows China to play one game while the United States is playing another. The United States uses a globalist perspective that features trade without borders, international cooperation, and a balance of power between blocs (i.e., the West versus the Communist world). It also features international rules of transparency, corporate autonomy, free trade, open markets, property

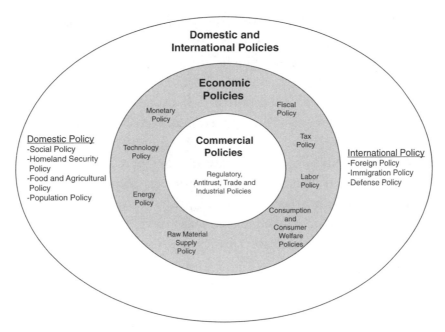

FIGURE 3.1 China Uses All Its Tools for Setting New Rules of Capitalism

rights, and the primacy of human rights for all people. This is a game of peaceful coexistence that includes not just trade but cultural exchange.

In contrast, China practices economic nationalism. Its leaders promote domestic firms, workers, and even the sustained power of the Chinese Communist Party at the expense of other countries and companies. It seeks to promote the unity, power, identity, and autonomy of the nation. It manipulates the rules of markets and trade to achieve the state's goals. The legal rights of foreigners are of secondary importance.

China's policies are incompatible with laissez-faire rules of competition. One of the clearest examples: Chinese banks pursue the interests of the nation, not the markets. Bankers don't maximize profits because they aim first to help the state build the economy, especially domestic manufacturing and exporting. The state-owned banks give SOEs three benefits that most companies cannot get:

ready loans even when an enterprise may not be creditworthy; debt forgiveness, in the form of writing off or perpetually rolling over loan principal; and access to loans at favorable rates.[19]

The 2011 report by the U.S.-China Economic and Security Review Commission noted that in 2010, China's prime lending rate was 5.36 percent. At the time, Sinopec received an average short-term interest rate of 2.7 percent, China Southern Airlines reported a maximum interest rate of 1.97 percent, and China Telecom received rates as low as 3.5 percent.[20] Since China Telecom's short-term borrowings totaled ¥20.7 billion ($3.1 billion)[21] during the period, it can be inferred that it saved up to $59 million in capital costs during 2010. This is the equivalent of 2.5 percent of net income.

Economic nationalism dictates that China bar free trade wherever it conflicts with its national mission. One example is China's treatment of Internet commerce. The most obvious example is the censoring of search-engine Internet traffic, which triggered Google's departure. More recently, the U.S. Trade Representative started an official inquiry under WTO rules in October 2011 to see, among other things, why China blocks foreign company websites in China. The sites blocked included those of firms seeking to provide customer service.[22]

Control of even minor rules by an economic nationalist can stymie foreign businesses' ability to function. A simple example: consider exports of steel, aluminum, soda ash, and other materials. China can manage trade volume by raising and lowering the VAT rebate upon export.[23] The opaqueness and complexity of the Chinese tax and regulatory processes related to this and other rules complicate planning and hinder profit making by foreign firms. Under pressure from other nations, China has ended many unfair practices, but it has miles to go to comply with the free-trade rules honored by firms in the West.

Because China takes so many actions that are driven by economic nationalism, the Chinese government controls the destiny of foreign corporations. As one Fortune 500 CEO doing business in

China told me under promises of anonymity, "No matter what percentage of our Chinese subsidiary we own, the Chinese government still knows everything about how our products are made and about how we manage our company. The government sets strict regulations and rules for us. For all intents and purposes, the government runs our subsidiary through directives. Our Chinese employees are beholden to this ruthless government. The government can close us down suddenly or it can help native Chinese firms to steal our technology and gradually replace us in the market. I don't know if there is any pot at the end of this rainbow, but we are forced by Wall Street's growth expectations to take the risk. It's quite scary. I hope it doesn't blow up in our face."[24]

State Coordination of Economic and Intellectual Property Policies

Chinese leaders support their robust form of managed capitalism with a slate of economic and intellectual property policies as well. Among them, several stand out as giving China an advantage that Western economies cannot match. The first is labor policy. China condones working conditions, factory safety rules, wage levels, and labor practices that are far below Western standards. It prohibits unions and collective bargaining. It holds down wages and suppresses unrest. It harasses and arrests strike leaders, suppresses protests with force, and bans the media from covering strikes. The net result is that China can produce labor-intensive goods at prices well below those in Western factories.

So long as China can continue to control labor unrest, it retains a strong advantage over other developed countries. The South Asia Analysis Group (SAAG) estimates that at least one strike of 1,000 workers erupts every day in the Pearl River Delta alone.[25] Strikes happen so often that a website outside China—chinastrikes .crowdmap.com—tracks the activity,[26] revealing a steady drumbeat of labor unrest across the country. Even so, strikes have not led to radical change to date. They appear to be mere drops rippling the surface of an otherwise calm ocean of economic activity.

Some observers suggest that the Chinese government may use strikes as a means of bolstering support for local Chinese firms. Inside the country, Chinese media do report on strikes at foreign companies—at plants owned by Japan's Toyota and Honda, the United States' Flextronics, and Taiwan's Foxconn, a unit of Hon Hai Precision Industry. This coverage stirs local people's discontent with foreign firms. Violence by authorities against striking Chinese workers fuels anger not against the government, but against company management, and, in turn, triggers boycotts against Japanese and Western goods. It may also galvanize general strikes by students, workers, and merchants in favor of the Communist regime.[27]

A second key standout policy that gives China an advantage is its coordinated energy policy. Unlike the United States, China has a comprehensive policy to provide manufacturers with cheap energy. According to reports by the U.S. Department of State, China's demand for energy is surging. China already consumes more energy than any other nation, and it also mines more coal than any other nation to satisfy its appetite for energy. Overall, it is the world's third largest net importer of crude oil and the second largest energy producer. Coal continues to top the list of Chinese fuels at 70 percent.[28]

China's growth plans require building more than $2 trillion in energy infrastructure to meet electricity demand by 2030. To meet this demand, China builds a new coal-fired plant every few days. The U.S. Department of State estimates that China will boost the share of electricity generated by nuclear power to 5 percent by 2020. Although there was a pause after the Fukushima Daiichi nuclear power plant disaster in Japan, China will presumably return to its pace of building one nuclear power plant every month.

China also leads the world in clean-energy development. It has plans for abundant hydroelectric production. The Three Gorges Dam is the world's largest hydroelectric dam, generating eight times the power of the United States' Hoover Dam. The country leads all countries but the United States in clean-energy investment, spending $47 billion in 2010, compared to the United States'

$56 billion.[29] During the next five years, China will spend more than $450 billion.[30] It now leads the world in installed hydropower capacity, with 213 gigawatts at the end of 2010. Solar, wind, and hydropower produced more than 250 gigawatts.[31]

China's push into renewables looks ready to speed up. Its 2011 renewable energy law requires that nonfossil fuels make up 15 percent of its energy sources by 2020. Chinese subsidies for clean-energy firms, forgiveness of company debts, and government purchases of clean-energy equipment from domestic firms are creating economies of scale that are putting Western clean-energy firms out of business.

China's current Five-Year Plan calls for greater energy conservation and efficiency, development of renewable-energy sources, greater use of nonfossil fuels, and increased attention to environmental protection. The government wants to move away from coal toward cleaner energy sources, including oil, natural and shale gas, renewable energy, and nuclear power.[32] In sum, China is preparing for its future, trying to build energy supplies and infrastructure to prevent any slowdown or stoppage in its industrial growth.

The third policy that stands out in giving China an advantage is its innovation and intellectual property policy. Implicit in this policy is the goal of reducing the cost and time of product development by copying proprietary foreign products. The most widely reported example in the last decade relates to automobiles. In June 2003, General Motors Corporation accused automaker Chery Automobile Company Ltd. of "design duplication" based on stolen trade secrets. GM filed suit in a Shanghai court during 2004. Chery, a Chinese state-owned enterprise founded in 1997, was accused of copying the Chevy Spark with its Chery QQ. The Chevy Spark was originally designed and sold by GM Korea as an affordable minicar and had been sold under the Daewoo Matiz brand since 1998.

Not only were the Chevy and Chery brand names strikingly similar, but GM claimed that the Chery QQ had the same snubby nose, bug-eyed headlights, and rounded high back. In addition, most components in the QQ could be easily interchanged with parts on the Spark. According to GM China Group, the two cars "shared remarkably identical body structure, exterior design, interior design and key components." Rob Leggat, vice president for corporate affairs at GM Daewoo (now GM Korea), said, "The cars are more than similar. It really approaches being an exact copy."[33] To make matters worse for GM's future sales, Chery released its version of the Chevy Spark six months earlier than GM did because of administrative delays imposed on GM China.

The Chinese government mounted a vigorous defense of Chery. One of the vice directors of the Chinese State Intellectual Property Office said that GM did not have a patent on its designs in China and thus the design was not protected according to Chinese law.[34] GM settled the suit in 2005. The terms were never released, but GM promised not to sue Chery again. Today the Chery QQ is the leading minicar in China, holding almost a 20 percent market share in the crowded Chinese minicar segment and outselling the Chevy Spark four to one. The Chery QQ has become a legend in the history of Chinese automobiles, with the highest cumulative unit sales of any car ever sold in China (800,000 within the first seven years).

The story is old, but the copycat practice persists. The Chinese imitation policy seems to have a simple implication for China outsiders: no matter what a company believes it "owns" in China, it has no proprietary right to its property. Once it signs off on doing business in China, the owner of a company's product designs is the Chinese government. In 2010, Jeffrey Immelt, CEO of General Electric, broke the silence of many CEOs when he spoke, in Rome, referring to China's protectionist actions, "I really worry about China. I am not sure that in the end they want any of us to win, or any of us to be successful."[35]

China's stated strategy is "enhancing original innovation through co-innovation and re-innovation."[36] That language translates into practices that in the West would be more commonly called theft. In the mid-2000s, China sought to develop a high-speed train system.

It solicited bids to make 200 trains, and four companies responded: Alstom of France, Siemens of Germany, Bombardier of Canada, and a Japanese consortium led by Kawasaki Heavy Industries. All four companies won a share of the business. Kawasaki got part of the job with joint-venture partner CSR Sifang Locomotive of Qingdao, China, to produce 480 train cars, some imported from Japan, some assembled in Qingdao, and some made in Qingdao.[37]

The joint venture delivered the train cars as promised. Kawasaki even took dozens of Chinese engineers to Japan for training. After the joint venture ended, however, the Japanese technology did not remain in Japanese hands. China began producing trains that looked and worked exactly like those from the Kawasaki group. China essentially appropriated its partner's technology. A Chinese official noted that Chinese engineers had "digested" the technology, and that the new Chinese trains had nothing at all to do with its former partner. The other suppliers on the original contract similarly lost control of their technology to the Chinese.

Although China has supposedly strengthened its intellectual property rights laws to comply with World Trade Organization rules, it remains a haven for knockoffs and clones. This is implicitly encouraged by China's Five-Year Plan, which mandates an import substitution policy. Chinese components are to replace foreign parts in all "core infrastructure." Specific components include integrated circuits, operating software, switches and routers, database management, and encryption systems used in industries like banking and telecommunications.[38]

According to a U.S. International Trade Commission study released in 2011, Chinese piracy and counterfeiting of intellectual property cost American businesses an estimated $48 billion in sales in 2009. The commission concluded that 2.1 million jobs would be created in the United States if China complied with international obligations to protect and enforce intellectual property rights. Of the total losses, $26 billion came from the information and service sectors, and $18 billion from the high-tech and heavy-manufacturing sectors.[39]

In its Five-Year Plan, China proposes to turn itself into a technology giant by 2020 and a world leader by 2050. It targets 11 sectors: energy, water and mineral resources, environment, agriculture, manufacturing, transportation, information and services, population and health, urbanization, public security, and national defense. It also enumerates 68 priority areas for breakthroughs in several specific fields: biotechnology, information technology, advanced materials, advanced manufacturing, energy, lasers, and aerospace.[40]

In a shot across the bows of foreign companies, the Five-Year Plan proposes new measures to stymie outside firms that wish to sell to China or protect their technology. Among them are product testing and approval hurdles that delay product introductions in China, patent laws that help Chinese firms defeat patent suits with trumped-up countersuits, tightened government procurement rules that lock out foreign firms, and new industrial and technology standards that erect barriers to foreign technology.[41]

China seems to offer short-term temptation and long-term risk for foreign firms, as it entices multinationals with the promise of a few years of good profits in a big market—only to be followed by forced displacement from the ranks of high-growth Chinese companies by administrative or legal maneuvering by insider SOEs.

State Coordination of Domestic and Social Policies

Along with aligning trade, commercial, economic, and intellectual property policies to support managed capitalism, China aligns social and other domestic policies to serve national goals. Here again, the choices help private Chinese entrepreneurs and SOEs drive growth. In contrast to the United States, China provides little in the way of social programs for the poor and needy. This bare-bones approach keeps government expenditures down, freeing up money for R&D, subsidies to SOEs, and loans to foreign governments. It also provides an incentive for people to save and, in turn, build the national pool of money that firms can borrow at below-market rates. This policy gives second priority to consumers who want to spend and employees who want to build a nest egg, but it gives the Chinese Communist Party a huge financial lever to propel growth.

Note that China avoids the social problems inherent in the laissez-faire and social-market capitalisms prevalent in the United States. There is no demand for maximizing stockholder wealth at the expense of society and workers, as described in the previous chapter. For example, Chinese banks are free to inject money into projects to build the economy rather than fueling shareholder returns and gilding executive bonuses. In addition, China is not forced by democratic means to overallocate funds to the needy. China's approach calls on the indulgence of the population as the country's leaders build the economy for the long term.

China Remakes the Global Rules of Capitalism

In spite of any internal disagreements, China's leaders have arranged their affairs to beat Western versions of capitalism. They have established enough focus on economic nationalism to get businesses working with the same goals: creating a competitive advantage over other countries and disrupting the Western rules of capitalism. They have aligned their commercial policies to bolster the ability of businesses to generate growth for the nation. And they have pursued social policies that favor growth over social welfare. In other words, whether by vision or by collective will, they have created a robust form of managed capitalism.

Many say that China has a bubble-up process that sends ideas to its supreme leaders, who then select the tactics that fit the goals of the Chinese Communist Party. Still, the leaders of the party set a strong direction, and once the decision is made at the top, execution is a simple matter: get it done fast, and get it right. In one recent case, the Chinese government decided that it wanted to redirect melamine production—a plastic used in making melamine board, dishware, wrinkle-free clothing, wallpaper, furniture, and many other products—for use in the energy-efficient building materials industry and in the oil industry. The government directive was achieved in just three days. And all the other industries in China that needed that melamine had to adjust to the decreased supply by finding new materials, which took only a few weeks longer. There were no delays caused by contract or labor disputes, no spikes in prices, and no lobbying by other industries to try to stop the shift. No approvals from the EPA or other government agencies were necessary. China's government has the advantage of speed compared with the United States, where major decisions can be slowed or stopped by the need for regulatory approvals or by lawsuits.

The top leaders of China have shown that they have the minds of disciplined strategists. One can argue that the leaders of any smart developing nation would take exactly the same course if they were trying to beat the West in the game of global competition. They would remake their central bureaucracy into a strong coordinating structure, able to direct the nation's businesses as they adopted capitalist principles. They would align trade, commercial and intellectual property, and economic policies to bolster the ability of businesses to generate growth for the nation. And they would pursue social policies that favor long-term growth over current social welfare. In other words, they would put their effort into managed capitalism rather than into a democratic, laissez-faire system or a micromanaged centrally planned economy, such as the Soviet economy. They would build industries, not government welfare systems, a lesson learned from watching the Soviets do the opposite.

China's leaders have turned the tables on Western capitalists masterfully.

China's success with managed capitalism has lured the United States into a weak competitive position. As Chinese manufacturers move down the experience curve, Chinese goods become cheaper and cheaper. These cheap goods stimulate consumption in the United States. But their low prices, which stimulate enduring trade deficits, come at the cost of lost jobs in the United States. In turn, the United States loses the income tax revenue from jobless Americans, and an indebted federal government falls deeper into debt. As the cycle continues, the United States moves into an ever-weaker position, increasingly less able to make payments on its debt. Eventually, foreign nations might refuse to keep lending the United States money.

China, meanwhile, continues to relentlessly ratchet down the United States' high standard of living. To be sure, this could hurt China in the near term. Its people's rising standard of living depends on exporting to U.S. consumers. But in the long term, China can win because increasingly affluent Chinese consumers will grow in number to replace the increasingly impoverished shoppers in the West. Moreover, China can support higher wages because it is acquiring the intellectual property to compete in higher-value-added products.

China is not the first country to follow a strategy for global hegemony. It is moving in the same way that Britain did when it rose to become an empire. The way forward is simple: the nation that works itself into being the global hub of manufacturing becomes the center of the world economy. Other nations supply it and buy vast quantities from it. With its growing wealth and ambition, it becomes the main repository of the world's technological knowledge. It gains a headlock on both manufacturing and technological leadership, and it creates wealth like no other nation.

China's economic dominance will become reminiscent of that in the United States. It will consume most of the world's goods, energy, and raw materials. It will produce most of the world's sophisticated products. It will set the pace for most of the world's most advanced R&D and knowledge-based, high-value products. Crucially, in the next few years, China will reach the tipping point where its domestic market will be sufficiently developed that it will no longer be reliant on Western consumers. Think about it. What will China do when it no longer needs the United States? Remember, too, that China accounts for about a fifth of the world's population. It will take decades, probably centuries, before China's consumer market is saturated and the United States can absorb the economic impact of China's impact on American employment and dislocation.

Meanwhile, as China takes market share in many industries, the U.S. standard of living will sink. China could create a lot of growth in demand for products from foreign companies, but it has so far controlled access to its home market with a tight fist.

Some commentators will argue that China's rise should not be compared to the rise of the British Empire because, unlike Britain, it is not a real leader in manufacturing. But this is merely wishful thinking, as is the standard critique of China that its educational system and political culture will make it hard for it to innovate effectively. China has already shown that it is a fast follower. Its strategy with intellectual property and knowledge transfer means that it does not need to make such huge investments in R&D. China already forces the transfer of knowledge as a condition of entry into its domestic market. That coercive power will only increase as Chinese consumerism rises.

China has effectively disrupted the advantages and strategy of America's capitalist system. Its leaders are doing an impressive job of growing a strong nation and increasing the standard of living of their people. They act like coaches, boosters, and even players in the economic game. This contrasts with U.S. leaders today, many of whom argue that the government should be a spectator only. U.S. leaders have dragged their feet in telling their constituents that the nation faces a new reality. U.S. politicians have instead perpetuated visions of revival without real reform. They have allowed China to play the United States for a fool, often reinforcing mistaken beliefs about how the global economy works.

American economists have argued that trade is good for everyone. All nations will rise together. Although trade theoretically raises total world production, it does not guarantee everyone an equal share. Centuries of history demonstrate this point. Laissez-faire economists want governments to stand on the sidelines of the economic game, acting at most as unbiased referees. They argue that if

China rises as a result, its ascent does not amount to a U.S. defeat. They ignore facts like a 2011 analysis by the Economic Policy Institute. Although criticized in some circles for its assumptions during the research process, EPI estimates that the growing U.S. trade deficit with China cost the United States 2.8 million jobs, including 1.9 million manufacturing jobs, between 2001 and 2010.[42]

Other economists tell us that only firms compete, and firms from the United States can outperform all others. But the evidence is piling up that U.S. companies can outperform others only by moving plants and jobs offshore, gradually becoming foreign corporations.

Free-trade traditionalists argue that everyone is better off with this system. Each country benefits from trading with others because each can buy the best in the world from countries that have natural advantages that allow their firms to specialize based on those advantages. One nation doesn't sink as others rise. They all get a better deal. As the textbooks suggest, based on the trade theory of David Ricardo (1772–1823), Portugal has sunshine and should grow grapes and make wine. Britain has lots of rain and green pastures, so it should raise sheep. Britain should also turn the sheep's wool into textiles. According to Ricardo, the ideal world would have the Portuguese trading their good wine for British textiles. Everyone would have access to the cheapest and highest-quality goods in the world—and so everyone would end up better off.

But what happened in reality? Britain got rich, and Portugal declined as a great power. Britain got the better deal because, in the era in which Ricardo wrote this theory of trade, textiles were a high-value-added, high-wage, high-profit industry. Portuguese consumers may have marveled at the cheap bolts of cloth that flooded to their shores from England, but their wages as vintners didn't rise, while the fortunes of British manufacturers did. Needless to say, Ricardo was English, not Portuguese.

The fallacy in Ricardo's free-trade theory lies in several realities. The foremost is that the theory assumes that world economies are static and in equilibrium. As today's experience shows, economies governed by people who want to improve their lives don't remain static. Nor do people accept equilibrium—particularly when their trading partner is getting the lion's share of the benefits. They seek to disrupt the equilibrium, change the rules of capitalism, and dethrone the leader who maintains the rules and equilibrium.

Ricardo's theory fails for another reason, as the case of China today shows abundantly. Some governments rig the rules of the game to their advantage. Others try to destroy their rivals' advantages. Still others build new advantages that surprise their rivals. The leaders of governments that have ambitions to rise in the world rankings are not sitting on the sidelines. They are shaking up the status quo.

Ricardo's theory also fails because people may buy more textiles than they do wine, creating trade imbalances and bleeding the wine producer dry (of cash, that is). Specialization can also cripple a country if it depends on foreign suppliers. For example, if an industrialized country trades its factory goods to an agrarian country in exchange for food, then a storm, a drought, or a war in the food-producing country may cause the industrial country to starve. The United States could learn from this principle: it is now dependent upon China for the rare earths used in most defense equipment and computers and for most goods sold in Walmart.

Finally, free trade can make a country dependent upon the buyer if the buyer purchases a big portion of the dominant country's output. Another CEO once told me that he had good news and bad news. When I asked about the good news, he said: "Walmart wants to put our product on its shelves, and it will finance the three new factories we need to build to handle Walmart's volume." When I asked what the bad news was, he said, "Walmart wants to put our product on its shelves, and it will finance the three new factories we need to build to handle Walmart's volume. That means it can close us down if we don't meet its future demands for lower prices." So, too, with China: as American corporations sell more to China, China will gain a lot of power over American firms.

The United States has gotten into a vulnerable position in part because the U.S. faith in globalism and free trade has been so hard to shake. That stems from a firm belief that free trade is a central element of what makes America unique. This belief, though reinforced regularly in political sound bites, has no basis in history. While U.S. leaders espouse globalism and free trade today, our founding fathers did not believe in them. Before the passage of the progressive income tax in the Sixteenth Amendment to the U.S. Constitution in 1913, most federal government revenues came from tariffs and duties on foreign goods. This did slow growth, but it made America self-reliant and less dependent. Despite the closed borders during the nineteenth century, the American economy grew. Imports and exports made up less than 10 percent of GDP until the 1930s.

The first secretary of the U.S. Treasury, Alexander Hamilton, believed in protectionism as a means of being sure that every American worker could be protected from cheap foreign competition. He didn't worry about whether the United States offered consumers the lowest prices in the world. He gave priority to preserving jobs for Americans. Hamilton believed that Americans would choose secure, higher-paying jobs (even if prices were a little higher) over scarce, insecure jobs with lower pay (even if this led to lower prices for goods). He would probably be mortified by the American habit today of glorifying consumption at the expense of production that creates jobs.

As the world's biggest economies compete for wealth using different capitalist systems, American companies are following the opportunities at hand. To amass market share and create growth in the short run, most of them go to China to take advantage of the fastest-growing market in the world. They may say otherwise, but the speed of Chinese growth puts them on track for a surprising future: eventually they will become Chinese-dominated companies because of the size of the Chinese market. KFC, arguably the most successful U.S. firm in China, runs 3,200 restaurants in 650 cities.

It opens one new restaurant in China every 18 hours. Its Chinese sales make up 36 percent of company revenue, a veritable gusher of cash compared to the firm's 19,000 restaurants in the United States. It holds 42 percent of the fast-food market. In China, not the West, lies its future.[43]

Other firms appear to be on the same track. Two examples are GM and Procter & Gamble. In spite of its bumpy ride getting established, GM sells more cars in China than it does in the United States. It is China's top-selling foreign brand, holding a 12.8 percent share of the car market. Procter & Gamble, in China since 1988, holds a 55 percent share of the Chinese hair-care market. [44] It has more than $5 billion in sales and 7,000 employees in China. It recently opened an $80 million innovation center in Beijing and plans to invest another $1 billion in China over five years.[45]

The trend is clear: certain American companies will become foreign ones. They may be incorporated in the United States, but when their sales in China become more than 50 percent of their total sales, they will bow to the pressures of the government running the market that sustains them. A few, like Google, will resist.[46] They will exit. But they will be rare. If U.S. companies don't morph into Chinese ones, there is another possibility: China may solicit their investment and technology but then launch competing SOEs to undermine the U.S. firms' success.

Danone, the French dairy and drinks group, formed a joint venture with the Chinese drinks giant Wahaha. Danone transferred part of its technology to the joint venture. Soon thereafter, Danone found a local competitor offering identical products. It was run by the same Chinese executive who had initiated the joint venture. Danone accused its partner of running a parallel set of companies and siphoning off $100 million from the partnership. The dispute erupted into a public feud that blackened Danone's reputation with Chinese consumers, as Wahaha orchestrated rallies to denounce its French partner. Danone settled with Wahaha in 2009, selling its 51 percent stake to its new competitor.[47]

Strangely, the biggest strategic dilemma that executives from Western firms face is, "What if we do well in China?" If an American corporation's Chinese division grows bigger than its home subsidiary, the power within the organization shifts to China. With recent changes in American court rulings that allow American firms to support political candidates and lobby without limit, we could see Chinese divisions (under the influence of the Chinese Communist Party) become so powerful that they can pressure their American parent company to donate money or advertise to sway elections, legislation, and referenda to protect Chinese interests. I am not saying that this is happening now, but the potential for the tail wagging the dog will grow.

And Chinese leaders, like good chess players, understand that Western firms want to enter Chinese markets because of China's big upside potential. However, this has reduced Western firms to pawns, easy to manipulate and easy to use as instruments of Chinese policies. Forced to protect their investments in China, Western firms have fallen into a trap that they now cannot get out of. Most ironically, Western firms may find that they are being manipulated by false dreams of future gold. There is some evidence to suggest that there is no pot of gold at the end of the Chinese rainbow. The Chinese government is already squeezing several foreign companies out of the market or containing them to small niches, while leaving domestic firms the lion's share of the Chinese market (except in the few cases of American success mentioned previously.)

By all appearances, China has used the West's devotion to free trade as its principal means of gaining advantage. Ironically, the primacy of free-trade thinking is enshrined in rules enforced by an organization that the United States has long supported: the World Trade Organization. Before China came on the scene, the WTO worked for the United States, prying open markets for U.S. goods. The WTO institutionalized the trade rules that had long made the United States a winner. The United States essentially imposed a part of its version of capitalism on many other nations.

However, what was once an advantage has now turned to a disadvantage with China's 2001 entry into the WTO. The United States continues to believe in the WTO. But China today plays on U.S. misconceptions—the WTO did not pry open China's markets, it merely opened Western markets to China. China competes in a free-trade world with managed-trade rules. The inability to control China's behavior by setting enforceable rules of trade is now obvious. It seems that the rules that the United States set for its own benefit 20 years ago are not the rules that will benefit America in the contest between capitalist systems that is occurring today.

China is playing to thwart free trade, just as America's founding fathers did during the United States' developmental stage in the 1800s. It is not in China's interest to open its markets until its home enterprises are strong enough to withstand global competition without government protection. The United States and the rest of the West will have to have to find a new solution to China's challenge. More free trade, by itself, just won't rejuvenate Western economies. In fact, it may sink the West as it continues to buy more than it sells to China.

China Challenges the World

What does the future of competition with China hold for U.S. and other Western leaders? I believe the West faces three possible scenarios.

The first is that China's advance simply stalls of its own accord. This seems doubtful for the reasons I will give next. The second is that China continues to compete vigorously with foreign nations and advances toward world leadership. This, I believe, is probable. The third is that China gains so much power that it establishes a global mercantilist empire, akin to the British Empire in the nineteenth century. This could happen, but Western leaders will probably rise to challenge and block it by economic, diplomatic, or military means.

Examining the first scenario, China's advance could stall for many reasons. One of them is a shortage of food, minerals, timber, farmland, or other resources. China needs to both feed its people and feed the manufacturing engine that continues to build wealth. It depends on a rapid GDP growth rate of around 8 percent or more to raise its people out of poverty. Any bottleneck in its supply lines could sharply slow its growth. Already China is short of oil, natural gas, copper, and gold. The challenge of staying ahead of the voracious demand of a country with 1.3 billion people is real.

The country's advance could also be stalled by a further global slowdown. At this point in its development, China relies heavily on Western markets. Should they dip too far, China remains vulnerable to catching the flu when the Western world catches a cold. China simply cannot sustain its growth without high exports of products and healthy levels of foreign direct investment. China's 2008 stimulus program of $586 billion seems to have helped the country bridge the downturn. Still, Western capital and consumers drive its economy, and China cannot thrive without them. In the long run, China's growing domestic market will replace exports, making China less dependent on the West.

Some observers believe that social unrest could slow China. The evidence of daily strikes suggests that there is plenty of discontent that can boil to the surface. Wages are low in some parts of China. Social benefits are nil. Working conditions are akin to those in the West 100 years ago. Freedom is limited. Unemployment, while officially about 4 percent in urban areas, actually exceeds 20 percent, according to some analysts, counting migrants to the cities from rural China. And the vast majority of Chinese in the western and central parts of China still live in poverty, under conditions no different from those 500 years ago. The twelfth Five-Year Plan calls for China to create 45 million new jobs over five years. It also calls for raising both urban and rural wages by 7 percent annually. Falling short of those goals could trigger demands for further stimulus that would drain government resources.

Despite the current evidence that China is entering a slower— but still good—growth period, no one expects the slowdown to become a recession. Any such slowdown is only temporary. Over the long run, China will probably extend its growth streak and maybe accelerate it. The structural conditions are set. China will keep pressing ahead with many managed-capitalist practices prohibited by the WTO. China's manufacturing prowess will continue to improve. It still has millions of low-cost laborers to bring into low-end manufacturing. It is acquiring capital, intellectual property, and business know-how to continue to grow. China still has a massive population that wants more goods and the latest luxuries. The WTO will continue to be too weak to control China. And the West is fearful of Chinese retaliation against its corporations operating in China.

In short, China's leaders will continue to increase the country's global market share and profits in just the way independent businesses would—aggressively. China will stay on the offensive, disrupting American and other Western capitalist systems. Meanwhile, unless its problems are fixed soon, the West will become too debt-laden to slow China's advance.

Examining the second scenario, China will play the heavyweight and continue its march toward world leadership. With its control over SOEs, Chinese leaders may direct domestic business executives to steadily usurp leading positions in every manufacturing and high-tech sector. They will continue leveraging the advantages of managed capitalism: state-underwritten capital, opaque bureaucratic rules that erect de facto nontariff trade barriers, joint ventures that drain technology from Western companies, concentration of market power in national champions, favoritism for domestic companies in access to natural resources, currency manipulation that keeps the Chinese official currency, the renminbi (RMB) artificially low, and social policies that give the state, rather than employees or consumers, the lion's share of state-generated wealth.

If recent history continues, China will continue to amass capital at the expense of its people—money that could be spent on social programs. It will continue building foreign cash reserves that amount to a war chest for global economic and political hegemony through continued loans to foreign governments. As China's leaders invest their capital in securities and infrastructure around the world, they may throw their weight around as the world's biggest investor and creditor nation. With the power of global bankers, they are capable of extracting economic and political concessions from every one of their debtors, especially if they near default. The foremost of their debtors is the United States. When push comes to shove, China will have the power to press the United States to back off on demands for fairer trade.

China may dangle over the heads of U.S. leaders the prospect of manipulating its foreign reserves—more than $2 trillion in U.S. dollars—to depress the value of the dollar to create inflation, or even threaten the United States with foreclosure by refusing to loan to the U.S. government in the future. However, this would hurt the Chinese as much as it would hurt the United States. Former U.S. Secretary of the Treasury Larry Summers has called this the "balance of financial terror." Nevertheless, China can reduce its dependence on U.S. trade, U.S. debt, U.S. markets, and U.S. currency over time, removing the balance of financial terror and creating the possibility of financial terror.

China will undoubtedly continue its policy of co-opting foreign firms. Pressing its low-wage advantage and the appeal of its large future market, it will draw more Western firms into business in China. It can hold the promise of high-margin, high-volume growth as an enticement to encourage U.S. and other Western companies to abandon their home territory and resettle on Chinese soil. And when they have consumed foreign capital to build domestic industries that were once unknown in China, they may close the door on further growth of foreign firms, as they did in the solar-panel industry. They will rout firms from the West not to be mean, but because the Chinese mean business—business according to the rules of state-managed capitalism.

The West will not have the option of escaping by moving up the value chain to make money in higher-value-added products. China will continue to leap up the chain of sophistication itself by copying, stealing, or openly appropriating Western technology from joint-venture partners. Forgoing the costs of R&D borne over decades by foreign firms, China will continue to take leading, low-cost positions after digesting and "reinnovating" to make Western technology its own. Like any hard-knuckled business, China will continue to press the limits of its trade partners' patience. It will not do right by complying with the capitalist rules of the West. It will do right for its nation, believing that it deserves to make up for two centuries of domination and humiliation by the West, starting in the early 1800s, when colonial powers interfered in China. This, I believe, is the most likely future that can be read clearly in the current trendlines.

Examining the third scenario, China will establish a global mercantilist empire, akin to the British Empire in the 1800s. If China continues its efforts to disrupt free trade by creating a mercantilist empire, it will stimulate resistance from several quarters using many methods. China has already begun laying the foundation for a mercantilist system in Africa, Southeast Asia, and Latin America. In the imperialist tradition, it has systematically gained control over billions of dollars of minerals, farmland, and transportation infrastructure around the world to avoid the shortages that could stall its economic growth.

China will go beyond co-opting businesses that set up shop in China. It will co-opt, and has co-opted, countries. With its huge foreign currency reserves, it can spend like a superpower to buy stockpiles of iron ore, oil, and other raw materials. But China does not just come as a buyer. It comes with its people to do the work, with engineers and workers to build the infrastructure, and with ships to carry the product. Peru, Bolivia, Argentina, Brazil, Angola, Congo, Nigeria, Sudan—they have all opened their doors to China's ready cash and aid. That China has such a large population can only work in its favor.

Note, however, that China is not just an average cash-flush customer. It has started to cement into place, as the British Empire did, three key assets: the world's central manufacturing hub, its most extensive global supply chain, and its most widespread global customer base. As in the example of Portugal and Britain, it is moving toward the position of high-value manufacturer, the trading party that stands to gain the most in trade transactions.

The winds of mercantilism fill China's sails. They allow China to corner the global market in surprising ways. Already, the country's companies have amassed quasi-monopoly power in some markets, reminiscent of the British East India Company. China International Marine Containers has a 56 percent share of the dry containers market. Galanz Enterprise Group (Guangdong) makes 40 percent of the world's microwave ovens. Acoustic Technology Corporation (Shenzen) has a 40 percent share of the world's cell-phone speaker production. And China has the scale to dump steel anywhere in the world and put local competitors out of business with a strategy of sequential predation.

Historically, if this kind of power is amassed, the world becomes restless because of fear of the superpower's purpose, creating incentives to build new military alliances, international institutions, and trade partnerships to counterbalance the power of the superpower.

The West Holds the Key

A win-win solution is not in China's interest. With its robust version of managed capitalism, it can win without cooperating. It has the structure, the strategy, the systems, and a critical mass of people and industry. But despite the challenges—or perhaps because of the immense national will to surmount them—I believe that the ability to win remains in the hands of the West.

Western countries, including the United States, have a window of opportunity in which to act. They can still disrupt China's superb capitalist strategy, still prevent its replacement of the United States as the world economic leader, still protect the economic and national freedoms of U.S. allies, and still prevent China from lowering Western standards of living. Time, however, is of the essence. If the United States and its allies do not understand the economic threat that China poses, or if they fail to develop a new strategy for addressing China, its momentum may become unstoppable.

One of the barriers to action is that businesspeople in many industries continue to support an obsolete view of business prospects in China. Looking at the short and medium terms, they believe that, as the global economy continues to develop and countries widely compete according to free-trade rules, China will eventually play along. But the evidence does not support the view that learning to dance with the Chinese dragon will eventually pay off. China's managed-capitalism policies are likely to continue to favor its SOEs and domestic companies for years. One by one, the dragon will quietly maneuver in a way that will squeeze out foreign companies.

The time has come for the West to retake the lead in this dance, not let the Chinese initiate the dance steps. U.S. leaders above all must avoid being drawn into temporary victories that end up in long-term defeats. They must recognize that any upticks in the American economy are only blips in a continuing decline driven by the rise of the dragon—unless Western governments change the way they respond to Chinese managed capitalism. The Chinese seem to offer gold at the end of their rainbow. But it is false gold. The real gold lies at home, in reinventing our system of capitalism so that it can respond to the Chinese challenge of managed capitalism.

4

Capturing Other Capitalist Nations

The Struggle for Strategic Supremacy and Economic Spheres of Influence

After the collapse of the Soviet Union, the United States tried to take on the role of being the world's economic leader, not just the leader of the free world. Many people expected a Pax Americana—global peace and economic cooperation enforced by the world's most powerful economic and military force. Some thought that America would be able to establish strategic supremacy everywhere, placing most of the world within its orbit.

The United States was in an enviable spot, as its strategic supremacy included many abilities:

- The ability to establish a basic set of rules of capitalism that everyone conformed to
- The ability to convince and help others to modify their version of capitalism to be compatible with the leader's system
- The ability to form an economic sphere of influence that operated for mutual economic and security benefit
- The ability to mold the economic spheres of rivals who wished to play by different rules of capitalism

- The ability to stake out the best markets for itself and its allies
- The ability to sustain its sphere as the most powerful on Earth
- The ability to influence global economic systems, including trade patterns, international currency and financial systems, and the rules of intellectual property ownership

Over decades, the United States had placed itself in a position to draw many other nations into its orbit by creating new international institutions that helped it establish the rules of capitalism, either globally or within its sphere of influence. Those institutions gave it the power to control the sphere's trade, currency, financial, and monetary systems.

But the United States' central geopolitical role has come into question. Though some may doubt this conclusion, let's look at some of China's actions that have affected America's ability to draw other nations and entities into its sphere of influence. China is disrupting the U.S. sphere by capturing new trading partners, international economic institutions, and international geopolitical institutions.

Capturing Other Nations Within the Leader's Orbit

Superpowers typically work to extend their capitalist systems to nations and industries that are critical suppliers and end markets, so that it has a reliable network of partners who are playing by the same rules. Think of the British Empire in the 1800s and early 1900s. To colonies such as India, Britain exported not just its legal system, but its cultural norms. The greatest modern exponent of economic influence, of course, is the United States. America does not "force" countries to join the World Trade Organization (WTO), but it has a great deal of influence.

The superpower facilitates trade among members of the sphere based on the superpower's system of capitalism. It also creates international institutions to control the sphere's trade, currency, financial, and monetary systems.

The game then becomes a question of which superpower can build the biggest and best sphere of influence by capturing the right collection of nations within its orbit and by taking control of or creating new international institutions that help it establish the rules of capitalism either globally or within its sphere of influence.

China is quietly and incrementally disrupting America's sphere of influence, reducing U.S. power one step at a time. Though some may doubt this conclusion, let's look at some of China's actions that have affected America's ability to capture other nations and entities within its sphere of influence. China is disrupting the U.S. sphere by capturing new trading partners, international economic institutions, and international geopolitical institutions.

Capturing New Trading Partners

As the flow of trade shifts, so does the flow of geopolitical and economic power. That raises the question of how vulnerable various countries within the U.S. sphere are to China's new trade power. A look at trade data reveals a surprising range in the various countries' vulnerability. Many of America's most important allies are what I term "dependent," "very dependent," or "extremely dependent" on trade for their economic survival. This makes them more or less pawns in the hands of a superpower that has the centralized power to direct or redirect trade in its direction.

Data from the International Monetary Fund's "2010 Direction of Trade, Cross Country Matrix" show that the United States (17 percent) and Brazil (20 percent) are among the least trade-dependent countries based on their percentage of trade relative to their GDP (in parentheses).[1] In contrast, South Korea (93 percent) and Indonesia (98 percent) are extremely dependent on trade. Dependent countries include Japan (29 percent), Turkey (32 percent), the United Kingdom and Spain (34 percent), Australia (35 percent), Argentina and India (38 percent), France (41 percent), Italy (43 percent), and Canada (48 percent). Very dependent countries include Russia (55 percent), China (58 percent), Sweden (67 percent), and Germany (74 percent).[2] Thus, many countries that are within America's sphere of influence can be influenced by changing trade patterns, indicating that America's sphere is weak unless much of the trade is with the United States.

Trade-dependent countries, especially very and extremely trade-dependent countries, cannot experience a shift, curtailment, or shutdown of trade without courting some degree of economic risk. Any country that can influence the trade flows of those dependent countries' can influence their geopolitical alliances. Only the United States and Brazil have maintained heavily domestic economies, but even they would face some degree of economic dislocation if someone could turn off the trade spigot.

The orbit of a country that is caught between the gravitational pull of two superpowers is influenced most by which superpower has more gravity—that is, which superpower trades more with the country. If one compares several key nations' trade with China and the United States, we can see which way these countries are leaning (see Figure 4-1).

In 2000, most countries traded much more heavily with the United States than they did with China. The big U.S. trading partners included Germany, Japan, Turkey, and the United Kingdom. We also see that many key nations—those in the center

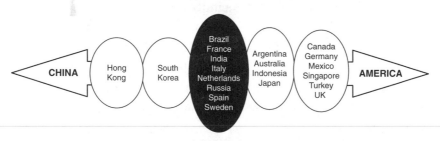

Key: * [(Imports plus Exports with China)/Nation's GDP] divided by same for the nation's trade with China from IMF trade data

Note: Black oval = approximately one-to-one ratio.

Source: Modified from a figure prepared by Raj Koganti under the supervision of Richard D'Aveni.

FIGURE 4.1 America's Strategic Supremacy in 2000: Trade Dependence of Key Nations on China versus America*

black oval—fell into a neutral zone, caught equally between the two superpowers. These included Brazil, France, India, Spain, and Sweden.[3]

By 2010, the trade data show a radical shift in the leanings of many countries that were once considered solid partners in America's sphere of influence (see Figure 4-2). France, Brazil, and Sweden remained in the neutral zone. But India, Russia, Spain, Germany, Indonesia, Italy, and Japan had moved into the Chinese economic sphere of influence. Only Canada, Mexico, and the United Kingdom remained firmly in the American sphere of influence.

The figures graphically illustrate the effect of China's economic growth and development. China's managed capitalism, the labor policies that support it, and the foreign direct investment (FDI) policies that strengthened it did not just move China to a new economic plateau; they shifted it to a new level of geopolitical and geoeconomic influence. In the two figures, the majority of countries have moved from the right side to the left, swinging almost like a pendulum from the U.S. economic sphere to the Chinese one.

The shift goes beyond what is shown in the figures. As mentioned in earlier chapters, China has forged relationships with supplier nations in Africa, the Middle East, and Latin America that are not shown in the figures. It has turned itself into a nexus for imported

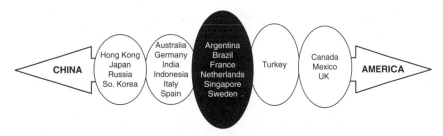

Key: * [(Imports plus Exports with China)/Nation's GDP] divided by same
for the nation's trade with China from IMF trade data

Note: Black oval = approximately one-to-one ratio.

Source: Modified from a figure prepared by Raj Koganti under the supervision of Richard D'Aveni.

FIGURE 4.2 The Rise of China's Strategic Supremacy in 2010: Trade Dependence of Key Nations on China versus America*

raw materials and exported finished goods. It is the world's only neomercantilist, with Chinese state-owned mines, arable land, buildings, infrastructure, water, and oil resources in several countries that China wants to be part of its sphere of influence.

Historically, the United States has tried to increase its influence through the use of military protection to keep several allies within its sphere of influence (including Japan, South Korea, Taiwan, Israel, and the NATO nations). But in many places, "geoeconomics" has supplanted geopolitics. Military power seems less useful because no major country is pushing for war. While military power has slowed the shift of power from West to East, the more important shift is from countries with weak capitalist systems to countries with stronger ones.

China's control over exports and imports based on its managed-capitalist system has markedly disrupted the U.S. sphere of influence. China was able to accelerate its economic growth by targeting trade with selected countries, such as Germany and Japan, so that they became dependent on exports to China, displacing products once exported to the United States. Trade-dependent economies that have trade surpluses with China are worried that they are dancing with a 900-pound gorilla and can't stop unless the gorilla allows them to. As China pulls more nations into its orbit, it is selectively dismembering America's sphere.

To be sure, China has not used its economic power to derail the U.S. economy in any overt, direct fashion. But it appears certain that it will continue to weaken the American sphere slowly and without fanfare. China is now the biggest exporter in the world, with more than $1.2 trillion in exports. Following it are Germany, with $1.2 trillion, and the United States, with slightly less than $1 trillion. Trade has become the carrot that entices countries to ally with China, and the United States has not adequately recognized that fact and used it to spur an effort to resecure its sphere.

Capturing International Economic Institutions

Another mechanism that China has used to disrupt the U.S. sphere of influence is to derail U.S. leadership of international institutions that were founded to help the West administer global trade, finance, and politics in ways that maintained Western rules of capitalism. Three such institutions are the most important: the World Trade Organization, the Group of Nations, and the International Monetary Fund (and related international financial institutions).

The World Trade Organization (WTO). Despite its ostensible aim of serving global best interests, in practice the WTO has tended to favor U.S. and Western interests. Ironically, China has stopped the WTO from working in the West's favor. In previous chapters, we discussed China's use of the WTO to operate by its own set of trade rules. That has given China a big advantage: access to world markets while protecting its home markets. But China has also used the WTO to give itself geopolitical advantage.

The United States focused on bringing China into the WTO in the hope that its entry would serve American interests: China would convert to the rules of capitalism and trade favored by the West. With its 153 members, representing more than 97 percent of the world's population, the WTO is the flagship organization of a U.S.-centered economic architecture. The goal was, in exchange for China's joining the world trade community, to guide China into acting like Western powers.

Some of the hoped-for results from China included the following: open trade through the elimination of tariff and nontariff barriers; Westerners' access to China's domestic market; free markets within China, without subsidies and intellectual property theft; allowance of for-profit businesses independent of the government; policies that integrated China into the world economic order; and binding dispute resolution by the WTO.

As it turned out, China fully exploited its negotiated entry deal, dating to 2001. This included taking advantage of exemptions granted to it as a developing economy. The exemptions made sense in 2001, but since then, China has turned into a developed economy in its coastal areas, which include more people and more acreage than most other countries in the world. Meanwhile, China has not lived up to the promises it made in return for WTO membership. Its delay in moving to parity with other countries in trade, its lack of protection of intellectual property, and its currency manipulation practices contribute to the economic power it uses to expand its sphere of influence.

Among other things, China has not limited subsidies for agricultural production to the agreed-to levels (8.5 percent of farm output value). It has not granted full trade and distribution rights to foreign firms. It has not protected intellectual property according to WTO agreements. And it has not opened its banking system to foreign financial institutions, as it was to have done within five years of WTO entry.[4] As previous chapters showed, China did not liberalize its trade regime to any significant extent, and to this day, its economy remains among the most protected in the world.

China has also become an active player in shaping new WTO negotiations to disrupt U.S. influence over the organization. In the Doha round of negotiations, started in 2001, the United States sought to lower trade barriers around the world. China played a role in delaying key negotiations by creating a "disagreement between exporters of agricultural bulk commodities and countries with large numbers of subsistence farmers on the precise terms of a 'special safeguard measure' to protect farmers from surges in imports."[5] By leading this debate, China essentially scuttled a Doha agreement on trade between developed and developing economies. Though many people yawn at the thought of WTO maneuvering, this behind-the-scenes action has allowed China to take some serious control of the WTO out of U.S. hands. The United States has lost a key tool for securing its sphere of influence.

The Group of Nations. With its entry into the Group of Nations, once the G-7, then the G-8 (including Russia), and now the G-20, China has disrupted the U.S. sphere of influence. After the financial crisis of 2008, the expansion of the group to the G-20 was supported by American leaders as part of its effort to "globalize" world trade and finance. The group includes finance ministers and central bank governors from 20 major economies, including 19 countries and the European Union (EU).

By admitting China and expanding the membership of the Group of Nations, the United States has granted many countries a platform for exercising political muscle over central banks. Though well-meaning, the transformation of the G-7 into the G-20 diluted America's influence over the group. As the G-20 studies, reviews, and promotes discussion, it addresses issues of international financial stability that go beyond the responsibilities of any one national banking system. Once again, with China's influence having grown, it can disrupt the Western bias in decisions made by the Group of Nations.

The United States once facilitated discussions among allies at G-7 meetings. Today, China coordinates a faction of countries that often oppose the original G-7, outmaneuvering the United States and other Western countries. In 2009, president Hu Jintao wouldn't agree to meet with France's President Nicolas Sarkozy at a G-20 meeting until France issued a statement saying that it did not support Tibetan independence in "any form."[6]

Without China in the G-20, Chinese and developing-country aspirations would have been less likely to interfere with U.S. goals. China's leadership as a protector of developing economies, bolstered by its economic aid to these economies, restricts U.S. maneuvering to implement changes that suit the West's financial interests.

International monetary and financial systems. China has disrupted the U.S. sphere of influence through its influence over the international monetary and financial system. As in the case of the WTO, the United States and its allies have largely controlled the institutions that facilitate and stabilize global banking, lending, and economic rebuilding of nations that are recovering from war or financial collapse. The West has also controlled global systems by keeping the dollar as the world's unchallenged reserve currency. Having taken a lead role in global finance, the United States has been able to secure a strong sphere of influence that includes nations in financial trouble.

One effort that has disrupted U.S. influence is China's manipulation of its currency. By undervaluing the renminbi in comparison to the dollar for years, China has spurred its exports by making its goods artificially cheaper. Even today, many observers believe that the renminbi, which China pegs to the dollar, remains at least

20 percent undervalued.[7] Given China's trillion-dollar export machine, this gives the country an extraordinary economic advantage that contributes to its sphere of influence.

The 2008 financial meltdown across the Western world gave China the opportunity to further disrupt the economic power of the United States by questioning the use of the dollar as the global reserve currency. Though the dollar won't lose its status any time soon, owing to its widespread integration into global trade and banking, China's suggestion that the world look to other options has undercut U.S. financial influence and could affect the value of the dollar. If the dollar stops being the reserve currency, demand for it will decrease, so its value will decrease, creating inflation within the United States.

China's central bank chief, Zhou Xiaochuan, has even floated the idea of moving the renminbi toward being a reserve currency. "The acceptance of credit-based national currencies as major international reserve currencies," said Zhou, "as is the case in the current system, is a rare special case in history."[8] Further, he said, "The [financial] crisis again calls for creative reform of the existing international monetary system towards an international reserve currency with a stable value, rule-based issuance and manageable supply, so as to achieve the objective of safeguarding global economic and financial stability."[9]

Many observers dismiss the Chinese suggestions of the renminbi as a reserve currency. Former Treasury secretary Henry Paulson, at a meeting in China, noted: "To me a reserve currency has got to be one that is liquid and is convertible and whose value is determined by the markets, not by governments." He noted that the U.S. dollar's reserve status was "earned . . . over many, many years [of] stable macroeconomic policies. . . . [With] the renminbi, there will need to be more reform, and it will have to earn reserve-currency status over time."[10]

China's ambitions for the renminbi represent a natural evolution for a growing world power. China could not become a world economic leader without reserve-currency status. But as it moves to exercise its growing strength, it is using its size, trade relationships, and credibility to undermine America's efforts to shore up the dollar. China's questioning can only lead to downward pressure on the dollar. If all nations decreased their demand for the dollar, the dollar would fall, making it more expensive for the United States to buy oil, raw materials, and finished goods from overseas.

As long as the dollar remains the world reserve currency, U.S. power over the monetary system is a threat to China's wealth. Some observers suggest that this could prompt China to use its own $2 trillion of dollar reserves to undercut the dollar. In a doomsday scenario, China could dump its dollars, creating an overnight currency fire sale and depressing the value of the greenback. China is unlikely to make such a move, since it would suffer a huge loss itself, but merely by floating the scenario, China puts pressure on the dollar. In Zimbabwe, dictator Robert Mugabe, who has given China almost carte blanche to exploit his country's platinum, gold, and diamond reserves, has reportedly taken the talk seriously. His allies in government have suggested replacing the local mix of currencies with the renminbi.[11]

While trying to undercut faith in the dollar, China has also taken greater control of affairs that were formerly mediated by the International Monetary Fund (IMF). The IMF was set up essentially to minimize harm to banks and governments in advanced nations that lent money to struggling countries that failed. The process of making loans through the IMF has long allowed the United States and its allies to impose restrictions on borrowers' government spending, tax policies, and economic practices. The IMF has also allowed the West to open trade avenues and convert backward economies to modern banking practices. In other words, the IMF could demand economic practices that were in line with Western standards.

But China has circumvented this U.S. power. It has started lending money directly to other nations, including debt-ridden U.S. allies in Europe, such as Greece, Italy, Spain, Portugal, and Ireland. As countries that contribute to the IMF have run low on funds, China has stepped in. This in part illustrates how much China's national goals differ from those of the West. With its huge reserves, one might expect China to redistribute wealth domestically, building a modern social safety net of pension and health benefits. But it has chosen instead to use its reserves to extend its trading network and sphere of influence.

Though China remains far from joining the global financial world by having a liquid, free-floating currency and an open banking system, and by taking a leadership role in helping countries that are in trouble, it has jockeyed into position to slash the ability of the United States to perpetuate its sphere of influence. It has even laid plans for adding to its clout in financial markets. It has created the Dagong Global Credit Rating agency, akin to U.S. agencies Moody's and Standard & Poor's. Though few Westerners will take a Communist-controlled agency's ratings seriously, China has nonetheless taken this step so that it can rate its own companies in order to influence their value on stock exchanges.

In just several years, developing nations led by the Chinese have realized a level of influence that they once only dreamed of. They are now able to push the United States around. China's coalition can do more than veto U.S. moves. It can actively pursue an agenda to undermine U.S. influence.

Capturing International Geopolitical Organizations

China uses the United Nations to disrupt the U.S. sphere of influence by taking greater control of the UN's policies. Just as with the WTO, the United States has steadily lost influence in an institution that was set up to favor its interests. The UN was founded in part to facilitate cooperation in international law and security (among other things). It was thus given military power and the right to intervene in conflicts and the affairs of sovereign nations through a vote of the Security Council. When mainland China supplanted Taiwan as the Chinese government represented at the UN in 1971, it brought another vision. Since 1954, it has pursued a foreign policy that stresses the equal, uninfringeable sovereignty of all states. This policy stems from its Five Principles of Peaceful Coexistence, which include mutual nonaggression, noninterference in each other's internal affairs, and mutual respect for sovereignty and territorial integrity.

The divergent visions of the UN and China have long created a conflict that, as China has grown more powerful, gives it more influence. China's view extends to all nations, large or small, Western or non-Western, rich or poor, democratic or authoritarian. It allows each nation to run its system without outside interference, whether its methods comply with UN standards or not. Since supplanting Taiwan at the UN, mainland China has used its vision to thwart the UN's goals. It has long ignored or rejected UN resolutions on Tibet's sovereignty and human rights. In 2011, it warned the UN to stay away during the so-called Jasmine Revolution as it carried out its largest roundup of dissidents in years to head off fears of an "Arab Spring" in China.

China also uses its vision to delay, weaken, or thwart UN efforts to rein in Iran's nuclear program. It has also thwarted efforts to stop North Korea's rogue actions threatening South Korea, including artillery barrages of South Korean territory and sinking or capturing ships. Though these policies may make sense for China, they further disrupt the U.S. sphere. China's foreign policy vision often serves it well in opposing U.S. influence in Africa, Latin America, and the Middle East, allowing it to use the UN as a platform for fostering divisiveness at the United States' expense.

China maintains that it "never seeks hegemony," according to a white paper issued in late 2011 by China's State Council.[12] Chinese officials use the term to refer to U.S. efforts to enforce the American government's will on other countries in such matters as trade practices, weapons proliferation, and human rights. But China's actions suggest that hegemony is on the minds of China's leaders. China has been effective in reining in U.S. attempts to limit sovereign states' efforts to develop and sell weapons of mass destruction, repress opposition and violate human rights, and pursue mercantilist economic policies that interfere with free trade.

Chinese support of rogue nations is also distracting U.S. attention from its long-term competition with China, and forcing the United States to waste funds to counter Chinese efforts to undermine U.S. influence in Asia, Africa, Latin America, and the Middle East.

China's Moves Add Up to a Logical Strategy Aimed at Regional and Then Global Hegemony

Whether by design or by happy accident, China's actions add up to what looks remarkably like a grand strategy for regional and then global dominance. (See Figure 4-3 for a summary.) Moreover, as China accumulates more wealth, it will have the ability to buy greater military and diplomatic power, and it will use this power to secure its place of influence as strongly as the United States once did. China shows no signs of reining in its moves toward gaining more influence. Nor would one expect it to. Logic suggests that China does not intend to cooperate further with the United States. It would make no sense to expect China, a nation that is on a winning streak with its current approach, to turn to a win-win strategy in either the economic or the geopolitical realm. China will not change unless the West actively pushes it to change its system to be more compatible with the West's capitalist system or the West provides China with more incentive to join Western capitalist systems.

The Weak U.S. Counterresponse

Today, the United States is a country that does not have the economic power needed to counter China's growing influence. Thus, the United States has moved to counter China's growing influence with military power. In early 2012, the president announced fresh initiatives in Asia. The United States will install a military base in Australia, and also improve relations with China's neighbors, Vietnam and Burma. The president also proposed spending less on ground troops and more on projecting power through Special Operations, the U.S. Navy, the Air Force, and unmanned drones

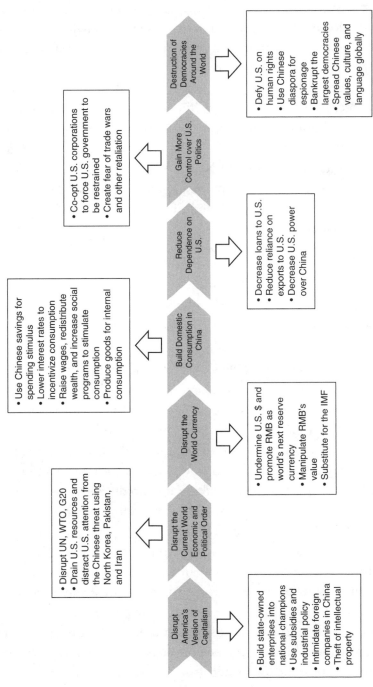

FIGURE 4.3 China's Incremental, Hidden Strategy to Dethrone America as the World Leader

operated by the CIA. These alternative approaches create options for pressuring and containing China's regional and national ambitions. However, the magnitude of these moves will not materially change the balance of power with China, nor will they force China to spend a lot of money in response.

The United States has not acted in a bold manner overall. For instance, it did not react to Chinese ally North Korea's artillery barrage of South Korea. Nor did it respond aggressively to the deadly sinking of a South Korean ship or the revelations of a uranium enrichment facility in North Korea. China has offered symbolic concessions on some points, and has promised to reform, but its moves appear to be targeted mainly at placating Washington. As China continues down this path, the United States has an uphill battle to further prevent deterioration of its sphere.

Anticipating China's Next Moves—Reducing Interdependence with the United States

Assuming that China is seeking hegemony over the United States, China cannot act immediately to secure such a leadership position. It is too interdependent with the United States to do so. For example, if China moves to hurt the value of the U.S. dollar, it inflicts harm on its own financial standing. If it cuts off loans to America, it harms itself similarly. If it engages in a trade war with the United States, it, too, risks being adversely affected trade-wise. In order to win in a contest for strategic supremacy, China must reduce its interdependence with America beforehand, so that it has more freedom to escalate the game of brinksmanship that it often plays with the United States.

This suggests that China may take three actions to reduce its interdependence with the United States. First, it could try to decrease its reliance on exports to the United States. Second, it could continue to build its mercantilist connections overseas to control both its financial position and its access to raw materials. Third, it could build enough technology and know-how to become an innovator in its own right, free of reliance on the West.

Reducing reliance on exports to the United States. China has a tremendous amount of leeway to reduce its dependence on exports. It could do so simply by spurring consumption of its goods by its own citizens instead of by Western consumers. The ratio of household consumption to GDP in China is only 37 percent, compared to roughly 50 percent or more in industrial and other emerging-market countries. China's production-oriented rather than consumption-oriented economy reflects its model of growing via high savings, high investment, and heavy exporting. But it could—and has started to—increasingly stress consumption at home.

The challenge for China is keeping wages growing so that it can support increased consumption. Most recent job growth has taken place in coastal provinces, where the private sector has flourished. China is expected to spur employment, and thus consumption, inland, encouraging low-cost, high-tech manufacturing to migrate west from the coast. China would then be able to replace the jobs that have moved west with higher-paying ones in sophisticated manufacturing on the coast—not a promising development for manufacturers in the Western world.

China also hopes to increase consumption by keeping a lid on inflation. One means of doing so is by managing interest rates. The chief of the Jinan branch of the People's Bank of China wrote in an opinion piece, "On the one hand, deposit rates should be raised to eliminate negative interest rates and reduce inflation expectations. On the other hand, lending rates should be left unchanged to lower lenders' interest margins and force them to improve their risk management."[13] If China succeeds in achieving the right balance, it will keep goods and services affordable to pull more consumption into the domestic economy.

China can also spur consumption by increasing spending on social security, healthcare, and pensions. It is expected to raise social security benefits, according to the recent Five-Year Plan. The Ministry of Finance proposed raising yearly social security expenditures in 2011 by the central and local governments to RMB 5.2 trillion (U.S. $824 billion), an increase of 14.8 percent over

2010.[14] On top of the increased benefits, China plans to lower taxes on Chinese households. All told, China's efforts may well stimulate consumption sufficiently to reduce its export dependence on the United States.

Reducing resource interdependence. Though China and the United States will remain interdependent when it comes to financing, raw materials, and energy, China can be expected to reduce its dependence where it can. Its sovereign wealth fund, the China Investment Company, manages more money—$300 billion in assets—than any other in the world. Among its investments to date is $498 million in Brazilian miner Vale SA. This and other investments by state-owned enterprises (SOEs) in mining and processing plants around the world guarantee China the raw materials to remain independent of the United States and other Western countries.

China's foreign direct investment (FDI) reveals a strong desire to build a Chinese economic base around the world. From about $2 billion annually in the 1990s, outward FDI rose to $12.3 billion by 2005 and $57.5 billion in 2009. Although China spreads its investments worldwide, it has focused mainly on acquiring access to resources in Africa, Latin America, and Australia, and on finances, services, and technology in Europe and East Asia. Assuming that the heavy flow of FDI funds continues, China will steadily increase its independence from the United States.

Reducing dependence on U.S. technology. China will presumably continue its policy of absorbing foreign technology. This will rapidly reduce its dependence on the United States and the West. Both its domestic R&D centers and those built by foreign firms will remove China's need to court technology transfers. Shanghai GM and Chang'an Ford are two examples of firms that are building China's technology muscle. Shanghai GM has a joint research center and funds research in Chinese universities. Chang'an Ford has an internal research center and, in partnership with the National Science Foundation of China, funds university research as well.

Shaping a New World Order

With China's growing ability to disrupt the U.S. sphere of influence, and with its increasing ability to operate independently of the United States, a new world order is about to emerge. The job of the United States and its key allies is to shape this new world order so that it retains a strong Western and democratic sphere and to create some sort of balance of power that does not leave the United States and its allies out in the cold. When shaping the new world order, U.S. and Western leaders can be expected to address three major issues.

The Balance of Power and Interaction Between Rival Spheres of Influence

China's power to overturn capitalist and geopolitical rules that were cemented in place after World War II is impressive. The post-Soviet world order based on one superpower setting the standard around the world has crumbled. A new bipolar world is emerging. My view is that the United States faces a geopolitical model like that in Figure 4-4. The United States and China occupy the poles. India and the European Union hang in the balance, able to change the balance of power between the two superpowers. India and the EU can stay neutral, straddling the superpowers' spheres of influence, or move into a preferred sphere. They may also remove themselves from playing roles as balancers between the poles. Both could fail to grow sufficiently through bad economic strategy, and the European Union could disintegrate through overspending by member nations that worsens the Euro-debt crisis. This highlights the challenge for the United States when constructing a twenty-first-century world order.

China is contesting any U.S. move to reform or bolster the U.S. sphere. This is true in every corner of the world, including Latin America, where under the Monroe Doctrine, the United States has historically held superpower sway. To counteract China's rise, the

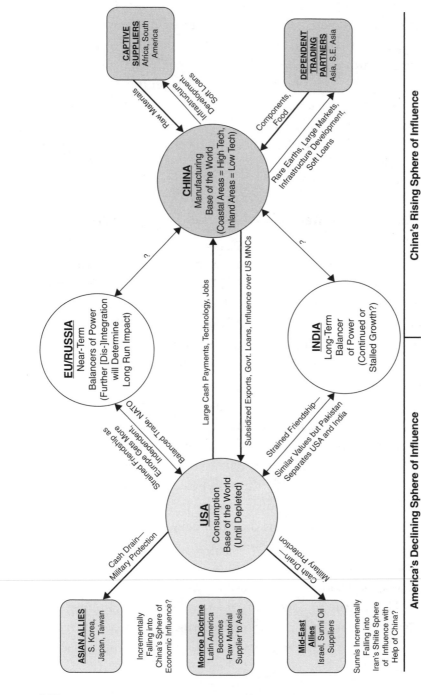

FIGURE 4.4 If China's Strategy Works, the Balance of Power Will Tip and a New China-centric World Economic Order Will Come About

108

United States may look to options such as bringing India into its sphere or pressing the EU members, Japan, and South Korea to choose a side. No one knows for sure which countries will move into which bloc—Japan, South Korea, Brazil, and so on. But we do know that the world is in play. Even in the United States' long-time geopolitical backyard in Europe, China is courting Germany, Sweden, and EU countries with debt problems. Allegiances to the United States may waver.

We also don't know how much military maneuvering will figure in as a complement to economic maneuvering. Both the United States and China suspect the worst of the other, and hawks in both countries are proposing more military action. Each country suspects that the other is pursing a strategy for long-term hegemony, tipping the balance of power not just in its favor, but significantly in its favor. The results are tensions and radical proposals on both sides.

From China, for example, came a comment from one strategist about breaking up India in order to pull that part of South Asia into the Chinese sphere. "To split India, China can bring into its fold countries like Pakistan, Nepal and Bhutan, support Ulfa in attaining its goal for Assam's independence, back aspirations of Indian ethnic groups like the Tamils and the Nagas, encourage Bangladesh to give a push to the independence of West Bengal and lastly recover the 90,000 sq km territory in southern Tibet."[15]

Pruning and Selecting New Members for America's Sphere of Influence

How big should the U.S. sphere of influence be, and how should its members be selected? Does it make sense to spend so much on military protection for so many countries when many of them have divided loyalties? Should the United States accept a smaller sphere of influence, containing only loyal partners, but costing less to maintain and yielding better returns? Will the carrying costs of military expenditures for too many countries overstretch U.S. resources?

As a way of answering these questions, national leaders would do well to look at the data for various countries to see whether they had trade surpluses or deficits with the United States and China. Putting countries in a matrix, as in Figures 4-5 and 4-6, can be revealing. The first figure shows the situation in 2005, the second in 2010.[16]

Comparing the two, we see that the most stable members of the U.S. sphere are Mexico, Turkey, and the Netherlands, which had surpluses with the United States in both 2005 and 2010. We also see that India, Indonesia, and Russia moved. In 2005, their surpluses with both the United States and China suggested that they straddled the two superpowers' spheres of influence. By 2010, their surpluses with China had disappeared and they were leaning toward the U.S. sphere. The trade data alone suggest that these three countries might make good candidates for growing the U.S. sphere of influence, if they are amenable. They would certainly add some large potential markets for countries in the American sphere of influence.

Trade Incentives to be Part of the Economic Spheres of China and/or the USA 2005		
	Trade Surplus with China	Trade Deficit with China
Trade Surplus with USA	*Surpluses with Both Superpowers* Japan South Korea Australia India Indonesia Russian Federation Sweden	*Surplus with USA Only* France Germany Italy Mexico Netherlands Singapore Spain Turkey United Kingdom
Trade Deficit with USA	*Surplus with China Only* Argentina Brazil	*Deficits with Both Superpowers* Canada

Note: China has a large trade surplus with the United States of America.
Source: IMF Direction of Trade—Cross Country Matrix (http://www2.imfstatistics.org/DOT)

FIGURE 4.5 Which Team Did Key Nations Play on in 2005?

Note also the movement of Sweden and Germany, which seem to have migrated into the Chinese economic sphere. Sweden went from a trade surplus to a deficit with the United States, while retaining a surplus with China. Germany went from a trade deficit with China and a surplus with the United States to just the reverse, a deficit with the United States and a surplus with China. Thus, Sweden and Germany, by virtue of trade flows alone, could be candidates for a shift out of the U.S. economic sphere. Note also that there are a few members (France, Italy, and Spain) that could be influenced by loans and trade offers to shift either way.

Trade is only one indicator of economic and geopolitical influence and allegiances. Many other factors, such as culture, national security goals, and human rights, affect allegiances. However, these two figures illustrate how some old U.S. allies are changing allegiances, economically speaking.

As for strategy, U.S. leaders would naturally want to consider aligning the funding of foreign military bases and deployments with the selection of countries in the U.S. sphere of influence. The

Trade Incentives to be Part of the Economic Spheres of China and/or the USA 2010		
	Trade Surplus with China	**Trade Deficit with China**
Trade Surplus with USA	*Surpluses with Both Superpowers* Japan South Korea Australia India Argentina	*Surplus with USA Only* Turkey Netherlands Mexico India Indonesia Singapore Russian Federation
Trade Deficit with USA	*Surplus with China Only* Germany Brazil Sweden	*Deficits with Both Superpowers* Canada France Italy Spain United Kingdom

Note: China has a large trade surplus with the United States of America.

Source: IMF Direction of Trade—Cross Country Matrix (http://www2.imfstatistics.org/DOT)

FIGURE 4.6 Which Team Did Key Nations Play on in 2010?

United States might want to run trade deficits with countries that contribute to the protection of U.S. interests. Additionally, the United States might want to make money from trade to defray some of the costs it incurs for the defense of certain countries. In 2010, many of the NATO countries ran trade deficits with the United States, a logical geoeconomic relationship. But Japan and South Korea do not seem to be paying for the U.S. military that is protecting them. Both ran surpluses in trade with the United States. An alternative view is that the United States needed to keep them inside the U.S. sphere, so it allowed South Korea and Japan to profit from the relationship with the U.S. economically and militarily. This practice may become less affordable or desirable for the United States as its national debt rises and the need to balance the budget becomes more critical. As it stands now, the United States funds its budget deficits by borrowing from the Chinese to defend Asian allies against the threats created or supported by China. Some might recognize this as running a scam on the United States to bury itself in debt.

A new stronger sphere that shifts power back to the West must take into account how countries are being economically repositioned by trade with China. To build a more powerful sphere of influence, careful consideration must be given to finding new members that counterbalance the size of rivals, provide the potential to strike at a rival's vital interests, or serve strategic purposes other than trade considerations. To build a tighter and more exclusive sphere, certain types of trade might by limited to members of the sphere. A sphere can be structured with exclusive trade deals to build value for key members of the sphere. For example, trade cycles like those of the British Empire can be created, where members of the empire traded rum for cotton, which was then traded for textiles and other manufactured goods involving machine-woven fabrics. And a successful sphere would require reliable international organizations run only by members of the sphere, enforcing rules and expelling noncompliant nations.

Figures 4-5 and 4-6 raise another issue of geoeconomic significance. Some countries do not fall into just one economic sphere. They straddle both the United States and China. The question that national leaders must ask is whether they want an open sphere or a closed sphere, as was the case in the Cold War with the USSR.

The Opposing Spheres

Western leaders will have to be prepared for an unexpected future. One way to do that is to consider "what ifs." What if Japan ends up in China's orbit? What if the EU falls apart? What if Latin America sides with the United States? What if India stays on the sidelines? What if the future pits East versus West? Or what if it pits democracies against dictatorships? What if nations shift sides constantly in an unstable and complex world? What if the world divides into exclusive U.S. and Chinese blocs separated by a new iron curtain?

Let's consider some specific possibilities about how opposing blocs may form. One of them is a north-south separation. The United States and the EU naturally ally with each other. Russia, to counter the economic advances of its ambitious southern neighbor, seeks to side with the United States and the EU. In response, China nurtures—in fact, today it is nurturing—a southern bloc. Countries that might move into the alliance of the south include Indonesia, the rest of Southeast Asia, India, Africa, and Brazil. The power of the southern bloc could exceed that of the northern.

Another possibility is an East-West separation. The United States, Latin America, and Europe (plus Japan, which is now a somewhat westernized democratic country) would stick with the United States. The Western bloc would hold together by virtue of its common European descent, laws, and culture. In this arrangement, the power of the United States and its allies could exceed that of the China-led Eastern world, including India and Indonesia.

A third possibility is a democracy-dictatorship separation. The United States, the EU, Latin America, and India would ally on the basis of sharing democratic values. The bloc would unite first-tier powers that have historical ties and shared concern over China's ambitions. China, Russia, and Africa would play the sole counterweight. Other countries would remain unaligned, open to straddling the superpowers' spheres.

During the Soviet Union–United States Cold War, the democratic and Communist spheres of influence had clear boundaries. The two seemed relatively stable and secure. After the fall of the Berlin Wall, everyone looked to the United States to provide global stability, as the sole superpower. With the rise of China, however, the boundaries have blurred, and future scenarios are not certain. Not all capitalists practice democracy, and not all capitalists welcome the U.S. sphere of influence. But one thing is certain: the United States does not have a strategy for fixing its deteriorating sphere of influence.

The Importance of Achieving Strategic Supremacy for the United States and Select Allies

The final "what if" that is worth considering is the worst case, or perhaps extreme case, for the United States and the West: What if China gains global hegemony? This would be a shock to the West, given that the fall of the USSR ushered in what many people took to be an enduring era of universal values, characterized by U.S.-style capitalism, Western democracy, and American-inspired modernity through globalization of trade, technology, ideals, and culture. But under China's hegemony, an era based on Chinese values and state capitalism would emerge. The countries of the world would take their economic and geopolitical cues from authoritarians.

As a practical matter, China would set performance, safety, and design standards for many products. Clean energy, heavy industry, railways, autos, electronics—China would set the prices and call the shots in every case. Because it would control the world's largest market, China would determine what the West would buy. Its economies of scale would also allow it to set cost benchmarks across an even broader array of industries than today, forcing Western companies to compete even more fiercely. Western companies would also feel even more pressure to cut wages, labor protections, work safety rules, and social benefits and services.

Based on China's actions to date, we can guess at the other extreme consequences of living under Chinese influence. China would have the incentive and the tendency to:

- Buy or control big chunks of the world's farmland, mines, water, and energy reserves to feed its people and its industries exclusively.
- Influence how much other countries spend on military or social programs, owing to China's influence on Western budgetary decisions as a big creditor nation.
- Depress Western social-spending standards to levels that fail to satisfy Westerners who have become accustomed to increasingly unaffordable social programs.
- Displace Western international institutions with Chinese-controlled institutions that sideline the United States and other Western nations as standard setters.
- Oblige countries around the world to accept Chinese immigration on a much larger scale, threatening domestic culture, public opinion, and even elections.
- Reduce privacy through electronic monitoring and increase fear of threats of retaliation against people and businesses that run afoul of Chinese norms.
- Chill public discourse as citizens, CEOs, university leaders, and politicians refuse to criticize China on any level to protect their interests in China.

Part 1 of this book presents a harsh picture: a China that is actively trying to disrupt and undermine the American capitalist system, a China that is ready and able to seize global economic leadership from the United States, a China that is willing to create a win-lose global economy through imbalanced trade, a China that willfully goes back on its word when it joins international organizations designed to foster cooperation and fair trade, a China that is taking advantage of American naïveté, and an America that is ill prepared to defend itself.

Many people would defend China, saying that China does not intend to disrupt the prosperity of America, become the world leader, or impose its will on any other nation. China is merely following the rules of development economics. There is no malicious intent to dominate the world. China's policies were chosen for good purposes—to bring a better life to its starving masses. And China's policies were built up over decades based on what its people needed at many different points in time, rather than as a single coherent and comprehensive plan. There was no intention, no goal, and no desire to overtake the United States in global economic influence or to bring down the U.S. economy. China is just a worthy competitor that has developed a superior form of capitalism. Western countries have only themselves to blame for economic decline and obsolete capitalist systems.

The problem is this: in the United States and elsewhere, the nation-states, corporations, and people must nevertheless deal with the damage that China causes them. They must move to counteract the detrimental effects of China's de facto strategy. It makes no difference whether China intended its strategy, or whether it put all the pieces together incrementally or in one giant moment of transformation. It makes no difference whether China's goals are based on good motives (feeding its people) or on malicious motives (establishing world hegemony). It even makes no difference whether China appears fated to be the world leader simply because of its size.

This book analyzes China's actions, not its words, and it has revealed a strategy of a type that strategists call realized and emergent. *Realized strategy* is the sum of one's actions, not one's intentions or one's words. It is the reality, not the aspirations, of a country or corporation. *Emergent strategy* is the accumulation of many actions, resource investments, and goals established over a long period of time. If these commitments are intentionally or inadvertently built toward an overarching common goal, the process of emergence becomes what my mentor James Brian Quinn identified as "logical incrementalism." A strategy does not have to be built all at once, or even be intentional, to become a strategy over time.

In reality, every corporation's and every country's strategy is realized and emergent over time. Few are able to make strategy work through a single comprehensive, logically consistent, and perfectly implemented plan. Therefore, the strategist looks at the facts—the realized and emergent strategy—and decides what to do based on those facts.

Welcome to the Capitalist Cold War

The shift of power to China will not go smoothly. Fights over currency manipulation, heightened trade barriers, intellectual property battles, disputes over climate change, dangerous investments in military one-upmanship, new tensions over North Korea, competition for global raw materials, increasing cyberespionage and hacking, fresh military operations in allied or rogue countries—the list of concerns related to an intensifying decline of the U.S. sphere of influence is long. The United States would face the dissolution of its vision of the world.

Based on the facts in this and previous chapters, my contention is that a capitalist cold war has started and will escalate in the future. While economists and politicians debate or deny the existence of such a cold war, China's actions fit the standard definition of the term remarkably well. The *Oxford Essential Dictionary of the US Military* defines *cold war* as "a state of international tension wherein political, economic, technological, sociological, psychological, paramilitary, and military measures short of overt armed conflict involving regular military forces are employed to achieve national objectives."

The United States has tried to avoid a capitalist cold war, but the delays in creating a strategy for facing up to the facts appear to be nearing an end. President Obama appointed a committee to recommend how to deal with the China question. Secretary of State Hillary Clinton said in New York that the United States wants "competitive neutrality" for world businesses. She noted that state-owned enterprises don't just go to market to make money. They "build and exercise power on behalf of the state."[17]

On the eve of the 2012 U.S. presidential election, not just Chamber of Commerce spokespeople, but presidential candidates and election pundits are talking of flexing U.S. muscle, exercising new resolve to fend off the decline of the United States. While many people ignored former Intel CEO Andy Grove in 2010, he essentially called for a "trade war" with China in a *Business Week* article that he wrote. Grove said that he backed a plan to rebuild the U.S. industrial commons with measures like a tax on offshored labor. He added: "If the result is a trade war, treat it like other wars—fight to win."[18]

These are the first real shots in the battle to modify the system of capitalism used by China. People are recognizing that the issue has become urgent. From a strategist's point of view, the United States, ironically, should take a page from China's leaders' play-book. Speak softly, but carry a big stick. Be stubborn and never give in to demands or threats, but make symbolic gestures to avoid appearing to be the provocateur. Act in small incremental steps and never retreat. Negotiate with deference and respect, continue with dialogue and goodwill, and act not out of any ill will, but use power silently to create the same fear of a retaliatory trade war that the Chinese have created. China's leaders believe that their first obligation is to their people and the goal of restoring national preeminence. Western leaders should do the same.

The United States needs a grand strategy to secure its position as a superpower. This is not a strategy that was useful for fighting the Cold War of our fathers. But it is a strategy for capturing nations and building a strong sphere of influence that defines the rules of capitalism. These new rules of capitalism will not be defined by the way the United States or the West has defined them for the last few decades. It is a strategy for playing the game of disruption, with each side fighting for a piece of the global economic and geo-political action to improve its nations. The live-and-let-live, open-market, free-trade concept, in which capitalism leads to democracy and better living standards for everyone in the world, has not materialized. The United States and its select allies must remain the rule makers of global capitalism and influence China to be a rule taker. Allowing China to become the rule maker would entail many hazards to Western democracy and standards of living.

That's why, in the second half of this book, I lay out a four-part approach for crafting a comprehensive national strategic plan. The plan includes reforming budgets and finances to restore U.S. financial power. It includes reconfiguring our capitalist system to strengthen our economy. It includes a plan for going on the offensive with constantly changing strategic moves to disrupt China's rise. And it includes taking actions in the geopolitical realm to ensure that the U.S. sphere stays strong. The plan is meant to be a discussion device to point out the issues. Many may disagree with the suggestions that follow, but few will disagree that these discussion are critical to the future of the United States and its allies.

Many policy makers and leaders around the world continue to search for a single silver-bullet tactic that can fix the U.S.'s capitalist system in one shot. Unfortunately, a great deal more is needed. Part 2 shows how to go beyond symbolic tactics to a long-term campaign for the restoration of American prosperity and world economic leadership. As in the former Soviet Union–United States Cold War, the battle in the capitalist cold war has many fronts. The task of winning is complicated—and many government, civil, and corporate leaders need to be involved. The United States and Western powers can—and will—win. The United States and Western Europe won the last Cold War with resolve and prag-matism. We will win this one in the same way.

Part 2

Crafting Capitalist Strategy
The Four Rs of Strategic Capitalism

Part 2 covers the four Rs of strategic capitalism:

- Rebalancing
- Reinventing
- Reenergizing
- Restructuring

The smart strategic capitalist takes charge of the four Cs from Part 1 by trying to guide competing, combining, controlling, and capturing behaviors to bring more wealth to his or her own country. Because capitalism is continuously changing as a result of the four Cs, capitalist strategy must be resilient and must constantly readjust to new circumstances and the moves of rivals. Resilience and constant readjustment come from the four Rs of capitalist strategy. Strategic capitalism constantly rebalances a nation's ambitions, resources, and threats to avoid overstretch and financial paralysis or collapse. A successful capitalist strategy also constantly reinvents the nation's capitalist system by combining and recombining the four generic types of capitalism to suit the nation's changing goals and competitive needs. Capitalist strategy anticipates that change will continue indefinitely, so capitalist strategists plan ways to prevent complacency and inactivity. Therefore, capitalist systems that win in the long term constantly reenergize themselves by being proactive and continually seizing and reseizing the initiative from their rivals. The best capitalist strategists give their capitalist system the right balance, reinvention, and energy to create the power to restructure the world economic order through perpetual struggles for economic leadership or influence.

5

Rebalancing Ambitions, Resources, and Threats

Constant Reallocation to Prevent Overstretch and Financial Paralysis or Collapse

Napoleon Bonaparte said in 1805: "All empires die of indigestion."[1] In trying to amass ever more territory, they consume more than they can handle. Napoleon got indigestion himself in Russia. After the French invasion of 1812, he retreated from Moscow, returning with only 5 percent of his forces. His catastrophic loss tipped the balance of power away from France. Yale historian Paul Kennedy calls this "imperial overstretch."[2] Empires often grow weak, he writes, "not always by defeat in battle, but paradoxically by the weight of their own strength."[3]

The United States is caught up in a classic overstretch today. It seems to run endless deficits and now faces a serious debt crisis. The cause is always the same: the United States does not think about the long run. Instead, national leaders scurry to create the annual budget as if only today matters. Politicians borrow more to fill the gap and show little thought for tomorrow. The result is that governments often operate inefficiently, take up too much of the economy, and leave potentially productive assets sitting idle for decades. Most important, they reduce the resources available for dealing with long-term ambitions and threats.

This overstretch means that the United States is now borrowing 42 cents of every dollar it spends to pay for its military and social programs. Its ambitions extend to policing, controlling, and operating armed forces in every region of the world. They also extend to providing ever-growing levels of services and benefits for a population that is accustomed to affluence. But the country's capitalist system no longer provides adequate resources to cover the costs of this rich menu of ambitions. It is also running up against an imminent shortage of resources for countering threats, especially as China becomes a major economic threat.

Constantly Rebalancing ART

What can leaders do to halt imperial overstretch? The political and public conversations about dealing with overstretch take an oversimplified approach: either find more tax revenue or cut spending. There is another way. Leaders have the option of taking a more strategic approach that uses more sophisticated logic to deal with imperial overstretch. That approach begins by viewing the problem as a question of balancing three factors: ambitions, resources, and threats (ART).

Let's step back for a moment to define these terms. When I talk about ambitions (A), I mean how much a nation seeks to accomplish: how much territory it controls, how many industries it supports, how many social services it provides, how rich its pension benefits are, how extensive its healthcare coverage is, how much income equality and economic freedom it provides, and how extensive its public works and infrastructure amenities are. When I talk about resources (R), I mean people, money, and even energy: how much will the government draw on the reserves of the nation in order to prevail? It also means how efficiently the nation uses those resources. When I talk about threats (T), I mean threats to the health, wealth, welfare, and security of a nation—military threats, diplomatic threats, supplier monopolies (e.g., OPEC), terrorism, internal unrest, and external economic threats.

The Roman Empire maintained a balance of its ART for five centuries. In the second century AD, Hadrian put a lid on its ambitions by stopping Rome's advance and building walls to define the edges of the empire. In the Republic period, Rome's leaders managed to reduce threats that consumed resources, eliminating them one at a time until the empire had no serious competitor for centuries. In a similar approach to managing ART, the British Empire extended its dominance for three centuries. As it lost one colony, it switched to another, focusing on India after losing America. At each turn, it changed its ambitions and abandoned certain threats (like revolutions in America) to prevent it from declining through a loss of balance.

The strategic lesson these empires illustrate is simple: deploying troops, funds, and materials to cover all corners of the world works fine as long as the empire has plenty of resources. But periods of such seemingly unlimited resources are rare. Leaders who take the approach of strategists will consider adjusting ambitions and threats rather than just spending their countries into decline, which can end in default on massive national debts.

Vaulting ambition is essential in the early days of empire, whether the empire is military or economic. But, over time, that ambition may need to be rolled back to match the changing circumstances. American capitalism has been very effective in the past—of that there is no question. The United States developed a form of capitalism that allowed it to become one of the greatest global powers the world has ever seen. For more than a century, U.S.-style capitalism reigned supreme. But today that model is no longer sustaining American ambitions. The U.S. model and rules of capitalism are under attack from a new version of capitalism as practiced by China. The logical response is for the United States to rebalance its ART to meet this new threat.

Rebalancing means adjusting to a new form of capitalism. It means scaling back the country's ambitions to match its resources. A lack of balance risks destroying a nation's capitalist system. Spending too much for too many ambitions or to fight too many threats creates debt, physical exhaustion, mental fatigue, and emotional frustration. As for the United States, a lack of ART balance has two consequences: both a decrease in affluence and an increase in vulnerability to today's prime economic threat, namely China. To get ready to compete with China and deal with other threats to the U.S. capitalist system, U.S. leaders will have to protect their capitalist system by:

- Generating, freeing up, or conserving the nation's resources
- Recalibrating the country's ambitions to reduce resource needs at home or abroad
- Sidestepping or eliminating threats to reduce the need for resources, or selecting a few critical threats to focus on

Constant rebalancing is also necessary because disruptive nations, such as China, seek to keep their rivals off balance (as discussed in Part 1). They take steps to reduce their competitors' resources, to encourage competitors to overextend their ambitions, and to increase threats that waste or divert competitors' resources. National leaders who simply try to maintain a balanced budget and accept trade imbalances, ignoring the way their competitors shift the ART equation, will find that they lose the ability to manage overstretch.

To maintain a competitive advantage, established countries recalibrate their long-term ambitions, reducing the scope of those ambitions so that the country can focus on and win against impending threats that require more effort. They investigate marshaling more resources, but they look beyond raising taxes to building a capable, motivated bureaucracy and reducing bloat and waste. And they select the right threats and counter them, seeking to avoid or neutralize other threats through cooperation or co-optation.

Leaders of successful, well-established, world-leading capitalist systems stay on the lookout for signs of disruption that may cause an imbalance in ART and hence a long-term decline. Sadly, few national leaders today have done so. Greek and Italian leaders have instead made themselves poster children for a lack of strategic thinking about ART. The United States has hardly provided a model in response. It has lost its balance with respect to ART, partially as a result of its own mistakes, but also partially as a result of China's strategy of disrupting the American capitalist system.

Overstretch and the Turnaround of America

The signs that the United States has lost its balance are obvious from the nation's bottom line and balance sheet. The nation now runs an annual deficit of $1.7 trillion. The balance sheet is loaded with more than $15.5 trillion in debt, even though the GDP is only $15 trillion. The fiscal future, to say the least, is clouded. Though on a delayed schedule, the United States faces the same pressures as Greece and Italy. It is in line for a superpower decline, just the same as the Soviet Union, because its ambitions have exceeded what the country can afford.

While we can't say where this approximately $50,000-per-person national debt will lead the United States, a cautionary tale of a country that didn't take decisive steps in a similar situation is Japan. The Japanese property bubble began to burst in the early 1990s. As observers watched incredulously, the manufacturing juggernaut of the 1980s slid from prosperity to crisis in just months during the mid-1990s. As debt soared, Japan came to have the highest ratio of debt to GDP in the Organization for Economic Cooperation and Development (OECD), today hitting 230 percent. Japanese banks didn't write off money-losing loans, but instead kept these zombie loans on the books, depressing credit and bank profits for years.

The message is hard to swallow but essential to digest: if the United States does not restore its financial fundamentals by downscaling its ambitions to what the nation can afford, our children and grandchildren will blame us not just for a cyclical downturn, but for a generational decline that may trap the United States for decades, like Japan.

As I write, the U.S. public debt–to-GDP ratio stands at 72 percent.[4] The gross debt ratio, including debt held by all government agencies, is more than 102 percent. Economists Carmen Reinhart and Kenneth Rogoff compiled data from more than 200 years of global economic history to show that in countries with public debt–to-GDP ratios above 90 percent, median GDP growth rates fall by 1 percent per year. Average growth falls even more.[5]

The urgency of cutting the debt cannot be overstated in any rational strategy to restore America's economic health. That's because the debt keeps growing so fast. The Government Accountability Office (GAO) estimates that with persistent and growing deficits, debt held by the public will exceed its post–World War II high of 109 percent of GDP by 2021, less than 10 years away.[6] At that point, we can expect to be long past the point of suppressing U.S. growth rates.[7]

How much does a 1 percent decline in GDP growth add up to? A 1 percent decline, compounded over 10 years, adds up to an economy that is more than 10 percent smaller. In the United States, with $15 trillion in GDP, that translates into more than $1.5 *trillion* less in GDP. That's enough to pay for 13 million jobs at today's wage and benefit rates. It is enough to fund the entire annual payroll for all of the more than 2 million civilian federal jobs *10 times over*. It is roughly equal to the entire annual GDP of Canada or South Korea. In other words, it would be as if a couple of large states in the United States disappeared.

Though some economists disagree over threat levels, we need to target a much lower debt-to-GDP level. The International Monetary Fund has suggested a target 60 percent gross debt–to-GDP ratio.[8] The European Union stipulates a 60 percent public debt–to-GDP ratio for countries that want to join the European Union. Of course, this threshold remains a minimum target. The IMF target would mean a mind-bending $6.2 trillion cut in the current U.S. debt levels, nearly $20,000 for every man, woman, and child in America (as of March 2012).

Government overspending shows that the United States is having terrible trouble exercising fiscal control. Borrowers who see a government that cannot summon the will to control itself are likely to lose faith in the United States as a safe place to invest money. The same goes for credit-rating agencies, which have been lowering rates on sovereign debt around the world. The uncertainty raises interest rates. That puts the United States in the hole even farther, as each time it refinances old debt with new debt, it has to replace old debt with securities that pay higher yields. This creates a vicious cycle that, if unstopped, becomes the mother of all overstretch, as the Greeks and Italians discovered in 2011.

If America is to have the strength to compete with China for world economic leadership, its first order of business must be to restore itself to economic health by balancing its ART. When dealing with overstretch, balancing ART is really a process of dealing with three imbalances:

- *Resources falling short of ambitions and threats.* The country has inadequate resources to carry out its national ambitions or deal with threats.
- *Ambitions outrunning resources and threats.* The country has broad ambitions that are unaffordable, especially given the magnitude and number of threats.
- *Threats overwhelming ambitions and resources.* The country faces powerful or unmanaged threats that exhaust its resources or leave inadequate resources to achieve its ambitions.

A good capitalist strategy must take all three imbalances into account simultaneously.

Increasing Resources to Match Ambitions and Threats

Perhaps the most fundamental aspect of a successful capitalist strategy is setting long-term economic goals that will increase or free up future resources. This requires tough choices about priorities. To guide those choices, successful leaders first establish quantitative benchmarks for their countries. Like leaders of corporations, they cannot strive for success without having a measure of what success looks like.

Setting National Economic Goals

Here is a list of economic and government benchmarks that nations—especially the United States—might follow over the long run to keep adequate resources available to pay for the ambitions of the capitalist system and to fend off threats to that system.

1. To ensure an evergreen fount of resources from the economy:
    -   *Prudent debt levels* of no more than 60 percent of GDP (gross national debt to GDP).[9]
    -   A *healthy GDP growth rate* of approximately 3.28 percent, the average growth rate of the United States from 1947 to 2011.[10]
    -   A *modest unemployment rate* of less than 5 percent, or the "natural" rate of unemployment.[11]
2. To conserve resources by managing the efficiency of government:
    -   *Efficient operation of government social programs*, with at least 86 percent of the dedicated funds going directly to beneficiaries of the program, rather than to bureaucracy, management, overhead expenses, and costs of raising funds from Congress.[12]
    -   *Efficiency in public service*, in which government services take no more than 17 to 25 percent of GDP, compared to the 36 percent spent by the U.S. government today.[13]
3. To ensure future resources by not squeezing selected taxpayers too much:
    -   A *shared burden of taxes* spread across all citizens but the most indigent, rather than creating a divided nation of people who pay and people who get the benefits. Today, the top 10 percent of U.S. income tax filers pay 70 percent

of all income taxes. Meanwhile, the bottom 50 percent of filers pay less than 3 percent of all income taxes, and 70 percent of Americans take out more than they pay into the federal government. [14]

4. To create new resources—competitive advantages—for the nation:

- *Annual government investment* in R&D of at least 2.4 percent of GDP (equivalent to the 1964 U.S. peak). To match some of the world's leading R&D rates today, the United States would have to spend between 3.5 and 5 percent. [15]

- *Annual government investment* in infrastructure development of at least 6 percent (equivalent to the 1951 U.S. peak), compared to the current U.S. rate of 2.4 percent. To match the infrastructure development rates of competitors, the United States would have to spend 5 percent (Europe) to 9 percent (China) of GDP. [16]

- *A strong, self-sufficient manufacturing base*, with 20 percent of all jobs in the country being in the manufacturing sector. [17]

5. To shift the economy from spending money now to investing for the future:

- *A national savings rate* of approximately 14.6 percent—the U.S. (December 1, 1975) peak rate—compared to the current 4.6 percent (January 1, 2012). The U.S. savings rate had slipped to a low of 0.9 percent in 2001 (October 1). [18] A 14.6 percent goal is still lower than, for example, Germany's rate of more than 16 percent, [19] and far lower than China's savings rates during the early 2000s, which ranged from 38 percent to a whopping 53 percent. [20]

- *A personal consumption rate* of 88 percent of disposable income (the U.S. rate in 1980), compared to the U.S. peak of just over 95 percent in 2005. [21] If people spend everything they make, they will be living hand to mouth. The goal of an 88 percent consumption rate is still far higher than China's rate of 40 percent, where the government actively discourages consumption.[22] The goal is to encourage a shift from overconsumption in the short run to saving and investment in the long term.

Policy makers may argue over the measures and the benchmarks given here. But from the point of view of developing an effective strategy, all organizations need goals, and the people that run those organizations should be held accountable for delivering results.

Today, politicians get paid whether their country does well or not. The system encourages quick fixes—repeated doses of watered-down jobs programs and quick-hit jolts of stimulus that keep countries upright but in a wheelchair. Instead, the system's incentives could encourage the achievement of long-term goals that can be met with long-term plans. Congressional, presidential, and executive-level civil service salaries should include deferred compensation that rises if the nation achieves its stated goals in the future. Otherwise, politicians and governments will remain too shortsighted.

Redirecting and Freeing Up Government Resources

When the economy is not generating enough resources, successful leaders redirect existing government resources to achieve higher-priority national ambitions or fend off critical threats. In good times or bad, they also look at hidden and idle government assets that are being underutilized. These assets can be converted to cash or redirected to new uses. In a turnaround economy, the task of redirecting and freeing up resources remains one of the most urgent of all. Even in good times, it remains essential to competitive advantage.

I am not the first and I won't be the last to say that today's federal spending is not sustainable. It's a debate that's been raging for years. Suffice it to say here that this is now so urgent and so integral to the long-term future of the United States that the decision cannot be put off any longer. (Some of the specific tactics I would offer for discussion can be found at my website, www.radstrat .com.)

Many observers will object that revenue-raising and belt-tightening measures during a soft economy could slow job creation. They could also plunge the nation into another recession. People who lose jobs and go without raises stop consuming and slow the United States' consumption-based economy. Some risk of bogging down near-term economic recovery is real. And yet the nation's leaders who concern themselves with long-term strategy will have to consider the alternative: much more difficult cuts in the future as the debt balloons. The U.S. government and consumers are addicted to living on debt. Like addicts who are forced to kick a habit, the United States will have to go through near-term pain to achieve long-term gain; national leaders will have to help.

Matching Ambitions to Resources and Threats

Balancing ART can also involve cutting back on the nation's ambitions in order to reduce the nation's resource needs. This begins with questions such as: What ambitions can we fund? Which must we shrink? Many of our ambitions remain worthy, but our leaders would do well to consider how those things can be prioritized and sequenced. It is not easy to pare them back. But as in any turnaround, leaders will have to target those that drain the most resources from the U.S. Treasury and national trust funds and scale them back. They will then want to transfer money to those ambitions that will create fresh resources for the future, position the country for growth, or deal with the major threats of our times.

Shrink Ambitious Entitlement Programs

The largest item in the U.S. budget is entitlements. Social security, Medicare, Medicaid, and low-income assistance (welfare) add up to more than 50 percent of the federal government's expenditures.[23]

To be sure, cutting benefit programs for individuals cannot become a tool to reverse the United States' longstanding commitment to taking care of the poor—that would reduce our social safety net too much, adding a new level of worries for Americans. Nevertheless, there is no doubt that entitlements will have to be cut if the United States is to balance its budget.

The approach to trimming should follow a philosophy aimed at building the nation's capacity to compete in the future. To start with, leaders should consider favoring programs that serve the "deserving" rather than the "undeserving" poor: the weak and elderly rather than the young and able-bodied. The cuts should also encourage responsibility and not dependency, personal development and not personal indulgence. A leader's ambition should not just be to cut spending, but to cut it in a way that makes the nation stronger and its people more self-reliant.

Consider Singapore, one of the best-run countries (financially) in the world. The Singaporean government funnels up to 20 percent of every citizen's wages directly into a compulsory savings/retirement account, with up to a 16 percent employer match.[24] Singapore also requires additional savings of up to 9.5 percent for healthcare. People then take care of themselves with their own money. (Clearly, Singapore is not a template that the United States would want to follow in other areas—for example, I am not advocating Singapore's policy of mass sterilization of women—but the country does offer some financial pointers.)

The biggest opportunity for shrinking entitlements while making the nation stronger is in changing social security. Franklin Roosevelt started social security as a safety net. People today treat it as a retirement plan. Thus begins the problem. People don't save what they should for their later years. That's not entirely their fault. Uncle Sam discourages them from doing so by repeatedly promising more money and providing tax incentives for spending today what they should be saving for tomorrow. Meanwhile, the Federal Reserve discourages savings by keeping interest rates on savings low.

As a result, the United States should change the incentives in the program, returning the responsibility for managing retirement savings to the public. True, George W. Bush didn't have much luck selling social security privatization to the American people. But the nation would benefit from again brainstorming to figure out a better way to encourage people to take their retirement future in their own hands.

The benefits of moving in this direction would also include eliminating the fiscal drain created by the structure of social security. The government funds the program by taking from current contributors to pay for the retirement of earlier ones. This works only as long as more is coming in than going out. If more isn't coming in, the scheme collapses. Politicians have taken heat for calling social security a Ponzi scheme. But apart from its being backed by the federal government, social security has a funding mechanism that is similar to a Ponzi scheme. Today the U.S. social security program scoops up less money than it needs if it is to honor its promises in the future. As in all pyramid schemes, the con promising the gilded returns will eventually not make good on his promises. Nobody stands to lose everything he or she paid into social security, of course. Still, people younger than 60 can look forward to Uncle Sam slashing the promised payout.

In the long run, the United States will have to shift this pay-as-you-go program to a save-for-your-future plan. One idea is to move to adopt personal retirement accounts through which people fund their entire retirement. Think Singapore again. I don't advocate turning the average Joe and Jane of America into investment managers. The stock market often defeats them because it is hard to "beat the market," as many finance professors will tell you. Instead, the United States might consider requiring individuals to invest their money in government-guaranteed accounts and U.S. treasury bonds. The additional benefit would be that the funds could be used for U.S. bonds devoted entirely to funding infrastructure investments (such as roads, bridges, and water systems) that charge tolls or fees so that the money to pay the investors back could accumulate over time. The government could make the investments appealing to investors by having the bond interest be tax-free when withdrawn in retirement, and by offering bonds at reasonable interest rates that exceed the artificially reduced rates in public financial markets due to the policies of the Federal Reserve Bank.

The changeover could happen slowly. Recipients of social security today rely on current payments by workers, and the system would have to stay that way for years to come. As the save-for-your-future program is phased in for people under 40, the United States would restructure the pay-as-you-go program for everyone else. That means that the United States would have to reduce the promises made under the current system. The country can ill afford to wait to make this transition. People are living longer—on average 14 years longer than when Roosevelt signed the Social Security Act into law. People also want to retire earlier. So the costs are going up, and the number of payers is going down. In 1950, 16 workers paid for every beneficiary. Today, it's 3, and in 2025, it will be just 2.3.[25]

Many think tanks have laid out detailed plans for changes that might work for America. One workable approach appears in the report by the president's bipartisan deficit-reduction commission, led by former senator Alan Simpson and Erskine Bowles. Suffice it to say the commission recommended that the United States pare the cost-of-living adjustment, gradually increase the retirement age based on life expectancy, and increase the payroll tax cap to bring in more money. These changes will cause pain, but greater pain will result from putting a relentless drag on economic growth by repeatedly going to taxpayers to cough up more cash for unfunded liabilities. The United States does need social security as a safety net to catch people who fall off the economic bridge as they age. But we need to have fully funded government retirement programs to ensure the safe passage of seniors through retirement.

Cap or Cut Programs That Are Not Essential
In the United States, some low-hanging fruit for cuts includes subsidies for flood insurance. If people take the unreasonable risk of

living in a flood plain, they should take the risk themselves, without expecting the government to pay for rebuilding. According to the Third Way, a Washington, DC, think tank, cutting flood plain insurance subsidies would save $8.0 billion over 10 years, leaving $2 billion of the current subsidy for the poor.[26] Another example is the mortgage interest deduction on second homes, which applies to vacation properties and even yachts. Cutting the deduction, Third Way estimates, would save $8.9 billion over 10 years.[27] A third example is ceasing to subsidize waste in unemployment insurance, such as giving benefits to millionaires and to those who do not follow through on requirements to look for work. Third Way calculates that this would save $8.0 billion over 10 years.[28]

We should, of course, also consider consolidating overlapping benefit programs under one roof. As the Simpson-Bowles report notes, Congress often fails to cut outdated programs, instead creating new ones to solve the same problems. An example: "The government funds more than 44 job training programs across nine different federal agencies, at least 20 programs at 12 agencies dedicated to the study of invasive species, and 105 programs meant to encourage participation in science, technology, engineering, and math."[29]

Our rethinking needs to extend to benefit programs for businesses as well. Among the best examples are the accelerated depreciation provisions for specific non-income-producing frills. According to the Third Way, increasing corporate aircraft write-off periods from five years to the seven years required in the airline industry would yield $3 billion over 10 years.[30]

In the meantime, Congress needs the courage to adopt more measures for self-discipline. Alan Simpson and Erskine Bowles gave several of them in their report: Cap discretionary spending at precrisis levels for the next 10 years. Enforce the caps with strict new voting procedures in Congress. Require the president to set annual limits on war spending when there is no formal declaration of war approved by Congress. Budget for disasters honestly and stop the abuse of "emergency" funding. Require a "Cut and

Invest Committee" to annually identify 2 percent of spending that can be cut and transfer half the cuts to invest in science education, an infrastructure bank, and high-value R&D.[31] It may be time for Congress to give the president a line-item veto to remove budgetary items until the budget is balanced.

Again, I am aware of the many voices that are already engaged in this debate. It is absolutely vital that these issues be addressed, but this book is not the place for that. Suffice it to say that this problem is now too urgent and too damaging to ignore.

One obvious area is reforming the U.S. healthcare system. The Simpson-Bowles Commission identified billions in savings from reform in the administration of Medicare and Medicaid. The government would save $110 billion over 10 years by reforming Medicare deductible and coinsurance rules. It would save $49 billion over 10 years by extending drug rebates available to Medicaid beneficiaries to those who are eligible for Medicare's Part D program. It would save $60 billion over 10 years by reining in excess payments to hospitals for physician training.[32]

Some cost increases in healthcare have nothing to do with the system itself. They come simply from advances in medicine. Developing and deploying new drugs, tools, procedures, and therapies cost big money. That makes reform to eliminate the all-you-can-eat healthcare buffet essential. The lack of patient and physician restraint in healthcare usage drives up costs immeasurably. U.S. leaders would do well to act quickly to contain Americans' spending habits. They should consider crafting a strategy for reform that sidesteps the counterproductive lobbying of doctors, hospitals, and insurance companies. A high-level strategy is essential if the United States is to make low healthcare costs a competitive advantage for businesses operating in the United States.

Focusing on Threats to Match Resources and Ambitions

Strategic capitalists seek to reduce or avoid threats in order to balance them with ambitions and resources. In good times, a nation may take on new threats if they are the price to pay for expanding the ambitions of society. But in a turnaround, an economic leader's strategy will have to consider reducing or avoiding costly threats or targeting the threats that are most important. Let's look at a couple of essential threats that must be dealt with if the United States is to survive and thrive.

Fixing Threats from Within

Perhaps the most difficult threat to avoid in America is politics. The same is true in most democracies. Politicians tout populist policies or bicker over ideology rather than solving the problems. They play politics to embarrass members of the opposing party. Matters get worse during an economic downturn. As resources decline, the political debate becomes principally a squabble over how to divide the economic pie. The first casualty is often serious debate about how to make the pie bigger or readjust national ambitions. U.S. political leaders have repeatedly fallen into the politics of division. To create a rational strategy to balance ambitions, resources, and threats, the United States faces the challenge of reforming certain elements of its political system.

I draw a sharp distinction here between democracy, which is vital to the freedoms we enjoy as U.S. citizens, and the political system through which U.S. democracy is enacted, which is a major factor in the current impasse. Strategic capitalism would require bipartisanship on a scale probably seen only during times of world war and national emergency. But I believe that this is the scale of the crisis that we now face. To make rational strategic policies requires all parties to place the national interest first. How best to achieve that?

To begin with, as noted earlier, a strategist would suggest that the members of Congress have their pay tied to the achievement of national economic goals. No improvement, no bonus. Part of the members' pay should be deferred compensation, payable only if the long-term goals set today are met in the future. Citizens are not served well when their leaders' incentives revolve mainly around getting elected rather than around improving the country.

For this reason, the nation could also reconsider term limits, campaign financing reform, and a balanced-budget amendment. Term limits will usher in new thinking. Campaign financing reform will reduce the undue influence of special-interest lobbying, unions, and a small number of billionaires funneling money through super PACs. A balanced-budget amendment will force politicians to stop buying elections with a "chicken-in-every-pot" ruse.

The United States could consider reforms to prevent politicians from pushing extreme platforms, usually to satisfy vocal minorities. This requires a change in the primary system for nominating presidential and congressional candidates. During primaries, the turnout is low, and those who vote are mostly favorers of strident special interests and ideologues with views that are far to the left or right of the general public. The process forces candidates to pander to the ideologues and special interests. When the general election arrives, the mass of independent voters must choose among the partisan extremes. Primaries do not provide candidates that represent the country's wishes because party zealots and special interests are more motivated to participate. The United States could consider returning to the processes of the past, where party leaders, brokered conventions, or state legislatures nominate candidates. On the surface this seems less democratic, but historically it produced great leaders, from John Adams to Abraham Lincoln to Harry Truman. These methods actually produced more centrist candidates and gave a chance to candidates who were not wealthy and could not afford to spend millions of dollars to get nominated.

Another aspect of democracy also poses a threat. Congress takes too broad a reach in controlling U.S. commerce. Its members take it upon themselves to do something about every problem in America, often with unintended consequences. Vastly expanded regulatory burdens are the result.

As other countries have loosened regulatory strictures on their economies, aiming to support more business operations and start-ups, the United States has dropped in the rankings of the easiest countries to do business in. In the 2011 survey by the International

Finance Corporation and the World Bank, the United States ranked fifth, behind Singapore, Hong Kong, New Zealand, and the United Kingdom.[33]

"Doing business" rankings weigh a country's rules for property rights, resolving conflicts, contracting between partners, protections against abuse, and so on. The United States can improve in many ways, even if it already has a competitive advantage over most countries. It ranked especially low in "dealing with construction permits," where it was twenty-seventh, and in tax paperwork and tax rates, where it was sixty-second.[34] Although the United States still ranks well in the eyes of businesspeople, a smart capitalist strategy should lay out how the United States can do better— for example, cutting corporate tax rates and easing immigration for entrepreneurs and highly skilled labor or scientists.

Dealing with Threats from Without

America faces many threats from outside its borders: Iran, North Korea, Al Qaeda, pirates off Somalia, drug cartels in Mexico. But as Part 1 discusses, none are more important than those that emanate from China. Part 1 identified three big threats to the survival of the U.S. capitalist system, which set the stage for the capitalist cold war.

- China's disruptive attempts to undermine and ultimately replace the American capitalist system as world leader (see Chapter 1)
- China's rule-breaking competitive advantages based on managed capitalism and a vastly different capitalist system (see Chapters 2 and 3)
- China's growing economic sphere of influence (see Chapter 4)

These threats are so big that the survival of America's capitalist system is at stake. If the United States' capitalist system fares poorly, the country's ability to support a strong military will decrease. This would, in turn, put America's national security and welfare at stake. These threats from China are not ones that U.S. leaders can ignore, reduce, or sidestep. Rather than minimizing them, as the United States has been doing for more than a decade, it is time for leaders to sidestep the smaller ones and focus on the most critical threats of our time. That is, leaders would do well to narrow their focus and target U.S. resources toward China. And they should plan to deal with the secondary threats when our economy can afford them, or deal with the secondary threats by creating international consortia that pay some of the burden if these threats require immediate attention.

If U.S. leaders do not act with courage, they can look for a future of accelerated decline, as has already been set in motion in Europe. Without leaders who will tell their people that they must accept some pain now to avoid more later, the members of the public will protect their berths on the economic ship, and they will ride the ship down, just as people have done in declining empires over the millennia. They will accept overstretch and lose the chance of a future that promises constantly rising standards of living. How sad it would be if this were to happen to all that has been achieved by the most advanced nations on earth today, leaving them submerged in debt, trapped in a downward spiral of economic decline, and reduced to lower standards of living.

The first aspect of finding a strategic solution is to recognize the historical trap of overstretch, to set new national goals for a financial turnaround, to abandon simplistic debates over taxing versus spending, and to reframe the challenge as balancing ambitions, resources, and threats. With a strategy that renews the resources of the nation, and with ambitions and threats on a tight rein, the United States will conduct global hypercompetition with a vigor that rivals that of any nation.

6

Reinventing Capitalism

Constant Rejuvenation and Revolution of Capitalist Systems

South Korea was one of the few developed countries to avoid a recession during the 2008 global financial crisis. Although its growth slowed to 0.2 percent in 2009, it rebounded to 6.1 percent in 2010, surpassing even the 5.1 percent rate prior to the crisis. What accounts for the vibrancy and resilience of Korea's economy? Most observers would point to the country's enviable position in Asia. After all, a rising Asian tide can lift all boats. But another explanation warrants more attention: the Korean government has guided its economy into a succession of ever more advanced industries.[1]

Working together, politicians, scholars, business leaders, and technocrats have created the strong Korean economy. They did not stumble into a resilient portfolio of industries accidentally. They developed a long-term strategy, a strategy that made the 1960s the decade of textiles, fertilizer, and cement; the 1970s, the decade of steel, shipbuilding, and chemicals; the 1980s, the decade of semiconductors, cars, and small aircraft; the 1990s, the decade of information technology; and the 2000s, the decade of biotechnology, materials, nuclear energy, and similar fields.

Korean leaders nursed these industries from infants to giants using a federal industrial policy. They took advantage of managed capitalism, in other words, to give birth to and protect industries within large conglomerates, or *chaebol*. To detail their intentions, they rolled out a series of five-year development plans over five decades. They then supported the selected industries with low interest rates, trade protections, subsidies, and other incentives. A number of Korean multinationals have since become household words: Samsung, Hyundai, LG, and SK Group. And by global standards, Korean citizens have become affluent. While per capita GDP was $7,960 in 1990, in 2010 it hit $29,004.[2]

Of course, South Korea has stumbled at times. Its economy nearly collapsed during the 1997 Asian financial crisis, in large part because banks lent too much to the *chaebol*, which in turn built too much capacity. The International Monetary Fund (IMF) came to the rescue with $58 billion. But the trouble lasted only about 18 months, and rapid growth thereafter ensured that Korea rose quickly on the roster of global exporters. By 2007, the information technology sector, for instance, made up more than one-third of GDP. It helped Korea become the largest exporter of dynamic random-access memory (DRAM), code division multiple access (CDMA) telecom equipment, and liquid crystal displays (LCDs) in the world.

The 1997 crisis was a turning point. The country's leaders restructured the economy and opened up the financial sector to foreign firms. They injected elements of laissez-faire into the economy. They continued to improve on social programs developed largely in the 1970s and 1980s to create a small social safety net, injecting more social-market capitalism into the economy. In 2007, Korea and the United States signed a free-trade agreement (ratified in 2011). While Korea has not deregulated its industries the way the United States has, it has been discussing the introduction of more laissez-faire capitalism. One thing is for sure: Korean leaders learned that dedicating a country to one form of capitalism does not ensure its success forever. To put the country on a par with the G-7 countries—their stated goal—they had to change their capitalist system.

Korea's rags-to-riches experience holds lessons for all countries. The most important one is that a commitment to one form of capitalism, in the face of an ever-changing global economic landscape, cannot bring a country perpetual wealth. It will bring distress. The most effective way to structure a capitalist system changes with the times. In the same way that companies that stick to one strategy forever eventually file for bankruptcy, nations that stick to one form of capitalism eventually file for help with the IMF.

Korea today has remixed laissez-faire, social-market, and managed capitalism so well that it has commandeered a spot among the leading countries in the most complex industries and cutting-edge technologies in the world. It has, in turn, become an export powerhouse, with trade surpluses with both the United States and China. It has become a job-creation machine in the process, turning out 260,000 new jobs in 2011, yielding a 2011 unemployment rate of only 3.7 percent. It has gained so much momentum that some Chinese manufacturers fear Korea's manufacturing muscle the way U.S. manufacturers fear the Chinese. And all this has come from a national plan to apply the most appropriate capitalist principles at just the right time, in just the right measure, in just the right way.

Remixing the Four Generic Types of Capitalism

The Korean experience reflects one of the key messages of this book: leaders who try to use just one of the generic types of capitalism to manage a capitalist system will eventually lose because they will come up against other leaders who are more imaginative. Winners craft a strategy after analyzing their particular situation. They create a competitive advantage with that strategy by weaving together the right mix of laissez-faire, social-market, managed, and philanthropic capitalism. They don't simply stick to traditional ideologies. They are pragmatic.

The range of possible mixtures of the generic types of capitalism begs the question: how do you choose the mix, and how do you make the resulting capitalist system successful? Here's a list of critical success factors that I observed when examining the capitalist systems of the 15 countries listed in Figure 2-2:

1. Formulation of successful capitalist systems
   - *Start with goals.* A successful capitalist system is designed to achieve explicit goals (as shown in Figure 2-1).
   - *Depoliticize the process.* Technocrats craft better capitalist systems than politicians do.
   - *Trade off the four types of capitalism.* Good systems explicitly trade off the pluses and minuses of the four types of capitalism.
   - *Create a working synthesis.* Good strategists find complementarities and resolve conflicts among the four types of capitalism.
   - *Retain some degree of free-market incentives.* All good systems retain some laissez-faire incentives for people to work, pursue growth, and accept personal responsibility.
   - *Focus on the long term.* Good systems mix laissez-faire short-termism with the long-term planning of managed capitalism.
   - *Favor economic nationalism.* Successful systems favor the domestic economy and exporting, as opposed to the global economy and open trade.
   - *Use trade to heat up or slow down growth and competitiveness.* Trade can be treated as a throttle that is moved up or down depending upon the profitability and competitiveness of domestic markets.
   - *Benchmark others.* The choice of system comes from benchmarking and improving on competing systems.
2. Ongoing management of a successful capitalist system
   - *Experiment with new mixtures.* Never stop evolving the capitalist system. Continuously adjust it to the changing needs of competition.
   - *Mitigate weaknesses as they are discovered.* Most good systems mitigate weaknesses. For example, the concen-

tration of wealth that results from laissez-faire capitalism can be mitigated with social-market wealth redistribution to prevent social unrest.

- *Mitigate externalities as they are discovered.* Good systems also mitigate laissez-faire "externalities" with social-market regulation, but they emphasize prevention over punishment and work to keep the costs to industry minimal. For example, the permitting process for building new industrial plants, electric power generators, or oil pipelines is quick, concentrated in one agency, and based on clear rules.

- *Create continuous improvement.* Good systems include mechanisms for continuous remixing to fit the changing needs of the country's citizens.

- *Monitor the implementation of plans and goals.* Tie the incentives offered by the government to the strategic goals and milestones contained within the strategy.

- *Build an innovation cycle into the system.* Use managed capitalism to pay for basic research, laissez-faire capitalism to help commercialize the basic research when it is ripe, and managed capitalism again to protect or shut down mature industries.

Reinventing the American Capitalist System

If managing a mix of capitalisms has worked for other countries, will it work for the biggest economy on the planet? The evidence indicates that the United States hasn't done a good job at strategically managing its mix in the recent past. The current mixture of capitalisms in the United States has resulted from piecemeal decisions, changing administrations, legacy agencies, experiments, and politics over more than 200 years. Until recently, this has served America well.

The form of capitalism that emerged, based initially on laissez-faire and self-reliance principles, was well suited to the early development of American commerce for two reasons. First, the U.S. economy benefited from a number of competitive advantages: plentiful natural resources, a good supply of hardworking immigrant labor, and, crucially, a large and growing domestic market. Second, the United States did not have large commitments in the form of federally funded social welfare programs, an international military presence, or very high standards of living to maintain. The mix was chosen based on U.S. advantages without regard to competition from rival nations, such as the European powers. In short, by good fortune rather than strategic design, U.S. capitalism was well suited to U.S. circumstances. The benefits in terms of economic growth and wealth creation are clear for all to see.

However, we are now in a different situation. The U.S. model of capitalism is out of step—and out of kilter—with the country's circumstances. This might eventually be able to correct itself (U.S. capitalism has always evolved), but unfortunately it coincides with the rise of a new model of capitalism. To use a metaphor from earlier in the book, the United States is like a champion boxer who has put on a few pounds and lost some of his speed. In time, the champion might be able to adjust his style to accommodate these changes (think of Muhammad Ali, for example). But unfortunately for the champion, he finds himself in the ring with the most dangerous contender he has ever faced, an opponent who is bigger, faster, and stronger, and is executing on a fight strategy designed to bring the champion to his knees.

There is no time for gradually evolution. The champion must adjust his fighting style and adopt a strategy quickly (think of Ali versus George Foreman).

Metaphors go only so far, of course. The point is that what has served the United States very well up until now will not work going forward. The evolutionary approach to capitalism is not sustainable in the face of the current threat. What was a strength has become a weakness that can be exploited by more strategic capitalists. The United States must now come to grips with a more managed—more strategic—approach to capitalism. This involves an industrial policy that protects national rather than corporate interests. For example, we must identify strategic industries and ensure that they remain strong so that America does not become reliant on foreign exports or know-how. But this is alien to current U.S. thinking.

In fact, the United States hasn't done much at all to choose industries to develop in the last decade. Furthermore, the United States hasn't offered anything but ad hoc help to industries, except in the cases of agriculture, defense/aerospace, pharmaceuticals, computing, telecom, and software systems for government needs.

How does the United States apply a mix of capitalisms to fix its struggling capitalist system? Like any organization that seeks to set its course rather than have someone else set it, it starts with a new competitive strategy. Politics aside, the evidence suggests that the right strategy for the United States has four parts: reduce the emphasis on two forms of capitalism, social-market and laissez-faire, and increase it on the two others, managed and philanthropic capitalism. By crafting and properly executing a strategy involving this kind of mix, the United States can regain its footing as the world's leading economy.

Reduce the Cost of Social-Market Capitalism

The place to start reinventing America's capitalist system is with social-market capitalism. Social programs, including social security, make up more than 58 percent of the U.S. government's expenditures.[3] The benefits and services of social-market capitalism, though meant to mitigate the income inequality created by laissez-faire capitalism, have overtaxed the U.S. capitalist system. As in Germany in the early 2000s, the number and form of benefits in the United States create a disincentive to work. The confiscatory level of taxes needed to provide social benefits also dulls the incentives for the entrepreneurial and professional class to invest in new businesses and self-education.

China spends 5 percent of its GDP on social programs, whereas the United States spends 20 percent.[4] This disparity makes it hard to close the manufacturing cost gap. As the overview of other countries in Chapter 2 showed, the United States has plenty of room to make different trade-offs to both restore greater work incentives and make the United States more fiscally competitive. Like people in Singapore, Germany, and South Korea, Americans can accept different trade-offs and find new ways for social-market and laissez-faire capitalism to complement each other.

Here are four options for change. I offer these as conversation starters. I hope they will redirect today's conversation about social-market capitalism. The conversation has become unproductive because of inflexible partisan positions. A lively debate about these tactics can lead the United States in taking the necessary steps to formulate a new overarching capitalist strategy.

Reset Expectations for Leaner Benefits

The United States can change the social contract to provide less. Americans are accustomed to government services getting better and better. This was only natural as the country's wealth grew. But its wealth is no longer growing, and the United States is sending a lot of its wealth overseas in the form of investments, foreign aid, and military support. The government can give individuals more responsibility for financing their lives. U.S. leaders can preach a new ethic: you get back what you put in, unless you are extremely indigent or ill.

When it comes to payouts for social benefits, many people feel that they deserve a healthy payout no matter what they put in. Also, many people believe that they have paid in far more than they have. A two-earner couple retiring today will have paid in roughly $529,000 in social security and Medicare benefits, but will take out roughly $833,000.[5] In times of worker shortages and depressed economies, the default thinking for large benefits must be that the U.S. government can pay out only what the elderly paid into the system. Failing that, families will need to step in to help one another more.

Require Everyone to Pay Some Portion of His Benefits

All people need to pay something for government services as a way to create an incentive to spend money wisely. When people get services for "free," they slip into thinking that they have no obligation to pay back the provider. Healthcare is an example. If it is given freely, people will not shop for the best prices, and they will not think twice before asking for services that are not necessary. Everyone who receives a government benefit should have a significant copay or should have to repay the government to the extent possible. The new ethic should be: everyone contributes something to cover the services that she receives.

The goal is to give people a sense that they are spending real dollars. As described in Chapter 5, one option for making sure that people have a nest egg is to require them to accumulate health and retirement monies in personal accounts. They would then draw from those accounts, with full knowledge that they have control of a limited purse. This is the practice used in Singapore. In the United States, benefits programs could require beneficiaries to cover significant copayments at the time of service. With the exceptions of the very needy and the very sick, everyone would then take some responsibility for his needs, discouraging people from applying for unlimited amounts.

Means-Test All Benefits

Many people who are receiving benefits have accumulated a healthy net worth over the years, especially many older people who are receiving social security and Medicare benefits. Given the nation's indebtedness, these benefits may have to be rationed in the future. Americans have gotten used to an environment of abundance since the end of World War II. However, Americans now live in a world of relative scarcity, which forces citizens and leaders to think more about allocating resources in new ways. The new ethic should be: Everyone will not be entitled to everything, so hard choices will have to be made. This is clearly unfair to the part of society that worked hard and now has to pay for those who are less fortunate. Therefore, whenever means testing is required, benefits should be limited to bare-bones programs.

Direct Benefits to Job Creators

The strategic purpose of reducing benefits to the elderly and poor is to better manage and target the spending that currently goes to social-market capitalism. By freeing up money for managed capitalism, the United States can create economic growth that will increase the government's tax revenues. In the long run, this will enable the government to provide more benefits. The United States urgently needs to move the balance of spending away from programs that redistribute the country's wealth and move toward those that create it—to fund the advances made possible by engineers, scientists, doctors, moviemakers, computer programmers, and entrepreneurs. The goal would be to use government money to invest in creating and supporting industries, creating competitive advantage, and building productive resources, so that the nation will stimulate a constantly higher standard of living.

Reduce the Excesses of Laissez-Faire Capitalism

The next step in reinventing American capitalism would be to cut back our commitment to laissez-faire capitalism. The moves by U.S. leaders to champion this philosophy since the Reagan administration have gone too far. Unlike many other countries, the United States has sought the efficient use of capital (maximizing stockholder wealth) at the expense of job losses. This, in turn, has encouraged investors to move their capital offshore. Corporations, enticed by low labor costs, have spent that capital on moving plants and even R&D centers overseas.

The result has not been to the nation's advantage. When people wear their investor hat, they will say that they've won—corporate profits went up. When they wear their consumer hat, they will also say that they've won—prices of a lot of consumer goods have gone down (or stayed down). When they wear their employee hat, however, the story changes. Many have lost, and lost big. The question is whether the net gain to American workers was worth it: did the gains of investors and consumers outweigh the losses of people as workers? In the last decade, I believe the net affect has not been positive for most people in the United States.

When all is calculated and considered, the strategists leading the nation must make this evaluation. Casual observation suggests that most people would say that they prefer job security, even if they have to pay higher prices at the supermarket and earn a little less on their savings.[6] Consumers seem to vote otherwise with their purchases of cheap foreign merchandise, but few of them actually know the long-term, indirect, and often unintended costs. Put another way, a U.S. capitalist system that stresses laissez-faire capitalism has traded national health for the wealth of a small number of investors and the wealth of Wall Street bankers who help these investors in their quest for the efficient use of capital.

My contention is that the United States has allowed laissez-faire capitalism to go to extremes. When unrestrained, the efforts that champion the search for capital efficiency hijack the worthy aspects of laissez-faire capitalism for the benefit of a few. The main beneficiaries are not workers or professionals, but investors and the financial services industry. Two strains of laissez-faire capitalism are guilty of taking a good thing to dysfunctional extremes: shareholder capitalism and finance capitalism.

Modify Shareholder Capitalism

Shareholder capitalism is a concept that directs company executives to seek one main goal: to increase shareholder value, or stock prices. To be sure, CEOs are obligated to deliver competitive returns in order to attract capital from shareholders. That's a given. But many companies have taken the maximization of stock prices as a goal above all else. Economists justify this view because corporations create wealth most efficiently when they focus on just a single purpose. This is the approach championed by Milton Friedman and the Chicago school of economics, which came to the fore under Ronald Reagan. Economists argue that without this focus, CEOs will waste money and divert cash to overpaying workers, satisfying unneeded bondholder covenants, donating money to pet causes, or providing customers with too many benefits that they are not willing to pay for. Thus, the needs of other stakeholders divert money from the shareholders.

Shareholder power has been increased by the corporate governance movement, to the detriment of a national strategy that focuses on job creation. The power of boards of directors has increased. CEOs are more easily fired if the stock does not perform, and their compensation is often tied to stock performance. Proxy fights are more frequent. CEOs work under much more pressure to meet their quarterly numbers to satisfy investors and security analysts. On the one hand, these pressures have given lazy CEOs a kick in the pants. On the other, they distract CEOs from the long run and from noble goals like building the American economy. Exacerbating this distortion is the short tenure of CEOs. In today's world, they hold office only for approximately three years on average, making long-term thinking a quaint idea of yesteryear.

The unintended consequence of too great a shareholder orientation is that company CEOs are forced to ignore the distinction between creating value for foreign countries and creating value for the United States. So long as they are creating more money for shareholders, they are doing a good job. The irony for national leaders is hard to ignore: at a time of soaring national unemployment, corporations have enjoyed record corporate stock performance.

This distortion can put many CEOs in an awkward spot. By moving money to its "highest and best" use for stockholders, they can become powerful agents in making China (and other countries) more competitive. If they want to keep their jobs, many executives have little choice but to favor moving most of their corporate footprint to China. They have to export American jobs, give away technology, share product and process secrets, and mentor joint-venture partners in management know-how—all hard-earned American competitive advantages—just to make money for their shareholders.

When the time comes to develop a national strategy, leaders would do well to note that, strangely, neither the shareholder value nor the corporate governance movement reflects actual legal obligations of corporations. No statute of incorporation instructs CEOs to maximize shareholder value. When society created the legal entity called a corporation, the purpose was otherwise: to create public good. Each corporation was vetted by a state legislature to guarantee its worth to society. After the Massachusetts legislature rejected Alexander Graham Bell's application to found Ma Bell, he went to New York and got approval to start the telephone industry. Seeking to avoid such incidents in the future, the states created a simple registration process for new corporations that circumvented legislative approval.

Of course, the changes in the laws spurred an enormous amount of wealth creation in America. Still, something has been lost over time. In return for automatically limiting the liability of shareholders to just the value of their shares, corporations were expected to do social good, not maximize shareholder wealth. But as investors got the green light to invest capital without risking personal bankruptcy if the corporation failed, they seemed to lose the sense of obligation to return the favor by doing good for the nation.

As a remedy for this distortion, one obvious option to consider is to restore stakeholder management as a worthy means for corporations to create value for society and shareholders alike. Stockholders earned less during the years of stakeholder management in the United States, but the overall economy did very well. The goal for executives was to simultaneously, or at least sequentially, satisfy enough stakeholders to keep the corporation as a vital value-creating enterprise for the nation. The squeaky wheels of shareholders and unions usually got plenty of grease, but the moral obligation to society was paramount.

Stakeholder management remains common in Europe. CEOs are charged with creating value for shareholders, lenders, employees, communities, customers, suppliers, and so on. The idea is to create a pool of wealth within a corporation that everyone shares in, not just the stockholders. Stakeholder management is thus thought to build a healthier economy in the long term. People hold more and better jobs. Communities enjoy more stable labor markets and collect revenue from a more resilient tax base. Suppliers win steady sales. Lenders put the economy (and themselves) at less risk, as they approve loans at more prudent leverage levels. This approach has worked exceedingly well for German corporations.

Another option to consider in addressing the concern over shareholder capitalism is to champion corporate patriotism. Corporate patriotism puts national needs above the corporate needs. In the battle to win at globalization in the last 30 years, "economic nationalism," or loyalty to U.S. workers, communities, and institutions, became a dirty word in business. Corporate patriotism, however, can serve as a critical bulwark against China's predatory practices. Executives today, enamored with the notion of the globalized company, will find corporate patriotism a quaint idea from a bygone era. But just as corporations assiduously trained their senior executives to replace corporate patriotism with a "global mindset," they could retrain them to follow the needs of a new strategy for national prosperity.

When it comes to promoting corporate patriotism, using the tax code is an option. Here are some examples. Corporations could continue to be charged the full tax rate if they manufacture overseas and sell in the United States, but if they manufacture more than 60 percent of their global production in the United States, manufacture 100 percent of what they sell in the United States, or increase their U.S. payroll by more than 10 percent in one year, they could be given tax credits based on the amount spent to achieve these goals, leading to corporate tax reductions of up to 100 percent. Companies that repatriated profits from foreign operations and invested them in U.S. plant, property, or equipment could also earn a credit against their income taxes by up to an additional 15 percent of the tax, rather than paying additional taxes as they do now upon repatriation.

To prevent a short-term focus on quarterly earnings, companies that spend more than 5 percent of their revenues on R&D in the United States could be granted significant R&D tax credits. Large companies that earn more than 60 percent of their revenue in the United States could also get tax credits, and if more than half of their employees live in the United States, they would get yet more tax credits. Start-up firms could be discouraged from moving overseas when they begin manufacturing through the enticement of a government subsidy or grant, infrastructure concessions, or tax breaks during product development. Tough "clawback" provisions should be used. If a firm had more than half its employees, revenues, stockholders, or production overseas, even if it was incorporated or headquartered in the United States, it would be considered a quasi-foreign corporation and would not be granted the military or diplomatic support of the U.S. government in foreign sites.

The message to businesspeople would be simple: if you invest in things that create jobs and competitive advantage in America, or if you take steps to enhance the U.S. economy, you will get a big tax cut. The cuts should be so large that they allow firms to pay no U.S. taxes if they comply with most or all of the America-centric provisions. (Of course, firms should not be allowed to circumvent the rules by contracting with foreign companies for manufacturing in order to show that all their employees are American.) Naturally, the notion of downplaying shareholder orientation may worry some investors enough for them to leave the United States, but incentives for investment in the United States can be used to minimize this.

The multiple stakeholder approaches based on shared value and conscious capitalism are great starts for rebuilding the multiple stakeholder approach in the United States They will not really catch on, however, except as public relations efforts that are some-times euphemistically called corporate social responsibility, unless national leaders take measures to reduce the power of boards, shareholders and Wall Street. CEOs cannot operate in the nation's best interest if they continue to work under the sole pressure to maximize shareholder wealth and make the quarterly numbers.

Modify Finance Capitalism

Finance capitalism is a concept that asserts that financial markets allocate capital most efficiently, and it directs the financiers who are in control of capital allocation to maximize capital efficiency. Excessive finance capitalism causes distortions in the objectives of the economy. Starting in the 1980s, corporate raiders, private-equity managers, and investment bankers began to transfer huge amounts of value from employees, communities, suppliers, lenders, and even customers to shareholders (including themselves). Like the CEOs following the Chicago school of economics, the finan-ciers would do whatever it took to redeploy company assets to maximize what shareholders would earn.

Private-equity investors took over companies, ostensibly to fix them when they were in financial trouble. They would make tender offers, launch proxy fights, or pressure company CEOs to break up their companies or sell the companies' assets to release shareholder value. At first, some of this activity helped make companies more competitive, so it benefited the nation. But just as often, the finan-ciers would milk companies or transfer wealth from stakeholders to stockholders. This practice destroyed a lot of companies that might have been rejuvenated. In essence, some private-equity firms began the liquidation of America.

Many finance professors have speculated and have found evi-dence that the much-lauded climb in equity values from 1982 through 2000 resulted mainly from transfers of wealth from workers and bondholders to stockholders, rather than the cre-ation of wealth through Wall Street's efforts to reorganize indus-tries. Over two decades, financiers drained value that had once been allocated to employees by holding wages at 1980s' levels and gutting pension plans. They took value from lenders by overleveraging, cutting necessary funds for the long term, and taking excessive dividends to the point of causing bankruptcies. They drained resources from communities by demanding tax abatements and service giveaways. They took value from workers by closing plants and sending jobs overseas.

Despite this evidence, America's financiers, investment bankers, private-equity investors, and mutual fund managers believe that they rank at the top when it comes to creating value for the nation. This is understandable on the surface. By 2001, the financial industry generated 46 percent of corporate America's profits.[7] But this wealth-creating reputation was an illusion, as much of the profits of financial service firms reduced the profits of other sectors of the economy through excessive transaction fees. In addition, the wealth created for investors evaporated as the dot-com crash and the financial debacle of 2008–2009 showed. And the illusion did grave harm to the country. When the financiers lost what they had gained in the financial bloodbath of 2008, taxpayers were forced to bail them out. This was a double whammy for U.S. citizens.

Prior to the 1990s, financial institutions rarely made more than 20 percent of the total profits produced by U.S. companies. They have not regained their 46 percent share as of 2012. Still, even as the economy recovers from the virus spread by the financial sector's practices, the sector makes about 30 percent of domestic U.S. profits, while creating only 10 percent of the value in the American economy.[8] That's 10 percent of the value and 30 percent of the profits. In the wake of those lopsided results, the financial sector has left a string of companies that are limping, indebted, and short of money to survive the next downturn.

Remarkably, the power of Wall Street remains triumphant, even after its irresponsible subprime lending and private-equity practices. Here are some options to consider that would reduce the power of Wall Street.

Control fees. There are ways to rein in the power of Wall Street in order to better balance Wall Street's critical role in providing capital with the needs of the rest of the nation. As a start, the United States could rein in fees. Wall Street asset managers get paid a percentage of assets under management for a client. The fees do not change if the asset manager doesn't perform well (something that no asset managers would allow if they were talking about a CEO of a company within its investment portfolio). Fees could be tied to the performance of the asset portfolio. In other cases, Wall Street financiers are allowed to profit at the expense of their clients. This happens when Wall Street prices an initial public offering (IPO) and buys the stock from the owners in advance. Often investment bankers price the stock too low, so that when the Wall Street firm resells the stock to the public, it reaps a windfall. One option might be creating a market in which young companies could issue IPOs without going through Wall Street. This would eliminate the monopoly power of IPO firms.

Mergers and acquisitions (M&A) specialists who charge major fees to break up firms, only to put the pieces together again, have made a lot of mistakes. Research by McKinsey & Co. and many others has long shown that mergers do not typically create value, despite all the talk about synergies and efficiencies.[9] And yet M&A specialists earn tens of millions of dollars on deals while having no incentive to do a deal that creates value. Rather than receiving a fee based on the size of the divestiture or acquisition, M&A specialists could be paid based on the long-term performance of the deals that they sell to their clients. No synergies, no fees.

Rein in Wall Street's control over CEOs. There are many ways to reduce the power of Wall Street so that it cannot bully CEOs into focusing on shareholders and the short term at the expense of other stakeholders and the national interest. One option is to reduce Wall Street's ability to threaten CEOs with dismissal, proxy fights, hostile takeovers, greenmail, and other financial maneuvers. The U.S. government could give CEOs more freedom to reject tender offers or to fight off proxy battles and other abusive practices such as greenmail.

It could also use the tax code to rein in Wall Street fees. Bonuses for investment bankers and traders that exceed $10 million could be taxed more heavily than earned income, because at these levels, the fee would not have been earned. It would be a result of the oligopoly power of Wall Street firms over the supply of investment money.

Provide start-up and growth firms with new sources of financing. Venture capitalists have become a constraint on company growth. They charge entrepreneurs so much for funding that the entrepreneurs often refuse the capital. The venture capitalists sometimes end up with ownership of the vast majority of a company's stock, leaving only crumbs for the inventors and founders of the firm. Venture capitalists sometimes call the amount that they pay to entrepreneurs and inventors "the management carry," suggesting that the investors "carry" the people who created the value. National leaders could devise new ways of funding start-up and growth firms, so that the venture capitalists will have some competition that forces them to set their prices lower.

Restrict the riskiness of the major banks. Outsized risks taken by banks have plunged the nation into economic distress. Subprime loans and other risky financial instruments could be restricted if a bank's balance sheet reaches a certain risk level. U.S. banks are now given stringent stress tests to prevent a crisis in the future. The United States could also impose criminal penalties for misbehavior or misrepresentation as well as for taking on too much risk. The goal would be to set up some mechanism that would force irresponsible bankers to "settle up" their debt to society. Bankers should also be responsible for the long-term performance of their banks, and they should not be allowed to walk away scot-free after causing millions of others to lose everything they have.

Restrict detrimental Wall Street practices. The upshot of finance capitalism is frightening: financiers are gradually liquidating America. Sears is a good example. Sears was bought by a private-equity firm that aimed to turn the company around. However, the private-equity firm starved Sears of the money it needed to modernize its stores, while never following up on the successful "Softer

Side of Sears" repositioning effort. The result is that in 2012, Sears is declining at a rapid clip, and the private-equity firm is selling or exiting 1,200 store locations. No real turnaround is being attempted. There has been no clever reuse of the real estate and no major effort at funding or rebranding the company. The private-equity firm has not added value but instead has milked Sears over the years and is now liquidating the company piece by piece. Investors in the private-equity firm got their payoff through the larger dividends that resulted from skimping on store modernization.

To stop this type of liquidation, U.S. leaders could develop a strategy to retain the strengths of laissez-faire capitalism while reining in its excesses. Practices like the gradual liquidation of firms that can be turned around must be stopped. Sears could have been saved, if not rebranded.

None of the options just given will sit well with laissez-faire economists. They will argue that unfettered markets give Americans the best results. But this dogged belief in the free market rests on shaky empirical ground. A report by the U.S. Financial Crisis Inquiry Commission, which published its findings on the 2008 financial panic in January 2011, noted that the financial crisis was caused by the deregulation of the banking industry and by bankers who took big risks to earn big bonuses. The worst recession in 70 years stemmed from laissez-faire capitalism in its purest form.

Once again, these options for reinventing capitalism and ending the excesses of laissez-faire capitalism are meant to stimulate discussion. Many other options might be useful for a new national capitalist strategy.

Increase Managed Capitalism Judiciously

The third step in creating a more effective capitalist system for America is to increase managed capitalism. For years the United States has practiced some managed capitalism without admitting it (in some cases even to itself). And, at times, it has been spectacularly successful at creating new industries as a result of government interference in markets. People the world over benefit daily from this success. Witness the explosion of companies in integrated circuits, aeronautics, and satellite communications. Or, more recently, the emergence of industries in composite materials, supercomputing, and global positioning systems.

Divert Resources to R&D, Innovation, and STEM Education

As a first step in developing a strategy that employs the strengths of managed capitalism, U.S. leaders could address R&D. We have let our commitment to investing in R&D falter, slowing the birth of new industries. As other countries broaden their industrial scope, the United States has even lost the ability to make the materials, components, and software that go into new products. The United States can no longer produce compact fluorescent lights, (liquid crystal displays (LCDs) for monitors and phones, lithium-ion batteries for consumer electronics, laptops and hard drives, rare earth metals, and more. The United States is also in danger of losing the industrial "commons" that supports numerous important technologies and products, namely, the R&D centers, manufacturers, machine-tool makers, monitoring and testing equipment makers, and suppliers.[10]

The United States today faces a challenge from China and other competitors similar to the one it faced with the Soviet Union in the space race in the 1960s. The U.S. government spent 17 percent of discretionary spending on R&D to counter the advent of *Sputnik*. But by 2008, it was spending just 9 percent.[11] As a percentage of GDP, the United States now spends less than 1 percent on R&D. In the 1960s, it spent approximately 2 percent. This partly explains why the percentage of U.S.-origin patents granted by the U.S. Patent and Trademark Office has decreased from 82 percent in 1963 to 49 percent today.[12]

The United States has even skimped on research that is critical to national security. One example is new technology for the energy industry. Because energy companies largely rely on federal R&D, the energy sector as a whole spends on average just 0.3 percent of its sales on R&D. That's less than Microsoft spends on R&D in one year ($9.6 billion). The federal government, the only entity fit for long-term research on futuristic energy technology, does not fill the gap. The American Energy Innovation Council calls for the federal government to triple its spending to $16 billion.[13]

When designing a new capitalist system, successful strategists and national leaders are careful not to simply cut the nation's ambitions. They change its ambitions to focus on a selected set of economic ambitions that make sense over the long term. The Simpson-Bowles Commission recommended a "cut and invest" committee. If the United States reinvests money in areas where it delivers a competitive advantage for the nation, it will lay the groundwork for more jobs later. One such example would be to invest in means to exploit domestic coal, gas, and oil reserves safely. This would improve energy security and create jobs at home.

President Obama called for doubling the budgets of the National Science Foundation (NSF), the National Institute of Standards and Technology (NIST), and the Department of Energy's Office of Science. The United States needs this and more. U.S. scientists are ready. In 1998, the National Institutes of Health (NIH) received 24,151 applications for new research grants. It received 49,000 in 2007. In 1998, 19,000 scientists applied for awards; in 2007, 36,000 applied.

True, the return on R&D remains hard to measure. However, in a 2007 report, the Congressional Budget Office concluded, "Federal spending in support of basic research over the years has, on average, had a significantly positive return." That report drew on studies that suggested that research in chemistry, physics, and other scientific disciplines yields broad and unpredictable benefits for businesses of many kinds.[14]

The source of funding for long-term, basic R&D is always an issue. Only a few corporations, such as Corning and IBM, engage in this kind of research. So the government must be the main source of R&D funds. In this respect, the revenue from a value-added tax could be dedicated to expanding the federal government's commitment to funding R&D at 2.4 percent of GDP, the level of the 1950s, compared to the 0.8 percent ($126 billion) forecast for 2012 by *R&D Magazine.*[15] We need to restore the engines of innovation at the National Science Foundation, the National Institutes of Health, NASA, the Defense Advanced Research Projects Agency (DARPA), the Department of Defense, and ARPA-E (ARPA-Energy). Some people call NASA a waste, but few of those people have taken into account the job growth over decades from the R&D money spent by NASA years ago.

Another source of R&D funds is public-private partnerships. Companies are generally not good at basic research, but the U.S. government has shown time and time again that it is good at it. A lot of the growth in the United States in the 1980s and 1990s stemmed from loose public-private research partnerships at places like Xerox PARC and Bell Labs, yielding a steady stream of inventions. Bell Labs came out first with the technology for the fax, the transistor, the photovoltaic cell, and cellular telephony. Basic research is too risky for today's companies, but it creates a fertile field for new industries, new U.S.-based production, more U.S. exports, and, of course, more jobs. As recently as 2001, Bell Labs had 30,000 employees. Now (as part of Alcatel) it has just 1,000.[16] Supporting the rise of new corporate labs would be an excellent use of managed capitalism in America's reinvented capitalist system.

A potentially large source of funds for R&D is the public, who could invest billions in venture capital firms. The nation today focuses far too much on consumption. That lowers the savings and investment rates, starving the country of money for investment in venture capital for R&D and future job-creating industries. As the government redirects money into long-term investments, U.S. leaders should encourage citizens to do the same. Consumption might fuel short-run economic growth in the United States, but venture capital investment fuels the long-term advantage of the nation.

A huge source of funds available for investment is lost when consumers sink nearly all of their savings into homes. Encouraged by the mortgage interest deduction, Americans end up with a nest egg in a single illiquid asset—a big risk, especially when the real estate bubble burst and the financial crisis of 2008 resulted. Despite all the benefits of homeownership, people don't actually get a good financial deal. They often spend more than they would if they rented. They also lose the flexibility to move to take a new job easily. The money that the Treasury loses from the subsidy for homeownership would be better diverted to R&D that creates jobs. To make this happen, the government could discourage consumption, encourage savings, and discourage homeownership for those who really can't afford it. This would free up funds for savings that could be invested in R&D ventures and the commercialization of new technologies.

To support a fruitful new R&D effort, the United States needs a new crop of educated science, technology, engineering, and math (STEM) students. The United States will have to rededicate itself to delivering education in American schools that requires superior performance in the subjects that matter if we are to outinnovate the burgeoning ranks of Chinese, Indian, and other top students around the world. U.S. students today lag other countries in the STEM subjects, which are critical to economic growth. The lag shows up in graduate education as well. In the United States today, the majority of PhD degrees in STEM subjects are awarded to foreigners.[17] This calls into question U.S. readiness to compete based on innovation, and it begs the question as to why we haven't done more to date to catch up.

South Korea provides a good example of what works. The country has many special high schools for the best and brightest STEM students. The government gives these students more scholarships, guides them into the best STEM universities, and bankrolls the living expenses of those who will create the jobs of the future. The United States has only a few such schools in the entire nation, and instead has moved in the reverse direction. The only federal program for gifted students was eliminated in 2011. The nation relies heavily on foreign-born talent, especially in math and science fields, according to the National Association for Gifted Children.

The association identified only 26 states that mandate services for top achievers, and only 23 that set aside money for them. However, 16 states do have special residential high schools for math and science.[18]

Compare that to Korea, which has 19 special science high schools. If the United States were to have the same number of special STEM schools per capita as South Korea, it would need to build and staff at least 100 more special STEM schools nationwide. As U.S. competitors invest heavily in STEM schooling, the creation of new industries by talented entrepreneurs won't be far behind.

For students who are not college bound, the United States could consider another option: create programs to professionalize the workforce. Overall, 65 percent of Americans do not hold a college degree. But the United States can offer training, apprenticeships, and internships that can lead to certification at varying levels of expertise. In many blue-collar occupations, people have no formal way to gain officially sanctioned training credentials. A new system, perhaps similar to the German system, could provide that for people in a variety of new fields. German authorities accredit apprenticeships in 356 fields, ranging from bookkeeper to baker to hair stylist to bank clerk to video editor. Even university students may be apprentices, splitting their time between school and work in fields such as biotech or aerospace. The precise skills and theory used in these training programs are strictly regulated, and every student receiving certification is tested thoroughly. The German company Siemens alone has 10,000 apprentices and spends about $220 million on its training program.

But R&D, Innovation, and Education Are Not Enough

A prerequisite for reaping the benefits of increased R&D is to change shareholder and finance capitalism at the same time. It does no good to create new technology if American corporations transfer it to China in exchange for access to the Chinese market. And it makes no sense to the public if corporations develop their prototypes in America and then manufacture the products in China for export back to the United States. The United States cannot afford to give away so much to China, where over time the top 1 percent of achievers will be in excess of quadruple the number in the United States. The United States is going to have to become the best at exploiting its knowledge and innovation, something that the free-market approach has done poorly over the first decade of the twenty-first century.

R&D, innovation, and education are not enough for other reasons. How can 300 million Americans expect to beat 1.5 billion Chinese at innovation, once all the rural Chinese have been educated and are ready to compete in the global economy? In the long run, the number of people in China's top 1 percent will be four to five times as large as the number in America's top 1 percent, and they will be better (having been drawn from a much larger population). A lot of R&D is successful due to serendipity. If China takes four to five as many attempts at it as the does the United States, then China will be favored by sheer luck.

And how does the United States expect to outeducate students from Asia, where education is taken much more seriously? Tiger moms push their children to excellence, while many American parents are more concerned with the happiness and self-esteem of their children and coddle them more. Their goal is not so much education as it is protection of the child from stress so that the child can enjoy childhood. Add to that the number of television shows, cartoons, and movies that teach students that "attitude is cool" but "brainiacs are nerds." Thus, the United States will have to do much more than innovate and educate if it is to make its R&D effort pay off.

My view is that we must have more STEM students and larger R&D efforts, but our advantage will have to come from superior imagination. Today's advances in cell phones, handheld medical imaging equipment, and 3D printers come from the inspiration that young STEM students got from *Star Trek*'s communicator, tricorder, and replicators, respectively. As these young people grew up, they were constantly looking for how to build the devices they saw as children. The United States must teach its people to dream bigger, risk more, and dare to make the impossible possible. That means the United States will have to teach its children how to fail, how to learn from the failures, and how to get back up after setbacks and try again and again. This, in turn, means that schools must focus more on building character and encourage science fiction writing and thinking.

Establish a Federal Industrial Policy Board

Another option to consider is the creation of a national, autonomous, nonpartisan agency to guide industrial policy, a "Federal Industrial Policy (FIP) Board." Unlike the Federal Reserve Board, the FIP Board would be run by strategists, not economists. The president would nominate its chairman and six other members to six-year staggered terms with the consent of the Senate. They would include long-term thinkers: industry strategists, futurists, imagineers (who, like science fiction writers, predict the technological possibilities of new discoveries), engineers, and cutting-edge scientists. Like the Federal Reserve, it could have its own budget and set its own direction without direct meddling by elected officials. Autonomy would be important to prevent politicians from getting in the way of developing a rational policy. Success cannot come from simply divvying up funds to give every lawmaker's district a piece of the action. Nor can it come from turning industrial policy into a tool for wealth redistribution to unions or to politically connected or failing businesses.

One strategic approach would be to structure the FIP Board with three basic types of divisions:

Industry divisions. These divisions would be organized around industries, such as a Division of Heavy Industry, a Division of Consumer Goods, or a Division of Power Utilities. Each would contain all the regulators for that industry under one roof. This would change the fundamental organization of the government, making it "customer-focused" rather than having a set of departments that produce red tape without tailoring the regulations to industry-specific contexts.

Each industry division would reconsider how to regulate the industry effectively. Less-burdensome regulation would be one goal, but the United States would also need to regulate more intelligently. Instead of being a country in which it takes a decade to get permits to build a new power plant, the United States could take the approach of bundling many approvals, from environmental to safety approvals, together to meet the industry's (customer's) needs. Time limits might be placed on regulatory decisions. The idea is to decide more quickly than competitors. An organizational structure of this sort could help the United States compete with China's fast-track business approvals.

Reorganizing the government not by functions (such as safety, the environment, trade, consumer protection, and so on) but by industry will create a one-stop shop for business. The divisions could, in turn, call on other agencies as "centers of excellence" for relevant legal, science, or technology expertise. "Account executives" at the one-stop-shop regulator could handle all requests from the businesses they cover. The FIP Board would be responsible for making sure that applicants meet the required standards and can move forward on schedule. Auditors could act as watchdogs for lapses and corruption.

In most cases, the use of more industrial policy does not imply using more money or heavier regulation. It may, of course, require seed and R&D monies for selected industries. But it promises a means for streamlining industry regulations, devising protection from foreign competition, and redirecting government monies and corporations to more productive areas within each industry, rather than support of obsolete giants focused on the products and technologies of yesteryear. Industrial policy could also include other tactics, such as channeling more money to industry-specific education, loosening immigration policies to attract industry-specific scientific talent, and changing tax incentives to attract foreign direct investment into the industry. The policy changes would all depend on the needs of furthering industry growth.

MARPA. An additional option for the United States to consider is to create a manufacturing R&D agency like DARPA, the Defense Advanced Research Projects Agency. It might be called MARPA, the Manufacturing Advanced Research Projects Agency. This agency would be responsible for creating the next industrial revolution in America. MARPA would fund R&D on new manufacturing technology and processes of all kinds: information systems, robotics, distribution, automation, distributed manufacturing systems, advanced materials to replace inputs supplied by foreign countries, plastics, composite materials, energy efficiency (shale gas, nuclear power, clean coal, and so on), mass customization, wastewater-processing technologies, water-efficiency technologies, worker safety and environmental improvement, 3D printing (distributed manufacturing), modularization, continuous flow, and other manufacturing process innovations.

These technologies would be chosen on the basis of their usefulness to the future of American industries and the employment of the U.S. workforce. To ensure that the United States retains an advantage over other countries, MARPA could license the technology it funded only to U.S. companies running plants in the United States. The government could discourage technology transfer by penalizing technology exports. MARPA would then become a driver of inventions that build the long-term competitive advantage of U.S. manufacturing facilities.

Another MARPA responsibility might be to create special economic zones that specialize in manufacturing and enjoy special tax breaks. The zones could be sited in depressed cities like Detroit and Utica, giving payroll tax holidays and investment tax credits for all businesses in the zone. Another idea is to create American maquiladoras in U.S. towns along the Mexican border. In these special zones, U.S. companies could build plants, hire Mexican labor at maquiladora rates, give Mexican laborers green cards, and allow them to bring their families to the United States so that they would stay and spend money in U.S. stores. These plants would provide the United States with an inexpensive labor force to compete with China while avoiding the escalating taxes and drug-related corruption in current maquiladora locations in Mexico itself.

MARPA could also be responsible for programs and policies to spur enablers of innovation across all economic sectors. Enablers would include basic and applied research institutions, companies that do artistic design work or make rapid prototypes, firms that do product testing, and other enablers, such as producers of machine tools and software developers.

Observers will raise the objection that MARPA won't make good investments every time. This is not a valid criticism, as MARPA would operate no differently from DARPA. This is also no different from the venture capital industry. MARPA would simply place many small bets on different manufacturing technologies that experts believe will generate future wealth. With foresight, MARPA experts could plan sequences of technology developments that would coalesce into major breakthroughs in manufacturing technology—just as DARPA technologies did.

The Industry Portfolio Management Division. From the point of view of a strategist looking to develop a strong portfolio of industries for the future, the United States has too few stars and cash cows. It also has too many dogs and question marks. That was the conclusion from the analysis in Figure 6-1.

To explore this further, let's look at the portfolio of industries in the United States to see if unfettered evolution has led to a good portfolio.[19] A nation's industry portfolio can be viewed on a graph as shown in Figure 6-1. Each industry is mapped using its industry growth and profitability rates. The graph has four quadrants that can be analogized to the quadrants of the Boston Consulting Group (BCG) matrix.[20] Tracing counterclockwise (from the top right) the industries are termed question marks, dogs, cash cows, and stars.[21] The cutoffs between quadrants are based on the weighted industry average growth and profitability.

Some strategists liken the quadrants to industries in different stages of development: The question marks are often industries in their infancy, the stars are industries exploding in the growth

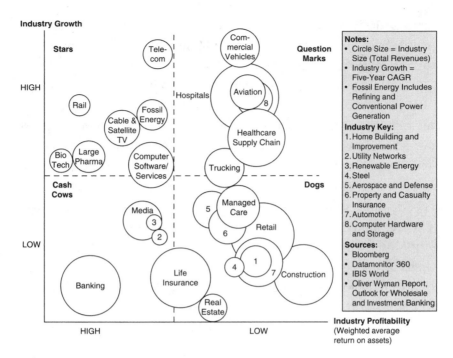

Industry Growth

Stars

Question Marks

Cash Cows

Dogs

HIGH

LOW

HIGH

LOW

Tele-com

Com-mercial Vehicles

Rail

Hospitals

Aviation

8

Fossil Energy

Cable & Satellite TV

Healthcare Supply Chain

Bio Tech

Large Pharma

Computer Software/Services

Trucking

Media

3

2

5

Managed Care

6

Retail

4

1

7

Construction

Banking

Life Insurance

Real Estate

Industry Profitability
(Weighted average return on assets)

Notes:
- Circle Size = Industry Size (Total Revenues)
- Industry Growth = Five-Year CAGR
- Fossil Energy Includes Refining and Conventional Power Generation

Industry Key:
1. Home Building and Improvement
2. Utility Networks
3. Renewable Energy
4. Steel
5. Aerospace and Defense
6. Property and Casualty Insurance
7. Automotive
8. Computer Hardware and Storage

Sources:
- Bloomberg
- Datamonitor 360
- IBIS World
- Oliver Wyman Report, Outlook for Wholesale and Investment Banking

FIGURE 6.1 U.S. Industry Portfolio 2010

phase, the cash cows are mature businesses, and the dogs are at the end stage of their life cycle. While many industries go through a life cycle and fall into the quadrants as predicted, many do not. An inspection of Figure 6-1 demonstrates that not all question marks are in their infancy, and not all dogs are at the end stage.

National strategy or industrial policy can be used to change the portfolio. For example, some dogs may be funded for strategic purposes, such as the defense of the nation or to keep a rival distracted, or to force a rival nation to defend its strongest industry. Some stars may be given subsidies or other incentives to stimulate growth or to create jobs, such as the biotechnology and software industries. Some industries may become cash cows because they are being protected from global competitors by tariffs or regulated in ways that keep prices high. And some question marks may simply be low on a nation's priority list and hence underfunded by government agencies. Question marks may be converted to stars if the government consolidates the industry to improve its profitability or creates a national champion ready to compete in the international market.

To evaluate a nation's industry portfolio, it is important to look at the present and the future. An economy's growth is driven by the number, size, and success of the stars. A country's current prosperity depends on the number, size, and success of its cash cows. The matrix oversimplifies reality, but you can see the point: to figure out which industries will deliver prosperity tomorrow, we need to understand the industries in the economy's portfolio today. The questions for national leaders are these: Do you know where your industries are? Do you have a plan to help them through their life cycle to create wealth for the nation? Have you prevented financial operators from taking them over, liquidating their assets for short-term gain, and sending jobs overseas?

So let's evaluate the industry portfolio of the United States shown in Figure 6-1. While an in-depth analysis is beyond the scope of this chapter, we can make a couple of important observations:

- *The United States is not winning the present.* There too few solid profit generators. Stars and cash cows have a smaller share of the total U.S. economy than the question marks and the dogs. The biggest cash cow, banking, is a volatile, crisis-prone industry. Plus, this industry makes its profits on the transaction costs from the rest of the economy rather than creating its own value by manufacturing products, so the U.S. economy does not generate enough profits. We have not carved out enough high-margin territory to pay the nation's growing bills.
- *The United States is not winning the future.* There are too few growth generators. The stars are too few and very small, and the growing question marks are mainly domestic industries. So we don't grow by trade that brings new wealth into the country. The industries in the star quadrant, key to U.S. profits and GDP growth, are mostly high-tech industries. This is a U.S. forte. And yet they are relatively small. In the

last decade, the United States has not put an impressive number of industries into the high-growth pipeline. So the stars are not aligned for future prosperity.

- *Too many dogs fighting over the same bone.* The United States has too many dogs, including the property and casualty insurance industry, as well as the automotive, retail, construction, and steel industries. We can speculate that the main reason for their poor performance is they are focused on the U.S. market and compete vigorously with foreign firms on a laissez-faire basis. Ironically, the very attractiveness of the wealthy U.S. market draws many global competitors, which in turn squeeze profits for everyone.

- *Too many question marks waiting to be answered.* The largest question marks are the healthcare supply chain and hospitals. Both are high growth but low profit. One can speculate that the low-profit problem is the result of a lack of true healthcare reform that increases the efficiency of operations and decreases the power of doctors and pharmaceutical companies to skim the profits from hospitals and health supply-chain managers.

Overall, the U.S. industry portfolio has not evolved into a promising portfolio because the forces of unfettered competition, global competition, and poor regulation have not positioned U.S. industries very well. Without a strategy, the United States has ignored the potential to:

- Create more stars through government-sponsored R&D
- Develop nonfinancial services–based cash cows that generate new profits (rather than skim the profits off other industries)
- Convert more question marks to stars
- Convert more dogs into cash cows
- Use dogs more strategically to fight off rival nations
- Stop liquidating dogs and question marks (giving up jobs) just to save consumers a few pennies on the dollar

Consequently, the manufacturing sector of the U.S. economy has been decimated. Offshoring has reduced the nation's manufacturing sector to less than half of what is needed to sustain a strong working and middle class. From a 1979 peak, manufacturing jobs have fallen from 19.7 million to only 11.6 million today. Less than 9 percent of Americans now work in manufacturing firms, and manufacturing is now just 11.2 percent of GDP. Today's manufacturing GDP share is down from 14.2 percent just a decade ago and over 25 percent in the decades after World War II. A strategy that addresses job and wealth creation would focus far more on industries that create basic manufacturing jobs. In July 2009, Jeffrey Immelt, CEO of GE, called for building the U.S. manufacturing base to the point where the manufacturing sector employed 20 percent of the workforce. Immelt maintains that the United States has offshored too much. The country cannot rely on financial services and consumer spending to drive job growth forever.

In sum, this industry portfolio analysis, though just a graphic tool for showing the composition of the U.S. economy in a new perspective, again calls into question whether the United States has been making smart choices. Or alternatively, has it failed to make the choices it should have because it is allowing unfettered market evolution to create the portfolio we have? To remedy this long-term drag on U.S. prosperity, a Portfolio Management Division could be responsible for creating a better portfolio by using protectionism, industrial policy, regulations, subsidies, and any other tools that the U.S. government can provide. The goal would be to build new stars, create cash cows, and reposition the dogs and question marks. This repositioning would create a more stable portfolio with better prospects for stable employment for workers and steady growth of GDP.

To see an example of a portfolio that has been managed well, consider Figure 6-2, the German industry portfolio.[22]

Germany has built a very different portfolio from that of the United States. It is much heavier in cash cows. Note, however, that Figure 6-2 divides the matrix into four quadrants with more

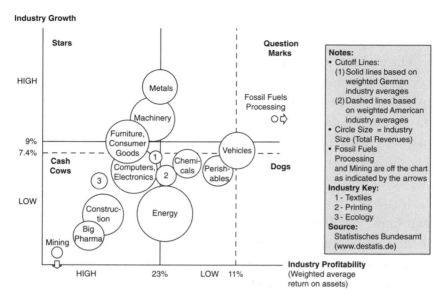

FIGURE 6.2 The German Industry Portfolio, 2011

ambitious growth and profitability percentages than those in Figure 6-1. These are based on the averages for German industries. If we superimpose the American percentages from Figure 6-1 (dashed lines), Germany would have all cash cows and stars. Germany, in other words, has achieved an enviable portfolio of national industries that capture the present and the future. Its use of managed capitalism has achieved just what a prosperous nation would consider a model approach.

Germany has achieved this model portfolio by using policies that support the *Mittelstand,* a group of midsize companies that occupy global niches, sell very high-quality products, and seek out new white space in sophisticated industries to compete in. Some of the *Mittelstand* companies that are recognizable in the United States include Stihl (chain saws), Jägermeister (spirits), and WMF (kitchen accessories and cutlery). Germany has also achieved this portfolio with the support of its world-class multinationals, such as Siemens, Daimler, BASF, Bayer, and Volkswagen, which benefit from the German capitalist system's focus on workmanship and engineering.

The multinational companies and the *Mittelstand* tend to avoid competing with each other, and the multinationals tend to expand in ways that do not overlap with others. This keeps profits high. As the best-quality manufacturer in the European Union (EU), Germany has enjoyed a boom in exports to the rest of Europe since the EU was founded. It is a big fish in a good-sized pond. As part of its portfolio approach, Germany focuses on heavy reinvestment in its cash cow industries. Because of family ownership and government and union involvement, industries get the reinvestment they need if they are to stay evergreen. Obsolete jobs and products are not supported, while new advantages are created for each industry to replace the old products and jobs. In the United States, the reverse often happens, as financiers abandon industries more readily than they fight to keep them evergreen.

How can the United States manage its industry portfolio to keep it evergreen? To start with, it would have to choose some industries to keep for strategic purposes. This would include those that protect national interests: defense, public safety, food, energy, and health. Next, it would choose to build industries that afford an advantage, such as infrastructure construction, materials, and universities. It would also choose industries that already enjoy a growth market at home: military equipment, healthcare, pharmaceuticals, computer chips, biosciences, telecommunications, software, and so on.

To create more stars, successful capitalist systems include what I call a "perpetual industry-creation machine." This machine churns out a string of technologies and start-ups. The United States has created such a machine before in defense, space, satellites, missile navigation, and other industries that stemmed from defense spending. When the machine works properly, the start-ups grow up and become the next Googles, Microsofts, Raytheons, and Genentechs of America. The United States could start with the "enabler" industries—the makers of equipment, materials, components, and manufacturing services—that make new industries possible. After the R&D phase is over, the Portfolio Management Division can coordinate the protection and subsidization of the industry until it has the economies of scale, the experience, the size, the skills, and the technologies to export. Just like big pharmaceutical firms, the nation needs a pipeline of technologies that can move into the commercialization and introduction phases of the life cycle.

To reposition industries so that they become stars or cash cows, the government can provide cradle-to-grave service for selected industries. As an industry goes through its life cycle, the government can provide help at every stage in the process. My research suggests that no single strategy fits an industry from cradle to grave. Successful strategic capitalists adjust the type of capitalism based on the industry's stage in the industry life cycle. At the birth of an industry, managed and philanthropic capitalism do a good job of funding universities and research institutes to conduct basic and applied research. The government can then provide grants, loans, investor incentives, and space at federal research centers and incubators. Without support, young firms have trouble overcoming the demands for short-term profit that can kill infant companies.

In the development phase of an industry, managed capitalism often does a good job of offering incentives to bring nascent ideas to the prototype stage. The government can protect young industries from outside competitors with tariffs, import restrictions, market access barriers, and standards that favor domestic firms. Without breaking World Trade Organization (WTO) rules, the United States can subsidize up to 75 percent of the costs of industry research or 50 percent of the cost of "precompetitive development activity." Thus, the United States can help underwrite everything up to the work on a commercial prototype.[23] This support can help companies avoid the early compromises that can result from responding to the short-term profit demands of venture investors, especially when another country that is more advanced in the field undercuts the start-up industry's quality and pricing.

During the commercialization phase, government can back off and let laissez-faire capitalism take over. As the government withdraws its protections and subsidies, it can allow the industry to rise to the challenge of global competition. At this point, it is appropriate for company goals to switch from development to profit making. The industry can now create wealth for the country, producing waves of new jobs.

In the maturity phase, the government can remain out of the picture. Companies can reinvest where they see the most promise. Their tax payments will support the government's social-market goals. With ongoing investment in late-stage R&D, companies can presumably contribute to society for many years as going enterprises. Eventually, most will decline, of course. At that point, the government can pursue a variety of strategies. Usually, it can remain out of the picture, refraining from using money that would be better spent on developing emerging industries than on supporting dying ones. However, it may want to intervene if an industry presents a way to revitalize the business for the future economy.

Nobody can accurately predict the path that new industries will travel. That means that government needs to keep a hand in guiding the industry's progress. A study by the McKinsey Global Institute found that the most effective help for each targeted industry varies. In some cases, an industry responds well to incubators or tax incentives; in other cases, it responds better to venture capital, special development zones, trade protection, or simply regulatory relief.[24] The trick is choosing the practices from the right form of capitalism to support an industry during each phase of its industry life cycle. Figure 6-3 shows how this worked during the creation of the Internet.[25]

Critics will say that that the government has tried this before, and that the government's record is pockmarked with failures. They will argue that bureaucrats in the government shouldn't have the power to pick winners and losers. They will argue that the United States should let the free market decide. And they will point to spectacular failures, such as the failed (if not fraudulent) loan of $535 million to Solyndra, the solar-panel maker that collapsed in 2011.

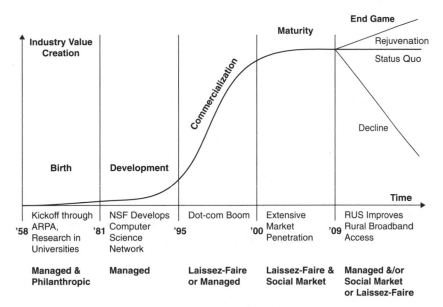

FIGURE 6.3 Adapting Capitalism to Building the Internet

But the logic of these criticisms is faulty. It stems from the once-burned, twice-shy syndrome, a meekness that seems inexplicable in a country of people that, once burned, have been known to try again and again until they succeed. To say that the government cannot do what entrepreneurs and venture capitalists do flies in the face of reality, as the case of DARPA shows. Loan guarantees, of course, may not be the best tool for industrial policy. But using a variety of government tools and accepting some failures couldn't be more in keeping with the American way.

The logic is no different from that in the business of baseball. A major league team needs a broad farm team if it is going to produce major league players. The fact that most farm-team players never make it to the major leagues doesn't signal failure. It shows that the system selects the most competitive players without making big bets on every single one. A few become superstars, and when they do, managers can reinvest some of the earnings from their performance to fund the farm-team cycle again.

All told, the purpose of the FIP Board would be to enhance the country's innovativeness, coordinate actions to build a coherent industry portfolio, reestablish a manufacturing base, create competitive advantage for the United States, and keep American government-funded R&D from migrating to China or other countries.

Harmonize Other Government Policies

As a final step in using managed capitalism more effectively, the United States should consider reforming policies in every branch of government to further the nation's industrial policy. This could include harmonizing policies for commerce, trade, education, energy, taxes, defense, homeland security, labor, and other areas to support what our number one goal must be: fix the economy by fixing our capitalist system. Even while staying laissez-faire in their thinking, U.S. leaders can align policies to give U.S. businesses a global advantage.

These suggestions are aimed at making managed capitalism more productive rather than an ad hoc element in the United States' overall capitalist strategy. Today, the United States relies largely on Congress and the president to make policy and strategy. These policies are often uncoordinated and distorted, to say the least. Sometimes they get articulated during crises, but this usually distorts the policies and limits their purpose to preventing the last crisis, rather than trying to set up organizations to create the future. They are also influenced by political considerations. But, as countries from Korea to Germany show, nations don't have to wait for a crisis and they can make their decisions in a less political way with the good of the nation in mind. They can grab the chance for more intelligent planning today.

As leaders trade off the pluses and minuses of managed capitalism with both laissez-faire and social-market capitalism, they need to study all policies for their consistency in creating national wealth. Trade policy, while normally associated with reducing trade barriers to create more of a free market, could instead become a tool for increasing the protection of fledgling industries—the question marks and cash cows. The United States could also more aggressively use many nontariff trade barriers related to health and safety to keep from violating other WTO rules. The health and safety rules might involve extra paperwork, detailed inspections, licenses, and changing quality standards that delay imports or make them more costly. (An alternative, discussed in Chapter 8, is to withdraw from the WTO altogether.)

Other policies that need strategies include energy, tax, and regulatory policies:

- *Energy policy.* Few observers disagree that the United States would benefit from energy self-sufficiency. One goal might be to target energy independence from all countries except Canada within 10 years. Renewable power will not be ready to fulfill the nation's needs for decades, so in the near and middle term, the United States could develop clean coal technology. It could also encourage investment and R&D to tap shale oil and natural gas more efficiently, develop mini-nuclear technology used in nuclear submarines without accident, and build efficient geothermal plants.

- *Tax policy.* As for taxes, the statutory U.S. corporate tax rate of 39 percent drives investment and jobs out of the country. So does the double taxation of corporate profits earned abroad. Recent moves by the administration to cut the corporate tax rate are moving in the right direction, but the goal should be to cut the statutory rate to below the percentage of most other countries in the world. Singapore's 17 percent rate might be a good target. While companies wait for such a change, U.S. leaders could encourage manufacturing by allowing a permanent 100 percent investment tax credit for all product and process R&D, building of manufacturing facilities, and purchase of factory equipment within the United States. They could also consider a limited payroll tax holiday for all companies hiring new people for manufacturing jobs. Like all other countries in the world, the United

States should also eliminate taxes on income earned, taxed in, and repatriated from foreign countries.

- *Regulatory policy.* As a further measure, the United States could make sure that America improves its ranking for ease of doing business. The United States must be the easiest country in the world in which to do business. That means relooking at the burden of regulatory compliance and permitting practices.

Increase Philanthropic Capitalism

The last part of reinventing capitalism in America would be to increase the U.S. commitment to philanthropic capitalism. Surprisingly, many countries around the world prohibit or tax charitable giving (to discourage the growth of uncontrollable nongovernmental organizations.) Others have no tradition of giving, preferring to pass family wealth on to their children. Although the United States has an unrivaled history of giving, Americans fall short of their potential in building the nation's long-term investment in itself. Moreover, as much as the United States needs more government support for R&D, the nation can compete more effectively if there is private funding that can go to work quickly, skipping the inevitable delays of federal bureaucracy. Philanthropic monies can also enable the United States to compete in many more niche fields—special technologies or rare diseases—that won't make the cut in spending programs with wide national interest.

By building an even larger lead in philanthropic capitalism, the United States can extend its advantage as the most powerful intellectual country in the world. A lot of corporate funding goes to short- and medium-term projects with big upside potentials. Only philanthropic capitalism will fund studies of niche diseases affecting just a small number of people. And only philanthropic capitalism can fund the longest-term, multigenerational advances of knowledge and technology. More emphasis on philanthropic capitalism would also help mitigate the downside of managed and social-market capitalism, in which the public comes to rely only on the government for bettering the world. Two broad options can be considered.

Champion More Giving by All Americans

The United States could shoot for annual charitable giving of 2.5 percent of GDP. That would be a 25 percent increase (about $75 billion) over the average 2 percent that Americans have sustained for decades. The most visible slice of that giving will come from the very wealthy donating to institutions during their lifetimes. But the United States could increase the desire of people at all levels of society to donate their time and money. A special emphasis could be put on greater tax deductions or credits for gifts to universities and research hospitals.

Reform Tax Incentives to Increase Giving by the Wealthy

Although charitable tax policy has undergone reform in the last decade, it has mostly focused on fraud prevention and nonprofit accountability. The United States can do more to increase the incentive for wealthy people and corporations to give money away to causes that will strengthen the U.S. economy. Many tycoons in the last decade have set an example by being major donors, such as Ted Turner, Bill Gates, and Warren Buffett. However, many of these gifts have been given to serve overseas causes. U.S. leaders can champion a philosophy that wealth generated within the American industrial system should be reinvested in the American system rather than in faraway lands. In addition, estate and corporate tax laws can be changed to make it easier to give to charities that create competitive advantage for the United States.

Reinventing Capitalist Systems Around the World

And what about other countries in the world? This chapter has demonstrated an approach that leaders anywhere can use. Every country must continually reinvent its form of capitalism to meet the times. That means adjusting the mix of the four generic types of capitalism—trying new mixes, new ways to execute, and new methods to capture complementarities and fix conflicts. After the fall of the Berlin Wall, everyone assumed that laissez-faire capitalism had won. But even the United States didn't win with unadulterated free-market thinking and practices. It won the Cold War with the Communists with a mix of capitalisms.

Today, some people are tied to the notion of laissez-faire capitalism—so much so that they suggest that countries of the world should resign themselves to a new normalcy, one in which free trade and laissez-faire capitalism leave each country at the mercy of free markets. The future that would follow is grim: for the United States, exports would continue to decline, imports would shoot up, unemployment would hit a new plateau, poverty rates would increase, and manufacturing would shrink even more. Some even advise that leaders accept a new normal in which everyone ends up with less.

But this is nonsense. Countries can craft strategies that mix different generic types of capitalism to achieve a "new" new normal. Korea shows the kind of new normal that most national leaders should seek for their country: quadrupling per capita GDP in 20 years. Other countries can do the same with a strategic mixture of laissez-faire, social-market, managed, and philanthropic capitalism. The notion is relatively simple, even if the execution remains a long-term process. The hard part for leaders is to drop their initial view that success requires one or another narrow form of capitalism. Once they are free of biases, they can get on with the real work—to imagine a new future, to craft a strategy with the four types of capitalism for getting there, and to rouse the citizens of their country to a new ambition for competing globally.

With the nation on this new track, the challenge then turns to the next chapter: how to outcompete rival nations with hypercompetitive strategies. Instead of looking inward to restructure the nation's capitalist system, the next step for leaders is to look outward, to a strategy for jousting with rival nations in a global field of play. In the same way that Korea showed it could develop a strategy to stay ahead of the Taiwanese and Japanese export machines, other countries can do the same. That's what it will take to prosper in the capitalist cold war. With the right mix of capitalisms to build on, the United States and its allies will seize the future.

7

Reenergizing the Capitalist System

Constant Proactive Strategies to Seize the Initiative

In its twelfth five-year economic plan, approved in March 2011, China made its growing ambitions clear. The country that is operating the world's manufacturing hub will now build a design hub as well. Products with labels reading "Made in China" will, in effect, soon read "Designed in China." China will become an end-to-end supplier to the world. It will do just about everything its trading partners now do—innovate, design, build, and deliver—and do it better.

This is no secret, of course. Nor is it a surprise, given that the twelfth plan has been in the making since 2008. What is a surprise is that national leaders around the world don't seem to fully grasp this picture. China is on the offensive, and it is seeking next to destroy the core competence of America: innovation and design.

Unlike in mere competition, in hypercompetition rivals constantly seek new advantages to overturn the lead of their rivals. They initiate moves and countermoves to escalate the competitive game. They seek not just to outdo their rivals, but to disrupt their rivals' advantages. China today is at the top of this game. And as it continues to transform itself, it promises to further undermine capitalist systems in nearly every country in the world.

My studies of corporate hypercompetition shed light on this evolution of competition among countries. I found that very different rules of competition apply today. Old notions of sustainable competitive advantage no longer fit the global economy and marketplace. Competitors have to prepare to gain a series of advantages that last only a short time. They build their weaknesses into strengths so that they can shift the basis of competition and create new advantages. They actively seek to make their rivals' advantages obsolete. They have to produce new strengths that both outmatch and neutralize the strengths of their competitors. And they do all these things in rapid-fire sequence.

Hypercompetition is hardball competition. Going on the offensive with hypercompetition does not take a big economy, as Korea and Germany have shown. It just takes a smart strategy that recognizes—and acts on—the facts of capitalist systems in conflict.

Some of my ideas will be controversial. I am aware of that. But my intention is to stimulate debate rather than cause offense. Sometimes, however, the two go together.

Most people recognize that a country will try to improve its competitive position over time in an attempt to raise the living standards of its people. The notion that a country might deliberately seek to disrupt the economy of another country in order to achieve the same end is more contentious. Some people may worry that by adopting a more aggressive capitalist stance the United States will diminish its standing in the eyes of the world. However, I believe that this is a risk worth taking—that, in truth, we have little choice. An aggressive stance is necessary to get the other side to cooperate and give in to U.S. rules. It may actually garner respect from natural allies as America declares its self-interest and shows its willingness and power to fight for its own interests. In reality, too, other nations are not fooled by U.S. claims to be acting in the best interests of the world. They expect America to act like a leader and find benefit from allying with a winner.

Most economic theories assume that international markets will achieve stability in the long run. This doesn't reflect the reality of how countries constantly strive to upset the equilibrium and dethrone one another. It also doesn't reflect the never-ending disruptive effects of shifts in demographics (aging and gender); mass migrations; regional wars; world wars; revolutions and coups d'état; famine and weather; plagues; shortages of raw materials and water; dependencies created by trade imbalances; growth of developing countries; indebtedness of consumers, workers, and youth in prosperous countries; or the mismanagement and economic mistakes of countries that never allow equilibrium to become reality.

My research also suggests that countries that want to keep up have to delegate current, near-term, and longer-term offensive planning to separate groups. One group runs the current strategy, another prepares the follow-on, yet another plans a third strategy, and a final one envisions a fourth-generation strategy. Successful leaders set the pace of change, allotting enough time between moves and countermoves to recoup their investment, though not so much time as to allow competitors to steal the lead.

One of the greatest challenges today is that China has adeptly turned the strength of democratic countries into weaknesses. Democracies are not quick to respond. Nor do they have the vision, coherence, or fact-based decision-making processes required to win. They get bogged down in politicking, short-term thinking, and a morass of hearings, lawsuits, and legal appeals. Politicians, rather than focusing on overarching goals, angle for votes and cave in to the pressure of the press. They operate without screening their decisions against the one and only critical test: "Does it help us win economically in the long run?" Or, more to the point, "Does this help us beat China?"

Countries in the global marketplace today face winner-take-all consequences, as we are seeing in manufacturing. Now is the time for national leaders to seize the hypercompetitive initiative. Now is the time for them to go on the offensive, to strengthen their economic fundamentals and forms of capitalism, and to disrupt China with superior strategy. Only with a plan to roll out a set of unpredictable one-two punches can they keep China off balance. Strategic capitalists who keep their rivals off balance with respect to their ART, and who take and keep the initiative in doing so, will be the ones that thrive.

Deng Xiaoping decided to take the approach of a strategic capitalist 40 years ago when he saw that his country was hobbled by Mao-era ideology. As Mao feared, Deng was truly a "capitalist roader" (putting his nation on the road to capitalism). Deng saw what the hard-line Communist ideologues could not. As a pragmatist armed with a smart strategy, he saw that economies were held hostage by political ideologues. My research on hypercompetition and seizing the initiative shows that successful organizations use five basic principles. In the case of the United States and China, these suggest that the United States should do the following:

- Reduce its dependence on China.
- Play on China's weaknesses to erode its strengths.
- Thwart China's future advantages.
- Disrupt China's current strategies and strengths.
- Undermine China's centers of gravity.

In the best case, these measures would force China to back down—force it to open its markets to U.S. exports and to play by fair free-trade rules followed by other nations in the world. Alternatively, they will reposition the United States to engage in successful hardball hypercompetition with China. Either way, the United States must take these measures to rebuild and maintain its economic superiority.

While this list sounds very aggressive, it is really only a defense against the extreme actions taken by China over the last decades (as discussed earlier in this chapter and in Part 1). The United States will not survive its boxing match with China if it continues to use a rope-a-dope strategy. It can't absorb the blows indefinitely and China does not appear to be getting tired. As they say, the only good defense is a good offense, especially when you are fighting with an opponent who won't play by the rules and won't cooperate or de-escalate the boxing match.

Reduce U.S. Dependence on China

Heavy U.S. dependence on China poses a barrier to implementing a hypercompetitive capitalist strategy. The amount of U.S. trade with China is so large that many U.S. leaders feel that they do not have a free hand to change policy. Chinese lending to the U.S. government is also hampering the United States from more proactive action. To remedy this situation, one of the first steps leaders could consider is reducing U.S. financial and trade dependence on China. This is a prerequisite for acting assertively on all fronts.

Reduce Trade Dependence

One way in which the United States might reduce its dependence is through a strategy of import substitution. Many vital industries have been taken over by the Chinese—including those that are critical to national security. As of 2010, among the imports from China were $91 billion of electrical machinery and equipment, $83 billion of power-generation equipment, $8 billion of iron and steel, and $7 billion of optics and medical equipment.[1] China's offering of goods for sale—from machine and welding tools to computers and cell phones to sewing machines and software—provides a rich menu of desirable products whose manufacture could bring jobs back to the United States.[2]

Another option is for the United States to draw up a list of 10 critical industries to promote U.S. job growth and national security. On the list would be food, defense, energy, robotics, industrial manufacturing, heavy machinery, electrical equipment, information technology, telecom, and software. The list would also include "enabling" industries like machine tools, which are linchpins for manufacturing excellence. And it would include enough of these industries to wipe out the $295 billion trade gap with China.

Critics will argue that import substitution is inefficient. They will say that it dampens innovation, raises costs, and hurts productivity. And they are right—but only partially so. If the United States gives reborn manufacturers incentives to export, domestic producers will have to compete internationally in order to grow. They will still feel pressure to innovate and run efficiently. Eventually, as the manufacturers regain a competitive footing, the U.S. government can open the doors to foreign competitors from friendly nations to keep U.S. firms on their toes.

Import substitution has worked before. In the nineteenth century, the United States sought self-sufficiency. By World War I, it had made its industrial base the envy of the world. Many other nations have benefited from the protection of jobs, the nurturing of domestic manufacturing capacity, and the improvement in national resilience to external economic shocks that stems from a policy of self-sufficiency. This is not to argue against trade, only against trade that makes the United States dependent on other nations for critical goods, especially on unfriendly challengers for global leadership and military supremacy.

The United States could adopt a new rule of thumb for manufacturing: what gets consumed in the United States should be made in the United States. "Buy American" can be revived as a legitimate way to channel American consumers' money back to other Americans. It would, meanwhile, prevent money from going to closed, undemocratic societies. The United States already has a Buy American law for federal purchases; it could expand it to cover purchases from critical industries that the country chooses to preserve in the private sector.

As an alternative, the United States could negotiate bilateral trade deals with friendly democratic countries, such as Brazil and India. This would be one way to diversify imports away from China and create trading blocs with mutually favorable trade policies.

The trade deals with South Korea, Colombia, and Panama in 2011 are a good way to start.

Reduce Financial Dependence

In tandem with sharply cutting imports from China, the United States could reduce its financial ties with China. This would involve sharply cutting the amount of U.S. debt held by the Chinese. Many Americans fear that the Chinese government, as our nation's banker, might gain control of U.S. fiscal and monetary policies. This could become a big risk should the United States threaten debt default. One option for the United States is to issue bonds with favorable interest rates, marketed by celebrities and civic leaders, to encourage Americans to buy back U.S. debt held by China.

The U.S. Treasury might also conduct a campaign to market Treasury bills, notes, long-term bonds, and savings bonds to the public. Savings bonds remain a poorly tapped source of funds. Investors used to be able to buy them at local banks, but no bank actually tried to sell them aggressively, because the banks make so little on them. The United States could instead engage the post office as its agent in marketing and selling bonds, and in any amounts. This would have the added benefit of helping to save the U.S. Postal Service from further cuts.

An option is requiring all Americans with 401(k) plans to invest a certain percentage of their savings in U.S. debt—50 percent, for example. If it were coupled with tax relief for income on the investment after retirement, this provision would give future retirees more assurance that investing in their country makes sense. Critics might argue that this would redirect investment funds from equities to government securities, in turn depressing stock prices. But this would be the cost of U.S. citizens regaining control of the country's destiny. (Note also that the Fed's low interest rates have been artificially reducing the value of savings to boost the stock market for years, so it is about time that savers get some relief from this artificial transfer of wealth.)

All these suggestions have two chief aims: get U.S. debt back into American hands, and get the manufacturing trade balance back to zero. When the United States does both, it will have regained its freedom of action. At that point, with China at arm's length, the United States can execute a true hypercompetitive strategy.

Play on China's Weaknesses to Erode Its Strengths

Sun Tzu, the famous Chinese strategist circa 500 BC, advocated winning without a frontal attack or, better yet, with no attack at all. His advice echoed the principles of the martial arts: use the least force necessary, outflank rivals with clever maneuvers, strike with quick, bold advances, maintain a lively tempo, use surprise, confuse rivals, stay flexible, and turn the weight and advantages of rivals against them. Contemporary authors have fittingly called this approach the "strategy of the indirect,"[3] "maneuver warfare,"[4] and "judo strategy."[5]

In the fashion of Sun Tzu, the United States could play on China's weaknesses to erode its strengths. All good strategists have at least a mental list of their opponents' weaknesses. Among China's weaknesses today are inadequate raw materials to fuel its growing economy and inadequate farmland and food to feed its people in the future. That gives the United States several targets for hypercompetitive action.

To compensate for its shortage of farmland, China has gone on a global hunt for agricultural land. In Africa, it has been negotiating a number of deals. For example, it has leased 6.9 million acres in the Democratic Republic of the Congo for the world's largest oil-palm plantation.[6] As well as its African interests, it has bought land in Southeast Asia and Brazil. As for raw materials, it has executed contracts across Africa to acquire oil and minerals. As described in Part 1, its moves recall those of the British Empire in the nineteenth century. The British established a global mercantilist system to feed their domestic manufacturing sector. Unlike former colonial powers, which took developing countries' resources by force, China has acquired raw materials in return for its investments in African infrastructure projects. China has used its economic power to require African nations to hire Chinese infrastructure firms and give visas to Chinese workers for construction jobs.

From the point of view of a strategist, this gives U.S. leaders an opening to disrupt China's robust raw materials supply chain. Via diplomacy, the bully pulpit, diplomatic deals, soft loans for infrastructure contracts with U.S. firms, and military influence, the United States could negotiate with supplier countries to keep China out. The United States could play on fears that China is just another imperialist nation, using land acquisition and debt to carry out its plan of creeping colonization.

Another option is for the United States to establish a sovereign wealth fund to buy up and control commodities. It could do the same by forming an OPEC-like cartel with friendly, democratic nations. The United States needs some way to break or periodically disrupt China's mercantilist ambitions—and the reliability of its supply lines—in Latin America, Africa, and the Middle East. This would also undercut China's reliability as the world's factory, discouraging Westerners from investing in the country.

A growing weakness in China is poor capital allocation. According to Reuters, financial corruption so plagues the country that in mid-2011, China slashed investments in high-priority projects, including those in high-speed rail and wind power. In addition, as a part of an economic retrenchment, it pared the $1.5 trillion it had planned to invest in seven high-priority industries.[7] It has encountered additional problems involving cities and towns that have amassed mountains of municipal debt from overbuilding infrastructure. The state may have to bail out overextended local governments. China has thus hit a weak patch, and the United States can undercut the Chinese economy by investing in the same industries that China wants to build, driving down Chinese profits and disrupting China's mercantilist ambitions.

Thwart China's Future Advantages

Sun Tzu inspired another competitive strategy that the United States could use: disrupt and thwart China's future advantages.

China has a number of goals for the future, and its plans offer multiple points where the United States could intercede and use hypercompetitive actions to prevent China from getting a further economic edge.

Become the Overwhelming Leader of Global Innovation

China's long-range plan is to become the world's central technological innovator by 2050. It is practicing what some commentators and *Star Trek* fans would call a "Borg" strategy, in which the collective absorbs all foreign knowledge in its path and resistance is futile. In the future, China will use this bank of knowledge, combined with an educated workforce of engineers and scientists, to supplant the United States as a birthing ground for new, profitable industries.

Recall the story of Japan. As it pushed its way into the U.S. manufacturing sector, Japanese firms saved time and money by acquiring U.S. know-how. In nearly 300 cases of links between U.S. and Japanese firms, more than 90 percent involved technology transfer to Japan, according to a report by the National Academy of Sciences. Japanese firms thereby spent 25 percent less time and 50 percent less money on innovation.[8] We can reasonably surmise that China plans to enjoy the same advantage for the foreseeable future.

China's stated strategy is "enhancing original innovation through co-innovation and re-innovation."[9] It has mandated that Chinese components replace foreign parts in "core infrastructure." Specific components include integrated circuits, operating software, switches and routers, database management, and encryption systems used in industries like banking and telecommunications.[10] To thwart this innovator strategy, the United States could create impediments to technology imitation and theft.

One option would be impeding technology transfer through technology pricing, trade secret controls, threats of retaliation, protection of patents, restrictive licensing, and other measures. In particular, the United States has the power under World Trade

Organization (WTO) rules to restrict the sale in the United States of products that contain stolen U.S. or European Union intellectual property. It could aggressively enforce the WTO rules and also allow U.S. firms to sue Chinese companies in U.S. courts, both to block the entry of products that contain stolen intellectual property and to recover lost profits from previous sales and encourage the European Union to do the same.

Another option would be to found a global world court to enforce intellectual property rules and create international antitrust laws for the court to enforce. Countries that did not participate in the world court—and China would have trouble doing so, given its current practices—would lose WTO membership. The court would have to have enough clout to seize assets outside China. The current U.S. approach is to write detailed rules and demand that other countries follow them. Effective, speedy, proactive enforcement mechanisms are not available. This is not working.

The United States could also consider the option of making the most of the human capital developed by the U.S. educational system. The United States remains the premier source of advanced degrees for promising scientists and entrepreneurs around the world. Overall, 34 percent of doctorates awarded in the United States in science and engineering go to temporary visa holders,[11] and many of these are Chinese.[12] Today the United States facilitates China's future advantage by training its young people and sending them back home. A new policy could quickly reverse the shifting advantage.

One idea is to make it easier for bright, aspiring students to get visas to study and, when they are finished, make it easy for them to get green cards to stay. Chinese students often study science, math, engineering, computer technology, software design, and other subjects in which the United States needs to keep an edge. If they trickle back home, they use this U.S.-acquired knowledge to undercut the United States' future. From the point of view of a strategy to build human capital, the United States might want to tap this brain trust on U.S. soil for U.S. companies.

A tactic to make this happen would be to require foreign students to remain U.S. residents for a certain period in return for access to a U.S. education. The residency requirement might be 10 years. If the students returned home earlier, they could be required to pay an educational fee or forfeit a surety bond. Nine out of ten Chinese stay in the United States for at least five years after earning their PhDs,[13] and the likelihood is that before ten years pass, many will have started families and decided to stay permanently. In this way, the United States would leverage its greatest resource—the best universities and research institutes in the world—to both attract the best and brightest and make them part of the U.S. economic engine. Despite what some critics suggest, the people who stay would not be those who would take American jobs. They would often be the ones who create them.

Disrupting China's future advantage as an innovator also demands that the United States do a better job of nurturing its homegrown brain trust. The United States must reform its own primary, middle, and high school education systems, especially in science, technology, education, and math. This is also a reason why we need to create more special high schools for talented young people, reward students based on merit, and divert funds from special needs and sports to developing the best and brightest.

Become the World Leader in Industries of the Future

China has designated seven industries as "strategic," meaning that they are key to the future of the global economy. These industries include clean-energy technology, next-generation information technology, biotechnology, high-tech manufacturing equipment, new energy (nuclear, wind, and solar), new materials (rare earths, nanomaterials, and carbon fiber), and new-energy cars (electric and hybrid). China has made it clear that it will support firms in these industries with below-market loans, cheap or free land, tax rebates, grants, R&D incentives, and artificially created demand for new technologies. Although these industries make up just 2 percent of China's GDP today, the country's leaders aim to raise that figure more than sevenfold to 15 percent by 2020.[14]

To remain competitive, U.S. firms in these industries will need help. Without it, China will devastate their profits, and the companies will either shift production to China or go bankrupt competing with Chinese firms. That's why, today, the United States should consider options to capture the growth of selected industries of the future. In addition, this might include the tactics used for slowing down Chinese innovation. It might also include specific measures fashioned for a U.S. industrial policy, as discussed in the previous chapter.

Become the World Leader in Manufacturing Technology and Equipment

Within a decade, China plans to go beyond its forte in basic, labor-intensive, and heavy manufacturing and acquire the capability of highly advanced manufacturers in the United States, Germany, Canada, France, Sweden, and other OECD countries. The need to thwart China's future role as a global manufacturing hub is urgent. Policies that continue to allow the migration of higher-technology manufacturing to China will destroy Western economies.

The United States has many options as it seeks to tailor its strategy to support manufacturing. Winners in manufacturing today succeed not just on price, but also on speed, reliability, design, service, customization, and so on. China does not hold the upper hand on many of these criteria. The United States can keep it that way. This is an instance where U.S. industrial policy could play a make-or-break role. Companies that are left to laissez-faire capitalism will not save American manufacturing on their own. They have shown over and over that they will give it away.

U.S. industrial policy could thus target the creation of the technologies mentioned in Chapter 6—robotics, rapid prototyping, seamless logistics, mass customization, 3D printing, and so on. Where a Chinese company might take two weeks to deliver, a U.S. company could deliver in two days. Where the Chinese might offer standard products, the United States could offer special-order parts and services. Once again, the United States could fund technology development with a new Manufacturing Advanced Research

Projects Agency, or MARPA. The use of technology developed by MARPA grants could be restricted to use in the United States.

Disrupt China's Current Strategies and Strengths

Sun Tzu's most important advice was to beat the enemy's strategy, not its army. While thwarting China's future advantages, the United States can also go the next step: disrupting China's current strategies and undermining its advantages. A number of China's current focuses emerge as important targets for U.S. attention.

Be the Best Through Mixing Managed with Laissez-Faire Capitalism

The overriding strength of the Chinese economy is managed capitalism. China's leaders work hard to make sure that Chinese companies get a leg up on the United States. The United States should consider doing the same: responding forcefully, with overwhelming strength, to help U.S. companies outcompete their Chinese rivals.

The clever and swift actions inspired by Sun Tzu are sometimes not decisive enough and take too long to provide victory. Strategists then look to principles outlined by Carl von Clausewitz, the Prussian soldier and military theorist. Von Clausewitz's thoughts appear in his book *On War*, published in 1832.[15] Clausewitz advocated unleashing massive, overwhelming force with relentless, extreme superiority at a given moment and a specific place—not necessarily everywhere, just at turning points in a battle. In modern times, George Stalk recommended this approach for competition in business in a *Harvard Business Review* article, "Hardball."[16]

China has taken a page from von Clausewitz by concentrating its economic forces in giant state-owned enterprises in key industries. Backed by China's finances and favoritism, the companies collectively unleash massive force to take domestic and global market share (e.g., in steel using its subsidies and economies of scale to drive out local players) and to strip the rest of the world of its natural resources, technology, and manufacturing base.

Guided by its five-year plans, with a relentless focus on honing its mercantile and industrial policies, China has single-mindedly knocked the United States back on its heels. Some people believe that the United States can respond to China by counting on independent American corporations to stand against a unified superior force. As we have discussed, they assume that free markets will win over managed capitalism. Since this has not worked against China in the past and holds little promise of working in the future, it allows China to bankrupt, hollow out, or co-opt independent American firms one at a time.

China will continue to use its autocratic bureaucracy to its advantage, moving quickly and decisively to triumph with its own industrial policy. Thus, the United States also needs a decision-making mechanism to match that speed and decisiveness. Once again, this suggests that the United States create a Federal Industrial Policy Board.

Ironically, U.S. strengths—namely, free trade, free markets, and democracy—have become an Achilles' heel in foresighted, rational economic planning. But the FIP Board would allow the United States to combine these traditional strengths with new ones. It would allow long-term thinkers to fill the U.S. pipeline of new industries with the help of the government's hand. It would then rely on the invisible hand to turn emerging entrepreneurial question marks into free-market corporate stars.

Build a Strong Heavy Industrial Sector at Home

In the same way that China aims to control many key heavy manufacturing industries at home through state-dominated firms—automotive, chemical, construction, iron and steel, and nonferrous metals—the United States needs to rebuild many industries that are critical to future American prosperity. While the U.S. Trade Representative's office can work to counter or negotiate the removal of Chinese subsidies, tariffs, and nontariff barriers that support Chinese firms, U.S. officials cannot win in this game. It must actively rebuild in the industries that China is planning to dominate. If the United States concedes too many industries, it will never be respected enough to deter entry. In fact, the United States is rapidly becoming the wimp on the block, attracting even more entry by those who know they can push the wimp around.

China also pursues this strategy with its companies abroad. It has announced that it will create 30 to 50 large, internationally competitive companies.[17] The infrastructure industry is one in which China has become a fearsome competitor. Today, Chinese infrastructure firms bid on energy, telecom, and transport projects around the world with the support of export credits, subsidized insurance, and favorable repayment terms, all offered by the Chinese government. By using lower costs to underbid other firms, it has cut out competitors in Africa, Southeast Asia, Eastern Europe, Russia, and Latin America.[18] China can engage in this subsidy for infrastructure firms openly because it has not ratified an OECD provision that prohibits such export credits.

As China builds its chosen industries at home and abroad, the United States faces pressure once again, if it is to succeed, to use an activist industrial policy. As we've discussed, other democratic countries have used industrial policy adeptly for decades, and the United States could put it to use to disrupt China's growing strength in industry after industry. This includes undermining the state-created advantages that so many Chinese firms—whether owned by the state or not—enjoy.

Modernize the U.S. Infrastructure and Neutralize China's Advantage

China has poured money into roads, bridges, rail lines, ports, and other infrastructure to turn the country into an efficient and attractive location for business. The country's current Five-Year Plan (the twelfth) calls for adding 9,000 kilometers (5,592 miles) of highways, expanding passenger rail to 45,000 kilometers (29,672 miles), installing light-rail systems in 21 cities, adding six new heavy-material ports (with four hundred forty 100,000-ton shipping births), developing 11 new regional airports, and constructing enough coal-fired power plants to increase electricity-generation capacity by 70 percent.[19] According to a report by the bipartisan Building America's Future Educational Fund, China is spending 9 percent of its GDP a year on transportation investment and maintenance, whereas the United States is spending only 1.7 percent.[20]

The United States can counter China's infrastructure effort with a dual strategy, in part upgrading the U.S. infrastructure to increase economic efficiency, and in part expanding the infrastructure to increase capacity. One priority could be speeding up the construction of next-generation power installations: nuclear, clean coal, solar, wind, and geothermal. Another could be redirecting money from resurfacing roads to widening roads to reduce congestion, adding airport runways to increase capacity, enlarging undersized ports, accelerating smart power-grid installation, deploying high-speed freight train networks, and expanding wireless Internet coverage and speed.

The top seven U.S. ports combined handle less container traffic than Shanghai does.[21] The United States has zero miles of high-speed train lines. China boasts 6,649 (and counting). Even Turkey has 466 miles.[22] According to the Building America's Future Educational Fund report, freight bottlenecks and congestion cost the United States $200 billion, or 1.6 percent of GDP, a year. It's no surprise that the U.S. infrastructure ranks sixteenth in the World Economic Forum's economic competitiveness ranking.[23] In the forum's Executive Opinion Survey, the United States ranked twentieth for the quality of its roads, twenty-third for the quality of its ports, and thirty-first for the quality of its air-transport infrastructure.[24]

The United States could neutralize China's position by developing a national infrastructure plan. Like those of many other developed countries, U.S. leaders could back that plan with funding from a national infrastructure bank. Moody's Analytics estimates that for every dollar spent on infrastructure, the United States would gain $1.59 in GDP. (That compares to just $0.29 for every dollar gained from revenue reduction via tax cuts.[25]) With its current "shovel-ready" spending approach, which plays political favorites, the United States does not create advantage and it risks losing its reputation as a prime site for advanced economic activity.

Counter China's Espionage Efforts in the United States

Sun Tzu once said: "One good spy is worth 10,000 soldiers." Though we cannot know the extent of U.S. and Chinese spy operations, we do know that U.S. strategy should be to counter Chinese espionage. According to Peter Brookes, a Heritage Foundation senior fellow and specialist in security issues: "Beijing is bent on China becoming an advanced technology economy as quickly as possible, and is putting a significant amount of resources into the effort, from spending on research and development to industrial espionage, using human assets or cyber operations." Brookes gave that testimony to the Committee on Foreign Affairs Subcommittee on Terrorism, Nonproliferation and Trade in the U.S. House of Representatives in 2011.[26] Brookes had earlier reported that as many as 3,500 Chinese "front companies" are involved in espionage on behalf of China.[27] The number of cyberattacks and Chinese spy cases reported in the news confirms that Brookes knows what he is talking about.

Undermine China's Centers of Gravity

As the United States and China slide deeper into hypercompetition, with one capitalist system pitted against the other, U.S. leaders may want to consider escalating to the ultimate step in hypercompetitive strategy: undermining China's center(s) of gravity. This option is available only if the United States has returned to financial health, as discussed in Chapter 5.

China has already taken this approach toward the United States, and it has done so in multiple ways. It has relentlessly attacked the United States' central source of wealth, the knowledge-based economy. It has undermined the effectiveness of the United States' central form of capitalism, laissez-faire. It has taken advantage of the United States' central vehicle for decision making, democracy, with faster and more decisive autocratic decision making. It has stolen so much intellectual property that it is undermining America's strategy of being a knowledge economy. And it has eroded one of the U.S. government's central sources of legitimacy: providing a decent standard of living for a broad middle class by paying high wages.

These Chinese body blows against the United States have worked, and the United States now faces sparks of unrest between rich and poor. U.S. leaders will want to evaluate at what point the United States will respond in kind to China's approach, deploying strategies to undermine China's centers of gravity.

As it is today, U.S. leaders remain embroiled in trade skirmishes, fighting over rules related to Chinese tires, frozen chicken, or steel. These are small steps, symbols, and signals. But U.S. leaders can choose to direct the nation's energy against China's three centers of gravity: (1) the Chinese Communist Party (CCP), (2) the industries that generate the bulk of the money, or "profit pools," for under-writing China's state goals, and (3) China's reliance on exports to generate economic power.

Undermining any one of these centers of gravity would cause disarray in China. Each is central to keeping China's economic engine on track. America's most powerful options are those that would knock these centers of gravity off kilter, potentially crip-pling the Chinese economy and capitalist system by permanently unbalancing China's ambitions, resources, and threats. At the least, taking action against these factors can slow China down and buy the United States and the European Union a decade to strengthen the finances of the Western world.

Undermine the Chinese Communist Party

Leaving aside a discussion of using covert operations to encourage the Chinese people, ethnic minorities, or religious sects to desta-bilize China's authoritarian regime, leaving aside a discussion of covert ways to get the members of the CCP to fight over policy differences or inflict purges on the more economically progressive members of the party, and leaving behind attempts to fund insurgents within China's allies or coups in some of China's neighbors, the United States has many options for discrediting or damaging the CCP. One option is to divide the CCP with offers that will split the party. Another is for the United States to secretly discredit Chinese leaders to remove those that are most resistant to cooperation with the United States. A third option is for the United States to provide information that delegitimizes the CCP to Chinese allies, citizens, labor unions, or other organizations to stimulate unrest. A fourth option is to play regions within China against each other. The goal of these options is to undermine the "harmony" of decision-making bodies in China.

Most important, the CCP's main claim to legitimacy is not its form of government. What Chinese citizens value is the government's ability to provide them with a better standard of living. The moment the economy turns down, support for the CCP will tumble. After all, China's leadership is not democratically elected, so people are already questioning the CCP's right to rule. If unrest in the streets becomes widespread, the Chinese will not have the resources to suppress open rebellion by 1.5 billion people. And if the CCP tries to maintain its authority, the cost of repression will divert money from building the economy and making loans to influence or control foreign nations.

Undermining China's Profit Pools

Among China's "pillar" industries are steel, cars, machinery, banking, software, computers, clothing, and petrochemicals. Among its most profitable industries today, largely state-owned, are energy, banking, petrochemicals, and mobile telecom.[28] All of the businesses in these industries are pouring or will pour money into China's profit pool. To the extent that the United States needs to buy from these industries today, it has another reason to embark on a strategy of import substitution. It could also instruct the U.S. Trade Representative to negotiate alternative bilateral trade deals with China's low-cost competitors to replace China's exports to the United States in China's most profitable industries. One option is to arrange everyone-but-China alliances with countries in Latin America, Southeast Asia, Africa, and India around key industries, cutting China out of a large part of global trade in the industries that matter the most.

Another option for the United States to consider is how to raise the costs for these industries or reduce the profits gained through their monopoly position in China's domestic markets. Concerted efforts to protect U.S. firms in China and to make them more aggressive might work. Rules that force American firms in China to pay better wages could also force the average wage up enough to compel Chinese firms to raise their wages. Wage increases would help make these firms less competitive.

To raise costs, the United States could apply pressure to achieve parity in labor laws. The United States passed the Thirteenth Amendment to abolish slavery. But in China, rural workers flock to the cities to work in slavelike conditions. This low-cost labor force gives China an edge not just at the expense of the United States but also at the expense of its own people. It enables companies to offer the rock-bottom "China price." The United States could take a firm stance against sweatshop conditions, indirectly attacking China's lowball labor costs and draconian work conditions. For higher-skilled labor, the United States could recruit talented people to leave China for higher wages in the United States.

The United States could also consider ways to fuel the dissatisfaction of Chinese workers and savers. Workers today regularly check the Internet to compare their wages with those of their overseas counterparts. Chinese savers increasingly find grating (in this case, in just the same way as Americans do) the depressed interest rates on savings and losses of principal to inflation. The United States could accelerate the desire of China's citizens to end this quiet transfer of personal net worth to banks and the state using well-placed propaganda.

Undermining China's Exports and Growth

China would have serious troubles if anyone were able to disrupt funding for China's growth, mainly in the form of reducing foreign direct investment (FDI) in China. In 2010, FDI in China totaled $106 billion.[29] One tactic to reduce this figure is to reveal just how risky that investment is. Educating securities analysts about risk levels could deter CEOs from increasing their Chinese investment exposure. If the United States could undercut confidence in the safety or profitability of investments in China, companies would slash their FDI. Many CEOs fear that U.S. tough talk about China's economic, trade, or military threat could hurt their stock prices. But national leaders would do well to change the conversation from what helps shareholders to what helps jobholders. Firms that diversify away from China could strengthen U.S. employment by returning manufacturing to the United States.

If nothing else, the president could take advantage of the bully pulpit. He (or she) could demand that the executives of companies that are highly invested in China pledge to pursue investments that do not undercut U.S. interests. A few questions aimed at CEOs would be revealing: Are you making things in China to import to the United States? Do you see your company as working for the United States or for China? With the help of the media, the president and other leaders could mount a campaign for more corporate patriotism, discouraging executives from writing checks in China.

Another option might be to use tax incentives to slash American foreign direct investment (FDI) in China. As an alternative to the various tax provisions suggested in the previous chapter, the United States could consider the notion of a 20-20-20-20-20 plan. A company might get to reduce its total income taxes by 20 percent by repatriating profits from operations overseas (with a minimum threshold based on firm revenues). It might get another 20 percent break for making in the United States everything that it sells in the United States. It might get a third 20 percent break for exporting things made in the United States with at least, let's say, 70 percent U.S. content. It might get a fourth 20 percent if more than, say, three-quarters of its workforce resided in the United States. It might get a fifth 20 percent if no more than 10 percent of its imported finished goods, components, or materials came from China. A tax scheme with this approach would aim to reward U.S. companies that direct their investment away from China.

The United States might also consider the option of including in its capitalist strategy a plan to force China to highlight the full scope of its threat. The next time North Korea fires on South Korea, the United States might treat it as a pretext to strike back against China, demanding tougher trade compromises in order to make China more helpful with North Korea. Tying trade to cooperation over Iran's nuclear program might be a good pretext for saying, in effect, "You aren't acting like a friend in the Middle East; here's the cost of not working with the United States." This kind of conflict would disrupt trade flows into and out of China.

As for directly undermining China's export machine, the United States might consider pushing the boundaries, as China does, on nontariff barriers. The options for nontariff trade barriers are many, including import bans, country-of-origin requirements, protection of sanitary and phytosanitary conditions, product-specific quotas, quality condition regulations, packaging and labeling requirements, product standards, complex regulations that require an insider's knowledge of how to get things done, trade documents like certificates of origin or certificates of authenticity, health and safety regulations, employment laws, import licenses, rules about subsidies or state ownership of the Chinese exporter, rules against export subsidies, minimum import price requirements, import quotas, intellectual property rules, restrictive licenses, and lengthy customer procedures. At first glance, some of these barriers would flout WTO rules, but the United States could work to test the limits of WTO enforcement, just as China does.

As Kevin Brady (R-TX), the Chair of the House Ways and Means Trade Subcommittee, says, "We will never win a battle to 'out-protectionist' China."[30] But the United States can use tough tactics as part of a stratagem in facing off with China to force

China to open its markets and to encourage Chinese leaders via hardball negotiating to reduce the constraints on American businesses operating in China. Only then will China think twice and ease up on its hardball protectionist game.

Another option to reduce Chinese imports would be for the United States to aggressively redefine and audit transfer pricing of goods made in China and sold in the United States. Transfer prices are normally set by companies to ensure that profits are booked, and thus taxes paid, mostly abroad. Because U.S. corporate tax rates are among the highest in the world, companies go to great lengths to set transfer pricing to favor overseas profits. New regulations could allow U.S. auditors to examine company books. Odds are that ending the transfer-pricing dodge would encourage more manufacturing at home and discourage companies from buying Chinese goods and selling them in the United States.

When Nations Are in Hypercompetition

Many national leaders in the developed world feel that they are caught in a downward spiral: if they lose more industry to China, they will become subservient to a larger power. But leaders can get their nations back on track by looking at the world as strategists who put the strength of their capitalist systems and global economic leadership above all else. They do not have to take guidance solely from economists or from business executives or from technocrats. They can take it from pragmatists who understand hypercompetition among capitalist systems.

Succeeding in a hypercompetitive world means acting early and often to throw rivals off balance and defeat their strategies. It means loosening politicians' frozen grip on one ideology or another and getting them to embrace strategies that put the United States on the offense. It means combining moves from business strategy, trade strategy, military strategy, and the strategy of diplomatic realpolitik. No country can succeed for long by simply sticking with the same strategy. Other countries will improve on that strategy or outmaneuver it. Nor can any country succeed by playing defensively, fending off attacks as they arise. More competitive countries, and especially China, will overwhelm their defenses through massive economic force.

Successful leaders prioritize plans and implement them in digestible chunks. They look ahead to craft a sequence of competitive moves—and then roll out one after another. They can conduct an aggressive offensive strategy today, set up for the next strategy, plan the strategy after that, and envision a strategy yet one further step out. And they can adjust as events unfold. This is a capability that is sorely lacking in many national capitals. It is especially lacking in Washington, DC, where leaders have little idea of what a capitalist strategy is, let alone how to break one down into digestible chunks and implement it in waves.

Only taking the offense reenergizes a team, corporation, military, or government. Proactivity begets more proactivity. In today's hypercompetition between capitalist systems, winners that have reduced their dependence on China will be able to relentlessly launch moves of the four kinds we have discussed in this chapter: they can play on rivals' weaknesses to erode their strengths, they can thwart rivals' future advantages, they can disrupt rivals' strategies and strengths, and they can undermine rivals' centers of gravity. Hypercompetitive nations will work to force the other side to back down in a game of brinkmanship, and to outmaneuver and outcompete the rival's hypercompetitive strategy. And they will do so before it is too late. As Leonardo da Vinci once said: "It is easier to resist in the beginning than at the end." The United States can't wait until China's economic and military power is unstoppable, and time is running out.

8

Restructuring the World Economic Order

Constant Struggle for Economic Leadership or Influence

Amerely leadership of the world economic order has been slipping. The veteran U.S. boxer has lost control of the ring and the momentum of the match. In some ways, the United States has been pursuing a rope-a-dope economic strategy, absorbing body blows from managed capitalism and waiting for the Chinese challenger to tire and succumb to U.S. rules of free-market capitalism. But this rope-a-dope approach has not worked. The Chinese pugilist has not tired. Instead, it has built up strength. And it has become emboldened to flex its geoeconomic muscle.

Given that China is not likely to be knocked out, how does the United States win? The first order of business is to define what winning looks like in the bipolar world of the future. That is, let's define success. In my view, success is control over the rules of capitalism (such as trade, property, antitrust, and contract rules). The rule maker gets to set rules that advantage itself and force the rule takers to live by those rules; the rule maker becomes the privilege taker. Based on this definition of winning, I believe a range of winning geoeconomic futures is possible for America:

- *The United States as a peacefully coexisting equal rival.* The United States could share power with China, resulting in two competing versions of capitalism that coevolve in two separate spheres.
- *The United States as a restraining force on China.* The United States could contain China's power and influence so that U.S. rules of capitalism prevail in most of the world, while China continues to operate with its own rules and exercises dominion over a small portion of the world.
- *The United States as a world leader.* The United States reduces China's power and influence and forces it to follow American rules of capitalism.
- *The United States as an omnipotent hegemon.* The United States eliminates China as a serious challenger to U.S. strategic supremacy. (Or China might implode on its own, in which case its economic power would disappear.)

The odds of the United States becoming a hegemon have slid considerably. However, the United States has the potential to secure any of the other three futures. To be successful in this endeavor, U.S. leaders will need to conceptualize how geopolitics and economics can be combined to greater effect. They will need to embrace political savvy, diplomatic pressure, military conduct, and economic power. The consequences of not acting decisively to guide the new world order in the United States' favor would leave the United States with another range of futures. These would define negligence and failure, and they would cause economic harm to the United States and its allies for decades:

- *The United States as satellite.* The United States might fall into China's sphere of influence, becoming subservient to Chinese rules of capitalism and becoming a part of China's sphere of influence.
- *The United States as a junior partner.* The United States could slip into having a valued number two position within

China's sphere of influence, able to influence Chinese rules of capitalism, but still under China's leadership.

- *The United States as a frenemy, engaged in co-opetition.* The United States might struggle as an equal world power with China, cooperating and competing to create a mixture of American and Chinese rules that spreads throughout the entire world.

If any of these three outcomes happen, American historians will look back at the current era and consider it a geoeconomic failure for America and its people. If U.S. leaders do act to change the future, they will press China to revise its overreaching and over-aggressive strategy. And they will ensure that the United States reclaims the center of the global economic boxing ring for decades.

Are Cooperation and a Win-Win Scenario Possible?

Is a cooperation-based win-win scenario possible for China and the United States? Indeed, yes, theoretically. But in creating a new world order, U.S. leaders would do well to bear in mind a number of factors that put the realism of cooperation and a win-win scenario into perspective.

The first factor is the notion that cooperation will solve all of our problems. The evidence does not support this. To date, U.S. government policy has been based on the hope for a prosperous free-market future realized through cooperation with China. But China hasn't cooperated in a way that raises the United States' fortunes along with those of the Chinese.

U.S. leaders have allowed this to happen by agreeing to give China a lopsided economic bargain. The United States' record $295 billion trade imbalance with China in 2011 is just one mea-sure of how bad this bargain has been. China remains unwilling to cooperate for mutual and equal gains, so much so that many people fear that the United States has been duped. Talking coop-eration while conducting competition, China has played the United

States for a fool. U.S. leaders need to reevaluate their focus. Cooperation, while it is a good thing in some walks of life, is not a good thing in all global trade. The reality is that the United States and China are "frenemies" that are engaged in co-opetition (the third failure scenario listed earlier).

Continued U.S. cooperation can morph into appeasement and co-optation. Co-optation can then turn into subservience and later into subjugation. Cooperating with China has deteriorated into a dysfunctional global relationship, with China as the exploiter and the United States as the exploited. U.S. leaders may want to play nice, sharing and creating wealth with China. But to date, playing nice has had the United States playing into the hands of a country with different goals. If the current trends run unchecked, as shown in Part 1, the United States will end up following China's rules of capitalism and living in China's sphere of influence.

The false promise of cooperation is related to the false notion of a win-win economic relationship. The win-win approach has not worked in the United States' relationship with China. Like many hard-nosed strategists, Chinese leaders have not played a win-win game. That is, they have played not for their share of the marbles, but for all the marbles they can get. This is a win-lose game, with the United States as the loser. U.S. citizens can blame Washington for unrealistically believing that the United States could convert China to pursuing a game that is contrary to its interests.

If the United States continues to seek a win-win result while China practices a win-lose strategy, China will win an even bigger share of the global economy. China presumably sees it as being in its interest to continue to beggar its neighbor because it is not seeking to maximize the world's total wealth. It is seeking wealth for China's citizens, to bring its poor out of poverty. For national leaders of any developing country, this is a worthy and defensible goal. U.S. leaders would do well to understand that China is playing a win-lose game. And it is seeking regional, or perhaps even global, hegemony over geopolitics and trade, hoping to make China truly the "Middle Kingdom"—the center of the world.

Is Chinese Dominance Inevitable?

Time is of the essence for U.S. leaders in creating a strategy for a new world economic order. China is solidifying its concept of world order at an alarming rate. It has warmed relations and cut deals with other developing countries across the "South," from Indonesia to Argentina to Nigeria. As shown in Chapter 4, it has curried economic and diplomatic favor with a host of former antagonists, such as Japan, South Korea, and India. It has even cozied up to the United States' neighbors—including Canada, a nation that is boosting its exports to China by leaps and bounds. Canada's growing exports to China include commodities like lumber and potash. Of late, the United States even seems to be giving China an assist, as President Obama refused to approve the Keystone pipeline from Canada to the Gulf Coast. The move opens the door for Canada to divert crude oil sales from the United States to China.

Incredibly, the United States has also lost to China its first-place position with first-tier trading partners like Germany, South Korea, Japan, and Brazil. It has largely stood still as China has co-opted countries by the dozens with contracts for infrastructure development. In exchange for soft loans for roads, ports, power lines, and railways, China has gained access to raw materials, energy resources, and local markets across the globe. It has also created geopolitical power. If the United States continues to pursue its current approach, it will fall even farther behind the curve in its geoeconomic influence.

The pessimistic view is that the United States has already hit a point of no return, and that China has an unbeatable lead in shaping the new world order. Some people even suggest that a world order dominated by China is unavoidable. Some CEOs have told me that China's global dominance is assured by virtue of the size of its population. Not only has power shifted to the East, these people say, but it will keep shifting, and we can't do anything to stop it. In short, demographics are destiny.

This is dangerous thinking. It leads to a *self-defeating, self-fulfilling prophecy* as U.S. investors and businesspeople flee the United States and bet their money on the demographic heavyweight, China. This accelerates the slide of the United States toward the status of a junior power to China. The reality, however, is that demographics are not destiny. People alone don't deliver global power. It is urgent that U.S. leaders express this message to stop Wall Street, business, and other investors with billions of investment dollars from making the prophecy come true.

When it comes to exercising its natural power to establish a new world order, the United States has not taken strategic actions. It has failed to use economic relationships to its advantage by using little discretion over whom it trades with. The United States goes on with a witless strategy of trading openly with almost everyone everywhere, including enemy nations. This strategy, lacking a truly most-favored-nation list, has cost the United States its economic edge. In addition, allowing other countries to run surpluses with the United States is justifiable only if the United States reaps critical geopolitical, military, raw material, or energy advantages. It certainly shouldn't build the power of unfriendly nations.

The United States' open-trade policies have only undermined its sphere of influence around the world, as Chapter 4 showed. Allies get scarcely any benefit compared to adversaries. When the United States wants to entice another power into its sphere of influence, it has little leverage. Why be part of the American sphere of influence if everyone can trade with the United States? The United States can buy loyalty by allowing some nations to run trade surpluses with it. But it can't run trade deficits with all countries. And buying loyalty through trade creates the weakest form of international ties, compared to, for example, having a threatening common enemy or sharing common values, culture, and language.

Many nations think that China will be benign because of its history as a counter to American power, insisting on a noninterventionist world. However, China's state-owned companies are interfering in foreign countries like never before. This is dragging the Chinese government into relations with unstable regimes and forcing China to abandon its traditional policy of nonintervention.

China still vetoes measures against interventions in pariah states, but this is now looking like pragmatic Chinese protection of its business interests rather than the philosophical high ground of protecting the sovereignty of all nations.

In 2011, China had 812,000 citizens working abroad. That huge expatriate community demands China's intervention to guarantee Chinese contractual rights, to evacuate people when needed (such as evacuating 35,860 Chinese from Libya when the civil war broke out), to deal with hundreds of kidnappings all over the world, and to protect Chinese assets.[1] China is being forced to assume the role of a superpower, flexing its muscle in foreign nations, as it implements its "going-out" policy. One reflection of this is China's proposed string of naval bases around the Indian Ocean to provide support for its interventions.

By acting with resolve, the United States can stop the Chinese from dominating the world, as discussed in Chapters 5 to 7. The United States has let China have its way too often. U.S. leaders have sought to avoid conflict—some would call this appeasement. The United States can win only by challenging China. Constructive conflict will allow the United States to negotiate fair compromises that yield better deals. The United States cannot shrink from pressing its economic, political, diplomatic, and military agendas. It must stand up to China at every turn.

Acting with greater resolve will occasionally force the United States and China into a game of brinkmanship. While brinkmanship can be scary, the Chinese have been playing this game all along. The United States remains the greater power, but in many instances, China has played this scary game better. It has bluffed, but it has not blinked. U.S. silence in response to aggressive acts against South Korea by North Korea, China's surrogate, is a good example of America blinking too easily.

Brinkmanship can be a dangerous game, as it can escalate military tensions along with economic ones. But the United States can limit it to economic brinkmanship over trade, and the United States stands in a position of relatively little military risk. The

Chinese today cannot go entirely to the brink either economically or militarily because they depend so much on U.S. markets and U.S. repayment of debt. The Chinese also have to worry about any military overtones scaring away the investment and technology inflows that remain the lifeblood of their economic growth and stability. Also, the Chinese economy still remains smaller than that of the United States, so China also knows that it cannot win by the use of deep pockets (especially if the United States gets its financial house in order, as discussed in Chapter 5).

A strong stance will reinforce a climate that encourages China to compromise. History shows that no one can hope for compromise from a rival who has no current incentive to do so. The United States must give China a reason to work more cooperatively with America. The United States could essentially take a two-step approach: escalate the tensions by refusing to compromise U.S. interests, and resolve the conflict when China blinks.

An Approach to a Grand Strategy

How does the United States prepare a geoeconomic strategy that will serve it in the future? How can the United States shape a new global economic order now that power is shifting steadily from West to East? What geoeconomic lines should the United States draw to define its and China's "turf"? How can these lines balance China's economic power?

The everyone-everywhere approach has fragmented and diluted the United States' influence. Focus is needed. The United States cannot include everyone in its sphere of influence, given its current imbalance in ambitions, resources, and threats (ART). Although the United States has long held a strong hand of geoeconomic cards, it hasn't played them to score the maximum number of economic points. It faces a rapacious, undemocratic power in a humble, developing-world guise. It needs to play its cards against that power like a geoeconomic pro.

Developing a grand strategy for the United States involves five parts:

- Planning a new U.S. economic sphere
- Building the institutions to govern a U.S. sphere
- Strengthening the United States' core and vital interests
- Isolating and containing China's economic sphere
- Tipping the balance of economic power toward the United States by geopolitical means

In the growing competition with China, the United States can use these steps to define whichever vision of success it chooses.

Planning a New U.S. Sphere

The first part of a new geoeconomic strategy for the United States would involve a plan to select the most critical geographies of the global chessboard and favorably position U.S. industries in those areas. The positions that the United States takes will indicate both where it proposes to gain control and where it proposes to disrupt its rival. Keeping geoeconomic factors in mind, good strategy would suggest that the United States attempt to simultaneously (1) control the fastest-growing or most profitable territories and (2) disrupt its rival's sphere of economic influence to weaken its economic power.

The task of constructing a geoeconomic chessboard strategy starts with dividing the world into geoindustry territories (see Figure 8-1) or into geoproduct territories (see Figure 8-2).[2]

The second step is to establish a strategic intent for each territory on the map. Typically, a nation chooses among six strategic intentions for each territory: core (C), vital interests (VI), buffer zones (BZ), pivotal zones (PZ), forward positions (FP), and power vacuums (PV). A choice of core ranks a region as being among the most important for that country (as shown in Figures 8-1 and 8-2). In the core, the central power sets the rules of the capitalist system.

Geographic Markets

Industrial Sector	North America	EU	Latin America	Mid-East	Japan and Asian Tigers	Russia Eastern Europe	Africa	India	Vietnam Indonesia	China
Low Value-Added Mfg			FP						FP	R/VI
High Value-Added Mfg	VI	VI	PZ		FP					R/PZ
Hardware Engineering/Innovation	Core	VI	VI		FP	PZ		PZ	FP	R/PZ
Software Engineering/Innovation	Core	VI	VI		FP	PZ		PZ		R/PZ
Financial Services	Core	VI	VI		VI					PZ
Extraction of Raw Materials, Metals, Forest Products, Energy, Rare Earths, Water	VI		VI	VI		PZ	PZ			R/PZ
Food	VI	VI	VI	VI	VI					
Defense/Aerospace	VI	VI	VI	VI	VI			VI		R

FIGURE 8.1 A Stylized Geoindustry U.S. Sphere of Influence, 2010

Product Markets

Geographic Markets	Financial Services	Valued-Added Services	High Tech Products	Industrial Products	Low Value-Added Products
USA	Core	Core	Core	VI	
Europe	VI	VI	VI	VI	
Latin America	BZ	BZ	BZ	BZ	
Raw Material/Oil Suppliers (Mid-East/ Africa)	VI	VI	VI	VI	
Far East and SE Asia (Vietnam, Thailand, Japan, South Korea, Taiwan)	FP	FP	VI	VI	
India	PZ	PZ	PZ	PZ	
China					

FIGURE 8.2 A Stylized Geoproduct U.S. Sphere of Influence, 2010

A choice of *vital interests* denotes territories that are critical to the continued success of the core, adding to the core's scope and scale. The central power influences the vital interests to modify their rules of capitalism so that they are the same as or compatible with the capitalist system of the central power.

Buffer zones insulate the core and the vital interests from incursions by competing nations and their capitalist systems. The buffer is a defensive position that can be sacrificed, but one in which the central power would prefer to hold its struggles over which capitalist system (and which nation's companies) win share.

Pivotal zones offer growth of such significance that the future will be determined by who controls those regions. Pivotal zones often become the core of the future. As old cores die off, they are replaced by successful pivotal zones that have grown so large that they can serve as a core. Ironically, many see China as a pivotal zone for the United States. However, this pivotal zone has grown so powerful and so resistant to U.S. rules of capitalism that it has turned into a rival challenging U.S. rules of capital as discussed in Part 1. The fear is that as Chinese markets continue to grow, they may become the core of many American corporations in the future.

Forward positions provide a place to counterattack rivals. They often sit near a rival's core or vital interests. One nation's forward position is often a rival's buffer zone. However, aggressive forward positions may be taken in a rival's vital or core interests. Forward positions can be used to threaten a rival with retaliation or to weaken a rival by attacking its core or vital interests, draining the rival of growth or profits and the power to set the rules of capitalism. Forward positions are also used to distract a rival's attention and resources, to throw a rival out of ART balance, to test the reaction of rivals to new initiatives, and to experiment or learn by acquiring the technologies or customer knowledge of the rival's competitors.

Power vacuums are regions that are free of control by major powers, sometimes creating a gold-rush mentality for nations to grab future opportunities. Boxes (or territories) left blank in Figures 8-1 and 8-2 represent conceded or abandoned positions, which may also be power vacuums if no rival occupies that square.

The strategic intent labels in the boxes in Figures 8-1 and 8-2 are inferred from U.S. government actions, as outsiders cannot know the intent of government leaders with certainty. (That's why I label the figures "stylized.") The figures were compiled from recent research on government policy and the presumed intentions of U.S. leaders. This is not to say that the U.S. government has actually taken such a methodical approach. U.S. leaders, as discussed, more often have relied on the evolution of open trade and the whims and exigencies of politics.

The U.S. chessboard contrasts with that of China, which again I infer from recent actions and likely intentions. China appears to have taken a much more thoughtful and strategic approach (see Figures 8-3 [China 1990] and 8-4 [China 2010]). As I have no inside information on China's secret intentions, the labels again

Product Markets

Geographic Markets	Financial Services	Valued-Added Services	High Tech Products	Industrial Products	Low Value-Added Products
USA					FP
Europe					FP
Latin America					FP
Raw Material/Oil Suppliers (Mid-East/ Africa)					VI
Far East (Japan, South Korea, Taiwan)			PZ	PZ	VI
South East Asia			PV	VI	VI
China	Core	BZ	PZ	Core	Core

FIGURE 8.3 A Stylized Geoproduct Chinese Sphere of Influence, 1990

Product Markets

Geographic Markets	Financial Services	Valued-Added Services	High Tech Products	Industrial Products	Low Value-Added Products
USA	FP		FP	FP	FP
Europe			PZ	PZ	FP
Latin America			FP	FP	FP
India			PZ	PZ	VI
Raw Material/Oil Suppliers (Mid-East/ Africa)			PZ	PZ	VI
Far East/ SE Asia (Vietnam, Japan, Thailand, South Korea, Taiwan)	BZ	BZ	VI	VI	VI
China	Core	VI	Core	Core	Core

FIGURE 8.4 A Stylized Geoproduct Chinese Sphere of Influence, 2010

represent a stylized summary, but they show an interesting game plan that China may have used to build its economic sphere of influence.

The main goal of these grids is to detail the strategic intentions that would facilitate a country's growth while disrupting that of rivals. Another critical goal is to focus leaders on the highest strategic priorities for where they wish to set the rules of capitalism, and at the same time avoid the expenditure of resources on industries (or products) and geographies that are not compatible with rules of the central power. Historically, territories on the chessboard can be exchanged through political horse trading, taken in war, converted through incentives, or won over through internal changes that lead national leaders to favor one capitalist system over another.

A third goal of the grids is to narrow the nation's intentions to what's affordable, so that ART stays in balance. Decisions about which territories to select require detailed knowledge of every corner of the globe. U.S. leaders cannot draw up universal economic rules of thumb and apply them everywhere equally. Nor can they ignore the need to construct a reasonable industry portfolio, as noted in Chapter 7. In the same way that a business divides up a marketplace and executes its growth strategy to match local conditions, nations can divide up the world into regions and plan their geoeconomic incursions accordingly.

The chessboard might strike open-trade policy makers as heresy. Today corporations decide where to grow without regard to the needs of the United States. But the chessboard allows the government to prevent investment in places that do not serve the national interest—such as the former USSR or today's Iran. It allows a way to visualize the world's current and desired future economic order. Without reasoning through choices in this way, the world order emerges chaotically through uncoordinated actions by firms, the government, and international institutions.

The battle for economic gains is fought not nation by nation or region by region, but box by box on the global chessboard. The United States may be very influential in several industries or products within a nation such as Germany, but China can be strong in others. China may also carry a lot of weight in trade with countries like Japan and South Korea, while the United States carries weight politically and militarily. With the grids, leaders do not approach other countries with a fuzzy notion of the balance of economic power. They approach them with a detailed map of targets for action.

Building a sphere requires a program for formal alliances. The key is to build the sphere with a smaller number of truly valuable, trustworthy, and reliable allies. The alliances should depend on both economic and military capabilities. History shows that the strongest allies have at least one of three things in common: common values, common interests, and common enemies. Common values and a common history are the strongest glue for an alliance. Common enemies are the next strongest, although this is temporary and can be easy to defeat because a common enemy can split off these allies by making them friends. Common interests (e.g., mutual trade flows) are the weakest, since the allies remain loyal only so long as they are earning money through their allegiance.

The United States already has geoeconomic and geopolitical alliances, of course, such as the Mutual Cooperation and Security Treaty with Japan, the North Atlantic Treaty Organization (NATO) in Europe, and the North American Free Trade Agreement (NAFTA) with Mexico and Canada. But U.S. leaders should consider creating a master plan to update and secure economic alliances, given that U.S. dominance and leverage will decline as China's rises. The United States can remain stronger by securing a few good allies, rather than having many allies that walk away when the United States needs them. The United States doesn't benefit from a sphere full of fair-weather friends, as it discovered during the war in Iraq.

Particularly important is strengthening U.S. relations with Europe. China has been currying favor with one country after another. It invested $1 billion in Greece to upgrade the port at Piraeus, receiving a 35-year concession on operating two container terminals.³ It has bought more than 10 percent of Spain's debt, and in 2011 it agreed to buy nearly $8 billion more, so much that the Spanish daily *El Pais* dubbed a Chinese vice premier the new "Mr. Marshall,"⁴ referring to American General George Marshall, who masterminded the plan to rebuild Europe after World War II. It has cut so many deals in Hungary that Hungarian leaders are trying to sell their country as a gateway for Chinese goods entering Europe.⁵

In the end, a nation's economic sphere of influence reflects its leaders' worldview and ambitions. It is determined by answering questions such as: Where are the boundaries of the nation's economic influence? What are the desired relationships with certain countries? How should the sphere be positioned to capture the best territories on the chessboard? How should the sphere be positioned to deal with rival spheres? How does the positioning of the spheres balance the distribution of economic power?

U.S. leaders need to both react to the competition between economic spheres and anticipate how that competition will develop—and get ready to head off the moves of rivals on each territory on the global chessboard. History has shown that the best solution for an ambitious nation is, on the one hand, to grab great wealth, and, on the other, to restrict the acquisition of wealth by rivals. Ironically, the ability to shift economic fortunes in these two ways gives the challenger greater relative power.

At any time, a country can change the configuration of its sphere of influence. National leaders who are vying for global economic leadership continually create, use, share, distribute, stabilize, counter, circumvent, and redirect their nation's economic power or the power of its main rivals and allies to tip the balance of power in their direction. This demands a process for planning how to control the playing field. In the Cold War against the Communists, the process was a lot simpler. Entire nations were at play: Poland was in the Soviet economic and military camp, and Britain was not. Each country had an economic system that was compatible with the rest of its economic sphere of influence.

In the Cold War against the Communists, a nation was on one side or the other, pure and simple. But even though President George W. Bush said after the September 11, 2001, attack, "You're either with us or against us," this is simply not the case in today's world. Nations have many more split loyalties than they did in the past. A single country may be in the U.S. economic camp with certain industries but not with others. A nation may also have split loyalties based on its needs for trade and military protection. Today's capitalist cold war requires more strategic thinking—and by many more parts of the government than the military-industrial complex of the Cold War against the Communists.

Getting spread too thin is one aspect of overstretch. Given that the United States cannot deal with everyone everywhere, it might be a good idea to build America's sphere on the principle that it is better to be a big fish in a moderate-size pond full of friendly fish than to be constantly fighting with a larger fish in a very large pond full of piranha and alligators.

Governing a New U.S. Sphere

Once an economic sphere has been conceptualized and built, the leaders in the sphere have to find a way to govern it. Typically, they create an international institution to do so, a group of decision makers to enforce the rules of capitalism in the sphere. As discussed in Chapter 4, today's world's economic institutions no longer serve the interests of the United States. They have not constrained China from taking advantage of other nations, and in some cases, they have aided China's rising economic and geopolitical power. To govern a sphere without Chinese interference, the United States needs an "out with the old, in with the new" policy.

Out with the old. From the perspective of a strategist, the United States could take some radical options as the first steps in building a set of new international organizations that could serve the purpose of governing an economic sphere built around the United States:

- *Pull out of the World Trade Organization.* The World Trade Organization (WTO) does not have the teeth to pry open Chinese markets. It does not end cheating through nontariff trade barriers. It does not stop the theft of intellectual property. It does not root out abusive business practices by which Chinese partners commandeer technology from foreign subsidiaries in China. And it does not stop Chinese state-owned companies from engaging in predatory or anticompetitive practices that were long ago outlawed in the United States. The United States may need to sever its ties with the organization to build an economic sphere that is not overrun by China.

- *Pull out of the United Nations.* Here again, the UN does not serve the interests of the United States in governing an American-led sphere of influence. Though it has done a great deal of good geopolitically, it offers little control over China's economic actions, the greatest long-run danger to the U.S. sphere. The UN worked best in moderating conflicts between Eastern European Communist countries and Western European U.S. allies during the Cold War. When it first replaced Taiwan as a permanent member of the UN Security Council in 1971, China rarely used its veto power to interfere with U.S. policies. But recently it has been much more active, using its veto power to stop UN involvement in Syria's civil war during 2012 and to hinder U.S. efforts to contain the nuclear ambitions of Iran. The United States could replace the UN with an institution without China and Russia on the Permanent Security Council, excluding all nations that disrupt democratic nations from working with the United States.

- *Pull out of the North Atlantic Treaty Organization.* NATO once gave the United States a counterbalance against the Soviet sphere, which has disintegrated. If the European Union pays for U.S. expenses, the United States should by all means stick with it. The influence is important. But today, the United States earns little economic influence or respect for all the money it spends.

All of these suggestions will meet with cries of heresy. But they deserve discussion as a starting point for brainstorming workable strategies for the future. As for the WTO, it fails not just for the reasons mentioned. It fails because no courts exist—as they do in individual nations—to stop global antitrust and anticompetitive business practices or open-trade violations. That means that there is no legal entity to restrain China from monopolizing global markets and putting local players out of business. Meanwhile, China has free access to one of the world's most prized business assets—the U.S. consumer market—without paying for it.

In with the new. By supporting the WTO, the United States continues to keep company with a handmaiden that takes the economy one step forward and two steps back. The WTO focuses on what often amounts to faux free trade and ties up global commerce in a web of distortions. This is true even when the trade agreements are struck with U.S. allies.

If the United States stays with the WTO, U.S. leaders should consider the option of working with the organization to fix two weaknesses: end loopholes that permit China to retain emerging-nation status, which allows it to trade with fewer restrictions than developed nations, and establish a world trade and antitrust court with real teeth. The court could break up global monopolies and cartels, including the monopoly that China has created in rare earth metals. The United States could also consider spearheading trade cartels of its own, benefiting all allies in the U.S. sphere.

As for the UN, the United States would be better served by an institution that placed India, Brazil, and Australia on a new Security Council. As it is, China vetoes too many measures that are in the United States' economic interest, especially measures that would rein in the trouble brewing in China's surrogates, Iran, North Korea, Syria, Pakistan, and North Korea, that is costing the United States billions to monitor and defend against.

As for NATO, the NATO nations have shown that they will not provide adequate support in carrying out allied operations. The United States does not have allies in NATO that will step up with money and manpower proportional to the benefit that they get from the United States. Their history of providing small numbers of troops to the NATO effort in Afghanistan suggests that our allies cannot be counted on, and from the economic point of view, they strain U.S. resources and weaken the United States.

Even during the NATO bombing campaign in Libya, NATO relied heavily on the United States, as NATO munitions ran out after just 11 weeks. U.S. leaders who are concerned about the economic strain of supporting NATO could heed the words of former U.S. secretary of defense Robert Gates upon his retirement in 2011: "The blunt reality is that there will be dwindling appetite and patience in the U.S. Congress—and in the American body politic writ large—to expend increasingly precious funds on behalf of nations that are apparently unwilling to . . . [be] capable partners in their own defense."[6]

Some options that the United States might consider to help it govern a cohesive economic sphere based on more than trade are:

- *Create an International Financial Supervisory Board (IFSB).* For countries within the U.S. sphere of influence, the United States could spearhead the creation of a body to rein in irresponsible financial management by member nations. The financial woes of the West show that central bankers and politicians cannot manage their economies. Strict regulations on the use of subprime mortgages, derivatives, and newly invented financial instruments by banks would be established worldwide. The IFSB would have the power to rein in nations that have budgets and deficits that run afoul of the sphere's standards. The IFSB could also become the repository for Western countries to pool funds, share the burden of bailing out countries in the U.S. sphere when they are in debt crises, and retain the bargaining power that comes with controlling the purse strings. This option sounds radical, but it is exactly what is happening in the Eurozone right now, as weak countries that have overspent and built up massive debts have turned to Germany and France to bail them out.

- *Create a Council for Democracies.* The United States could create a new institution to determine eligibility for entering and staying in the U.S. sphere of influence. The Council for Democracies would rate nations and certify them as democratic. Those that win certification would enjoy preferential trade with others in the sphere. Those that do not would face trade barriers or expulsion to encourage better human rights, the rule of law, property rights, and other elements of a strong economy and democracy. The council would exclude countries like China, whose low costs often stem from doing things that democracies cannot do. China can force its people to place their savings in state-run banks that give them a negative return, and in turn use the money to fund investments in foreign countries.

- *Create an International Fair Labor Council.* The United States could create an institution to remove unfair economic advantages based on human and labor rights practices that do not meet the standards of Western democracies. The council would rate and certify countries as being developed, developing, or undeveloped in terms of social-welfare benefits, labor costs, and working conditions. Countries that do not comply with Western standards would face import trade restrictions or tariffs. The council could rule out doing business with countries like China, which gains advantage by withholding from its people the social benefits offered in all the developed countries that it does business with.

- *Create a Democratic Sovereign Wealth Fund.* A fund for the democracies, like sovereign funds in many nations today, could buy up natural resources around the world to keep them available for democracies. The fund would use money from nations within the American sphere for foreign direct investment. It would allow the West to compete with China in buying up raw materials and mitigate China's efforts to withhold critical raw materials such as rare earth metals. The purchased assets would become the common property of the

U.S. sphere. Members of the sphere would not be able to cash out their shares of the assets, so they would have incentives to conform to the sphere's rules. The fund might even be funded by a small tariff on all imports into the sphere of democratic nations, creating a massive fund to thwart China's global mercantilist strategy.

While many people will disagree with these options, the important point is to find new ways to stabilize an American sphere of influence and to prevent irresponsible spending or banking from weakening the economy within the sphere. Even the United States would have to fix its budget and debt problems to remain a member. These kinds of institutions might raise the cost of doing business for member states, but they would also provide more financial security and strength. These options would require member nations to give up some sovereignty. They would also create the risk that certain nations or multicountry coalitions could hijack the institutions in the same way that China has done with the G-20. Yet the collective economic power created would counter China's growing economic strength. In sum, the goal is to seek free trade within a bloc of friendly nations with common values, enemies, and interests.

In the rivalry between China and the United States today, appeasement has been shifting the balance of power. The leading nation has largely acquiesced to the challenger's constant violation of WTO rules, hoping that when the challenger's growth reaches a certain point, it will join all other nations in participating fairly in a global marketplace. But since history suggests that the United States cannot count on that future, decision makers appear to face only one other choice: to fully engage the challenger in the capitalist cold war to stall the progress of history toward further Chinese growth at the expense of U.S. prosperity.

To be clear, the preferable option would be for a global compact in which all nations trade freely and fairly. How can anyone be against an economic tide that raises all boats? However, the option of everyone living happily ever after together is not currently on the table—in spite of the ideals of the WTO. Too many U.S. economic boats are hitting bottom because of China's actions, and the day of totally free, cooperative trade seems far off. For this reason, it is logical that U.S. leaders use tactics such as those discussed in Chapter 7 to change China's interests in conforming to Western rules of capitalism. In the meantime, the United States could anticipate and prepare for a future that preserves free trade for true allies. The U.S. free trade bloc would offer incentives for allies to separate economically from China and to cooperate economically with other members of the U.S. sphere.

Strengthening the United States' Core and Vital Interests

The next step in preparing for China's future efforts to undermine the economic power of the United States is to rebuild the strength of America's core and vital interests. The book has discussed two key aspects of strengthening the U.S. core in Chapters 5 and 6: reinventing the U.S. capitalist system and running a financially sound nation. A third option for strengthening the core and vital interests is nurturing relationships with our nearest neighbors and most important suppliers.

As for relationships with our nearest neighbors, two broad options might be considered:

- *Redouble our efforts to build trade with Mexico and Canada.* Nothing benefits the scale, scope, and strength of the core of a sphere of influence like strong relations with neighboring vital interests. While U.S. leaders focus on environmental and immigration issues, they forget the more important economic ones. China has made deep inroads into Mexico and Canada. The United States could launch new efforts to forge exclusive links with the two countries as resource suppliers and manufacturing partners. The United States might also consider paying particular attention to Mexico, which is China's third-largest trading partner in Latin America. A chaotic Mexico, undermined by corruption and a violent narcotics trade, and neglected by the United States, becomes an opportunity for China to make inroads with a vital interest.

- *Rededicate the United States to the Monroe Doctrine.* The Monroe Doctrine states that the United States should remain first among countries with relationships in the Americas. Nations from other hemispheres, in particular China, should not be allowed to wedge themselves between the United States and Latin American countries. Bit by bit, China has ramped up trade and investment to the United States' south, with billions of dollars of investment in countries ranging from Argentina to Brazil. The United States could launch a new effort to head off this development.

China has become the biggest foreign player in the Americas. The United States developed a bad reputation in South America by pressing for free-trade measures that gave U.S. exporters the upper hand, and by supporting Latin American dictators who were aligned with Washington for decades. But the United States could rewrite trade rules to balance trade with the South, cutting exclusive deals and focusing on a few industries where there is a genuine win-win for both the United States and Latin America. Latin America can become an alternative supplier for many low-labor-cost products that are now produced in China. Latin American countries have the skills, labor pool, and low-cost manufacturing base to do it.

As an example of countries in Latin America that have shifted toward China, take Brazil. The country has enjoyed brisk demand for commodities like soybeans and iron ore. It has attracted eye-popping investments from China, such as the $10 billion loan to Petrobras to develop its oil fields. It has built its annual trade with China to $30 billion. But the United States has some clear advantages in negotiations with Brazil. It shares Brazil's differences of opinion with China on issues ranging from human rights to nuclear nonproliferation to climate change to Brazil's bid for a role on the UN Security Council. It also shares the problem of losing manufacturing to China. Nearly all imports from China are manufactured goods, whereas four-fifths of Brazil's exports are commodities.

Brazil is in danger of becoming part of China's mercantilist system. Like most countries, it remains valuable to China mainly as a source of feedstocks for China's voracious manufacturing sector and as a consumer market to absorb Chinese-made products. A new port project, Superporto do Acu, has even been nicknamed the "highway to China."[7] Ten deepwater berths will be able to handle the largest vessels in the world. Ships carrying 400,000 tons of cargo will transfer a flood of grain, minerals, and oil to China.[8] Coming back will be finished steel and electronics that will undermine Brazil's indigenous manufacturing sector. This is a step back in time for Brazil. It began the transition to high-value-added manufacturing, but Chinese trade is gradually forcing it to revert to an agriculture- and raw material–based economy.

Leaders across Latin America face similar trade conditions. Their concern over too many win-lose deals with China offers the United States an opportunity. For example, the United States and each Latin American country might consider targeting a handful of industries to build trade cycles, where the United States buys a good from an supplier, adds value to it, and sells it back to the supplier nation, and then that nation adds more value and sells its product worldwide with American corporate assistance. Moreover, if Latin American countries cut their imports from China, the United States would regain the sphere of influence envisioned by the Monroe Doctrine.

Isolating and Containing China's Economic Sphere

The next important part of a U.S. grand strategy is to isolate America's most important rival. This is the step in which the world order evolves from an unstable and unequal economic battle between two superpowers into a more stable and more equal economic cold war, the capitalist cold war. The United States can choose to wage that economic war as it is doing today: with two overlapping blocs, in which some parts of each bloc straddle both sides. But as we have seen throughout this book, that overlapping and chaotic world yields a poor bargain for the United States In the long term, it is untenable.

Isolating China. If cooperation is not possible because China continues to disrupt America's capitalist system, the most logical world order would be a world that is divided clearly into two distinct blocs. Although this might sound radical, in fact it merely represents a formal recognition of the way in which economic affairs are heading today, given the United States' current economic policies. One possible configuration of a bipolar world order is based on two independent, exclusive blocs. Economic activity between the blocs would be minimal or carefully negotiated.

In this vision of the future world economic order, the greatest challenge would be to find ways to ensure that both blocs remain relatively equal in economic size. An imbalance could lead to complications, such as the more powerful economic bloc building and using military force to capture access to various markets or supplies. As Woodrow Wilson once said, "Only a peace between equals can last."[9]

A second option might be to have nonexclusive blocs. Many of the United States' allies and trading partners today straddle the United States and China tradewise, as illustrated by Figure 4-2. However, these dual loyalties promise to paralyze these nations if and when they have to choose between the two trading blocs. Blurring of economic loyalties in a nation's forward positions, buffer zones, or pivotal zones may be acceptable. But straddling will not be acceptable in the core and vital interests of a future American sphere, if it is to be a strong economic sphere. To prevent commingling of incompatible democratic and Communist ideals, as well as the constant struggle over the rules of capitalism, the United States might more logically prefer the first strategy: two entirely separate blocs.

A Free World Alliance or League of Democracies is the most likely result of restructuring the world order and replacing the out-of-date blocs created in the post–World War II era. This might include a core comprising the United States, the EU, and India. The three large democratic societies share a language, a legal outlook, a business culture, and a belief in individual freedom and human rights. They are logical allies.

A global reorganization into two blocs would meet a lot of resistance—and not just from China. Many Indians have mixed feelings about tighter relations with the United States because of India's desire for nonalignment and America's long-term support for Pakistan. At least some of the more than $1 billion in annual U.S. aid to Pakistan is thought to be diverted to supporting Pakistani troops who aid terrorists. But India remains an archrival of China, and this could facilitate gradual tightening of the U.S.-EU-India bloc. The United States could not build a Free World Alliance all at once, of course. The strategy would call for building the bloc in increments, in the same way that China has created the makings of a bloc of countries through gradual shifts in trade and military policy to serve as its suppliers and consumers.

Containing China. Another key part of the grand strategy is to contain the rival, gradually reducing its power over its neighbors. As the United States takes measures aimed at building an smaller, more exclusive sphere of influence, it could also attempt to contain China's sphere by firming alliances with Japan, South Korea, Taiwan, Vietnam, Thailand, Malaysia, Burma (Myanmar), and Indonesia. The goal would be to contain China's influence within its borders or the borders of its nearest neighbors. So far, the United States has been slow to check China's ambitions across Asia, owing to both the U.S. commitment to furthering free trade and the decade-long distraction of fighting terrorism.

There are four options for containing China that the United States and its allies might consider:

- *Cozy up to China's neighbors.* As the world migrates into blocs, the United States cannot sit and watch as China pulls all its Asian neighbors, by sheer economic power, into a regional sphere of influence. The United States could, for example, cut bilateral deals that favored mutually beneficial trade with countries that are now being co-opted by China, such as Japan, South Korea, Vietnam, Indonesia, and others. The United States would gradually cut off trade between China and its neighbors, preventing China from building a sphere with a regional core. The United States began by opening economic doors in Vietnam with a bilateral trade agreement in 2000. In 2007, the U.S. Congress approved Vietnam as a most-favored trading nation.

- *Isolate China with exclusionary trade deals.* Instead of WTO-style free-trade deals, the United States could arrange deals that were designed specifically to exclude China and countries using similar unfair trade practices. Initial baby steps were taken with the Trans-Pacific Partnership (TPP), the trade treaty initiated in 2005 by Chile, New Zealand, and Singapore that has so far excluded China. The TPP, which now includes 10 nations, has pursued such tight provisions on trade protection and subsidies for state-owned enterprises that it essentially locks China out.

- *Cut China's relationships with critical economies.* China's neighbors often serve as U.S. vital interests, forward positions, or buffer zones. U.S. leaders could split China from key partners to contain China's influence. Countries of prime geoeconomic importance include Russia, Japan, and India. The United States is capable of helping Russia, India and Japan with the many disputes that these countries have with China.

The Chinese feel that they have a right to build a sphere in their region. They were stripped of it during the early nineteenth century by the British Empire, and China has not regained its earlier glory. China, unchecked, would naturally want to create a modern version of its ancient tributary system, in which neighboring countries like Japan, Korea, Vietnam, and Indonesia were akin to vassals of China. The vassals paid their dominant neighbor the equivalent of protection money. This was justified by the emperors based on the

Confucian practice whereby younger sons looked after their parents. Many people in the region worry that the same kind of deference to a dominant China will be expected if financial difficulties force the United States to withdraw from its Pacific commitments.

As the United States sorts out the countries that belong in its sphere, it may be tempted to let Taiwan drift further into China's embrace. That might serve U.S. interests, as Taiwan's occasional threats to formally vote for political independence from China create outcries and threats of military action from China. If these threats were left for resolution solely between China and Taiwan, the turmoil could create a crisis that would scare foreign direct investment away from China, weakening China without U.S. involvement. However, Taiwan remains key to containing China and acts as a U.S. forward position that projects America's capitalist system and democratic values into the very heart of China.

Tipping the Balance of Economic Power Toward the United States

As a final part of America's strategy to build a new world order, a smart strategist would consider other tools to tilt the balance of economic power in the U.S. direction. This would include U.S. geopolitical and military maneuvering to strengthen its geoeconomic position. The Obama administration seems to have realized this in 2012. On the president's November 2011 Asian tour, he said that the United States would remain a Pacific nation. He announced the United States' "Pivot to the Pacific," including stationing troops in Darwin, Australia, and support a larger Philippine navy. He also initiated diplomatic moves to open the U.S. relationship with Burma (Myanmar), a critical land route for inland Chinese goods to Indian Ocean ports.

The United States also flexed its military strength in recent joint military exercises by the U.S. and South Korean governments in the Yellow Sea and the Sea of Japan in 2010. This was a signal to China about the limits of the power it exercises through its surrogate, North Korea. In 2011, the United States began visiting the former U.S. naval base at Cam Ranh Bay in Vietnam for ship repairs. This was possibly a signal that as China tries to claim sovereignty over shipping lanes in the South China Sea, the United States stands by Vietnam.

Here we shift gears away from economic options and turn to geopolitical options that are moves of last resort in a capitalist cold war. Options for a variety of military, diplomatic, and covert means exist. They can take one of two forms: (1) undermining China's capitalist system (as discussed in Chapter 7) or (2) undermining China's sphere of influence while building up the United States and its sphere.

Taking advantage of internal unrest. As unrest continues in China, the government will have to spend more to suppress internal protests. Covertly encouraging tensions among Tibetans, Uighurs, and other minorities living among the Han majority in China would put a steady drain on funds that China would otherwise spend on continued efforts to disrupt Western capitalist systems.

To the extent that China steps up repression, U.S. leaders need only express concern in public to dampen the ardor of U.S. CEOs for investing in China. A few words of concern from the president flashing across news screens nightly would quash investment enthusiasm.

Using proxy and covert military conflicts. Though looked down on by many in the American public, covert action to create instability that challenges rivals has a long history in the United States (for example, support for the Solidarity movement in Poland, funding for Contras to fight Communists in El Salvador, weapons for mujahedeen to fight the Soviets in Afghanistan, help to Libyan insurgents to overthrow Muammar Gaddafi, Special Operations forces to kill Osama bin Laden, and unmanned drones to eliminate other terrorists). China also has a long history of covert support for North Korea, Pakistan, and Iran. It has deftly forced the United States to spend money to counter the threats and proxy fights that it supports.

The U.S. military's recent success with operations against anti-American terrorists has opened the eyes of the American public and led people to accept covert options more readily. This is a positive development, as covert operations can save the United States billions of dollars and thousands of lives. In the Soviet Union-U.S. Cold War, the United States' covert operations helped bog down the Soviet Union in endless fighting in Afghanistan. Today, Russia and China surely see U.S. involvement in Afghanistan as playing an equally useful role in bogging down the United States. The war diverts American attention and funds from efforts to deal with China's and Russia's strategies.

The financial advantages of covert operations are large compared to running big U.S. military installations overseas. While the U.S. public thinks that the United States is in the driver's seat when it stations troops in forward positions to contain China, China is economically in the driver's seat. It spends only a paltry amount of money on troops, while forcing the United States to spend a bundle. Large bases and deployments overseas do give the United States a strong sphere of influence in the short term, but in the long term they can draw the country into military overstretch.

As for U.S. strategy, the goal is to drain China's resources with covert and proxy wars, rather than being drained by China. I am not suggesting that the United States participate in a war, but rather that it simply support guerrilla actions or insurgencies to force China to station troops in or near its far-flung sphere of supplier nations and Chinese government–owned assets in foreign locations. The cost of protecting the Chinese mercantile system could be enormous, considering the large number of mines, agricultural fields, and oil assets that China has bought in Africa and Southeast Asia.

Building the U.S. sphere by winning over the pivotal zones. The United States has the potential to enhance its geoeconomic sphere if it can use geopolitical means to attract the EU and India more securely into the U.S. sphere of influence. Think of the bipolar world illustrated in Figure 4-4; India and the EU are pivotal to tipping the scales in one direction or another.

As one means of tightening bonds with Europe, the United States might consider negotiating payments for its efforts in NATO so that Europe can retain its security interests outside of Europe, rather than simply dissolving NATO as discussed earlier. Or the United States might dissolve NATO in exchange for some very large concessions from Russia that would benefit both the United States and Europe, such as troop reductions or withdrawals beyond the Urals, nuclear reduction pacts that protect Europe, new trade agreements, or better Russian treatment of foreign corporations in Russia.

If NATO is kept or a new military alliance is formed, its purpose may be renegotiated to act as a counterbalance against China. The challenge would be convincing allies that NATO can or should become a counterweight to China, and it would be an even bigger challenge to convince Europe that it needs a military counterweight to China before China's military has been significantly modernized and enlarged. Repositioning NATO in this way might draw Russia closer to the free-world bloc, especially given Russia's worries over China.

On the surface, Russia might seem like a natural ally of China, and the two countries have closed ranks somewhat.[10] Russia now pumps 300,000 barrels of oil a day from Siberia to China through a pipeline that was opened in 2011. But the two disagree on many issues, even as cross-border trade grows toward $80 billion. And Russia is working on diversifying the sale of its oil to buyers other than China.

Russia has a long history of border clashes or tension with China. Russians fume over illegal, if overstated,[11] Chinese immigration. They even worry about gradual Chinese annexation of eastern Russia through immigration. They also are concerned about key differences in military policies, such as ballistic missile defense and military operations in space.[12] The United States is capable of playing on Russian concerns over China's ambitions. If the United States dissolves NATO, as discussed earlier, this might be used as a bargaining chip to encourage Russia to move troops away from the West to the East, containing China on the north and pinning down Chinese troops on its borders.

In any case, China's actions so far have encouraged European countries to turn East for leadership. The United States must devise a strategy to give Europe a reason to look West again, perhaps by preventing the political splintering that's occurring.

Thus, a good U.S. geopolitical strategy would include methods to prevent China from dividing and conquering Europe. This includes preventing Chinese businesses and state-owned enterprises from buying up pieces of the continent. Keeping the European Union together and boosting trade with it remains critical to having a counterweight to China. This is especially true given the current debt and currency crisis. The United States already has many other ways to work with Europe, and it needs to weigh further measures to support the EU.

An equally important strategy for tipping the balance of power toward the U.S. sphere of influence is to woo India. Despite India's antipathy for Pakistan and America's traditional support for that nation, the Indian public largely has a favorable view of the United States.[13] It fears Chinese hegemony in Pakistan and the Indian Ocean, and opposes China's territorial claims in Arunachal Pradesh on its northeastern border with China. China is funding projects like the deepwater port at Gwadar, Pakistan, one of the five "string of pearls" ports funded by China between Kyaukpyu, Myanmar (Burma), and Lamu, Kenya. The United States has the opportunity to form much tighter bonds with India. President Obama visited the country in 2010, and the United States launched fresh talks called the U.S.-India Strategic Dialogue. This is a good start.

The United States must capture India's interest soon. India has agreed to an initiative to expand trade with China by more than 50 percent in just a few years, signing $16 billion of deals in just one day in 2010. The two sides aim to boost trade to $100 billion by 2015. To the United States' advantage, India's antipathy for

China remains high. Expanding India-U.S. cooperation can yield many benefits for both countries. India need not become a close ally and seems to go out of its way to show its independence from the United States, yet the United States can find ways to keep the tilt of the country's economy away from China.

Also to the United States' advantage, India runs a massive trade imbalance with China and suffers the same worries as the United States over the loss of current or potential manufacturing jobs. The United States can use strategic dialogue to encourage India to remain a foe of China and continue to deploy forces along its borders to contain Chinese influence. However, the window of opportunity for the United States and India may close quickly if America does not accelerate the tightening of relations.

In the worst-case scenario, the EU breaks up and India and Russia side with China. This would contain the U.S. sphere to only a few allies. Just in case, the United States should anticipate this possibility, recognize that American rules of capitalism will not be prevalent in the world, and prepare itself for greater self-reliance and more isolation.

Managing the Capitalist Cold War

As the struggle between the United States and China for world leadership develops, the world is facing an age-old pattern of escalation. Two competing nations keep turning up the heat, and the key questions are: Will the tit-for-tat actions press one nation or the other toward checkmate? Will the escalation boil over into war? Consider France and Germany over the last few centuries. They were constantly vying for hegemony over continental Europe. They fought multiple times—the most recent series of conflicts started with the Napoleonic Wars and moved on to the wars of 1870, 1914, and 1940. Each time, the two superpowers escalated economic tensions into military conflict.

That pattern of the past is just one more reason that U.S. leaders today would do well to listen to the warnings and advice of this book. The goal is to wage a capitalist cold war to prevent a hot war. It is also one more reason that I predict that U.S. leaders will turn from ideology to economic strategy to win. They must not fall into the trap of using geopolitics or military power alone to win the geoeconomic game. They will win like true economic strategists facing worthy competitors, using financial renewal, a retooled capitalist system, a robust hypercompetitive economic strategy against China, and a hard-nosed geoeconomic approach to reaffirm the United States as world leader.

So many countries have become dependent on China that it has become the emperor in the room that nobody wants to insult. Brazil, India, Japan, South Korea, Indonesia, and until now the United States have been willing to stand up fully to the challenge that China has posed. None can easily do so today because breaking with China would cause them economic dislocation. But U.S. leaders will muster the will to block China's economic advances in each buffer zone, from Indonesia to Vietnam; to protect its core and vital interests, from Europe to the Americas; and to prevail in building a strong economic sphere based on a superior capitalist system.

Neither country is likely to checkmate the other. But the country that makes moves chosen by the most intelligent minds, executed in the most coordinated fashion, will take positions on the global chessboard that will give it an increasing competitive advantage. As in chess, so in the capitalist competition among nations: the winners will not succeed through luck or chance or trial-and-error experimentation. Nor can they succeed by random evolution with market conditions. They will use a sequence of strategic actions to their advantage in a game of hypercompetition. They will also act boldly. And they will recognize that, as chess grandmaster Garry Kasparov said, "A brilliant strategy is, certainly, a matter of intelligence, but intelligence without audaciousness is not enough. Given the opportunity, [the player] must have the guts to explode the game, to upend [the] opponent's thinking and, in so doing, unnerve him."[14]

Conclusion

Realizing Strategic Advantage

Grand Strategy Based on Realism

A joke that is making the rounds is: "We're all working for the Chinese; we just don't know it yet." There is more truth to this than people would like to admit. The good news is that if national leaders take this warning, and if they seriously turn to strategic capitalism to respond to the warning, they can create a solution that puts·their countries on a path to renewed growth and wealth.

Do You Want a Level Playing Field?

In his classic book *The Art of War*, military strategist Sun Tzu wrote that leaders need to cultivate their forces to fit the "situation" and the "configuration of power." The desired situation, Sun Tzu wrote, is like a mountaintop position. With downhill advantage, a leader's forces have the energy and momentum to succeed with certainty. "The strategic power . . . is comparable to rolling round boulders down a thousand-fathom mountain," Sun Tzu observed.[1]

Today, the United States is fighting an uphill battle against a well-organized rival. American CEOs are urging the government to establish a level playing field so that their corporations can compete with China. But China has not given up its advantages, nor should it give them up. And this book, as Sun Tzu did, argues that the United States should position itself at the top of the hill, taking advantage of the downhill momentum. Playing to win means establishing a tilted playing field, not a level one.

American CEOs would like to win entirely through the heroic efforts of their companies and their employees. However, they are learning that for global companies today, success comes not only from smart corporate strategy and execution. It also comes from the strategic advantage—the tilted playing field—provided by their national capitalist system. Corporate executives alone cannot be responsible for creating jobs and national prosperity. They have to build on their nation's advantage. The responsibility for crafting and executing a grand economic strategy to make a country's system the best in the world falls on the shoulders of the country's national leaders.

Do You Want Market Evolution to Control Your Destiny?

Believers in the alchemy of free markets have long argued that the natural evolution of those markets will make a nation more competitive. The market allocates capital most efficiently. But a quick look at the United States' industry portfolio in Figure 6-1 shows just how market evolution works. As a result of stockholder and finance capitalism, open trade, free markets, and commoditization, the United States has evolved to a place where most of its industries are earning low profits, falling into the dog and question mark quadrants identified by the portfolio matrix. Today, the largest industry that serves the role of cash cow is banking. Yet banking does not create value so much as it skims value off the top of other value-creating industries.

The question is: does the market evolution that has led to an industry portfolio shaped by finance capitalism best serve the long-term position of the United States? My answer, argued in this book, is that it does not. Compare the U.S. industry portfolio to that of Germany in Figure 6-2, for example. With a steady strategy using managed capitalism, Germany has developed several evergreen heavy industries that produce profits by creating value in their own right. The contrast with the United States couldn't be clearer. The U.S. portfolio has evolved, but it has evolved in the direction of extinction.

The nineteenth-century English economist David Ricardo argued that global trade, if left to run its natural evolutionary course, would maximize the world's production. He created the theory of "comparative advantage." Countries, Ricardo argued, would prosper by specializing in what they did best, even if other countries could do it better. Trade would allow others to buy best-in-the-world products that they could afford. Trade would also allow nations to create jobs when they sold what they made, given that they were making the optimal use of their resources, no matter how inferior they might be to the rest of the world. But the economic reasoning behind this approach didn't take into account that, while comparative advantage spurs total global growth through trade and more efficient use of assets, it does not bring about mutual and equal prosperity. Instead, competitive advantage—being the best in the world—is what wins.

The lack of mutual benefit is a critical part of the problem facing the United States and other Western nations. Open trade can enforce not first-rate but permanent second-rate economic status for a country with an inadequate capitalist system. The redistribution of wealth is something that Ricardo said nothing about. And no wonder. He was basically producing theory that justified the economic imperialism of the British Empire in its glory years, the 1800s. Global trade has always benefited countries with the globally best "competitive" advantage.

No national leader today should count on the theory of comparative advantage to provide prosperity. Free and global markets— "the invisible hand"—will not guide nations and their corporations to their most competitive position. Intelligent minds can guide an economy better than invisible hands. The evidence that this is true abounds—and not just in China. Managed capitalism has been effective even in America, as I've discussed in the previous chapters. Strategies conceived by intelligent minds that also harness the workings of the free market fare the best.

Do You Want to Be Ruled by Fear?

U.S. leaders are afraid to act because of eight myths that make it appear that America is caught in an inescapable trap. These myths and their supporters give China an air of invincibility and establish a fatalistic attitude in boardrooms, the halls of Congress, and White House meeting rooms. By dispelling these myths, U.S. leaders will mobilize the resources of the nation to action.

Eight Myths That Prevent U.S. Action on China

1. *China will inevitably be the biggest market.* Not true. Demographics are not destiny. In most of human history, populous nations have not ridden their national headcount to dominance.
2. *China will retaliate if U.S. leaders and corporations speak out.* Not true. Although executives may fear losing China's business, U.S. leaders should feel free to pound the podium for action. China will not retaliate because its economy depends on us (for now at least).
3. *China is a friendly power that the United States can cooperate with.* Not true. China has undertaken multiple economic measures to weaken the U.S. economy, and it continues to do so. China speaks softly but carries a big stick.
4. *China will become democratic if the United States engages the country.* Not true. The United States will instead lose its own freedom as companies acquiesce to China's undemo-

cratic ways (e.g., Microsoft) or exit (e.g., Google). We cannot expect China to embrace democracy or completely free markets because that would destabilize the country and its Communist Party leadership.

5. *The United States needs China too much to fight.* Not true. China needs the United States even more, owing to its manufacturers' dependence on the U.S. consumer market and the Chinese government's fear that the U.S. might devalue the dollar, undermining China's holdings of U.S. currency and debt.

6. *Investment in China will benefit the United States.* Not true. U.S. companies have trouble repatriating profits from China. Once China absorbs U.S. technology, it will replace foreign corporations with domestic ones, vaporizing the value of the United States' foreign investment.

7. *The United States should avoid a trade war with China.* Not true. We are already waging a trade war, and China is winning through subsidization, nontariff barriers, substandard labor practices, intellectual property theft, and other measures.

8. *The United States should seek a win-win solution with China.* Not true. While a mutual gain is a nice idea in business, it has hurt the United States in national competition. The win-win fantasy blocks aggressive action and ironically buys China time to gain even more power.

Americans must not fall into the trap of believing these myths. Not only are they falsehoods, but they are propaganda designed to make the United States fearful of undertaking hypercompetitive action and using its competitive advantages. The best strategy, as Sun Tzu would say, is a strategy where you win without firing a shot. So don't let the myths make China seem invincible. They are only trying to win using propaganda before the battle is fought to its conclusion. If the United States lets them, these myths will lead to a self-fulfilling, self-defeating prophecy: paralysis and decline.

Do You Want to Control Your Destiny?

Germany has stayed at the top of the economic heap in Europe amid the recent global slump because of its mixture of capitalisms. It created a mix of laissez-faire, managed, and social-market capitalism, all in moderation. It has built up superior engineering skills, systems, fiscal prudence, and technical training systems. Canada has clambered to one of the most stable positions in the Americas, in spite of its connection to the United States during the Great Recession. Canada's mixture of social-market, laissez-faire, and managed capitalism dictated fiscal prudence and a stable, well-capitalized banking system. China has leapt to the summit of the strategic mountain globally because of its state-managed capitalism.

China has won its place not because of the evolution of free markets and amazing businesses—which by themselves are not role models. China has won because the state manages a system that supports companies both at home and abroad in ways that disrupt America's capitalist system and keep the United States off balance. Sun Tzu couldn't have been more correct.

State-owned enterprises often are poorly run, use capital inefficiently, struggle to innovate, and suffer from corruption. Workers are exploited, toiling in conditions that create massive social unrest seething just under the surface. But China is smart: it is sacrificing in the short term, building the advantage of a managed economy, and undermining the United States' will to fight. China, despite its supposedly "inferior" enterprises and inefficient resource allocation methods, is steadily winning because of its pursuit of a long-term strategy that is stripping business from other countries.

If other nations are to keep up, their leaders need to consider remaking their capitalist systems. Over the course of the last eight chapters, I have suggested how leaders can undertake this transformation. It requires abandoning unquestioning faith in the economic ideologies of the past, whether laissez-faire capitalism, social-market capitalism, managed capitalism, or any other economic theory or formulation. It necessitates a fresh understanding of how competition works among nations today. And it demands a grand strategy based on mindful management of the levers of economic power, tailored to win in today's chaotic economic and geopolitical terrain.

Then Think Strategic Capitalism, Not Ideology

This book outlines a campaign for conducting the necessary transformation. It is based on strategy from the realms of business, geopolitics, and the military. It takes a methodical approach, starting with an analysis of the four Cs. This yields an understanding of how nations today are competing with their forms of capitalism, combining different types of capitalism to gain advantage, controlling capitalist rules, and capturing economic supremacy by spreading their capitalist systems around the globe. The result is a bracing image of the nature of competition today—in particular, the competition between China and the United States and its allies.

The analysis shows that we are not living in an either/or world. Countries do not practice either laissez-faire capitalism or managed capitalism or social-market capitalism. They practice a combination of these with different emphases. Laissez-faire capitalism works best to spur people to create value. Social-market capitalism works best to redistribute value, build a consumer class, and establish stability in downtimes. Managed capitalism works best to spur the invention of technology and build industries. Philanthropic capitalism provides seed money for progress for both a nation's society and its economy.

Each form of capitalism has its uses. When national leaders embrace this notion, giving up the idea that only one model works best, they free themselves to imagine and create new models of capitalism that can work better. Often the best thinking comes during the resolution of contradictions among models, using some of one *and* some of the others. China is rising because it has mixed two seemingly incompatible generic strategies: laissez-faire and managed capitalism.

This book builds on the four Cs with the four Rs, showing leaders ways of *rebalancing* their capitalist system, *reinventing* their forms of capitalism, *reenergizing* their capitalisms through hypercompetition, and *restructuring* the world order around those capitalisms. The four Rs are the four pillars of strategic capitalism. They guide leaders in crafting a strategy to outperform other economies. (For the recommended moves for crafting a strategy in the United States, see the box.)

The Four Rs of Strategic Capitalism: How the United States Can Use Them to Win

Rebalancing
- Recalibrate our ambitions for social and military spending.
- Adjust our resources to restore financial soundness.
- Select, neutralize, or avoid threats to prevent overstretch.

Reinventing
- Temper laissez-faire capitalism.
- Reduce social-market capitalism.
- Increase philanthropic capitalism.
- Formalize managed capitalism.

Reenergizing
- Go on the offense.
- Erode rivals' strengths by playing on their weaknesses.
- Thwart rivals' future advantages.
- Disrupt rivals' strategies and strengths.
- Undermine rivals' centers of gravity.

Restructuring
- Plan a new U.S. sphere of influence.

> - Govern the sphere with new institutions.
> - Strengthen the United States' core and vital interests.
> - Isolate and contain China's sphere.
> - Tip the balance of economic power toward the United States.

The task facing U.S. leaders is a big one. It cannot be accomplished all at once. It is a long-term plan, a strategy to pull the United States out of its short-term focus and provide America with substantial gains for years to come. No nation can win against a country like China unless it takes the long view. The Chinese draft five-year plans, one after another. The approach may be bureaucratic, but it also ensures that people think about a future that is decades away. This alone gives them a marked advantage.

And Think Hypercompetitively

The core principle guiding this book is hypercompetition. No nation can establish a sustainable competitive position—a spot so strong that leaders can turn their attention to other things. Instead, nations must vie continuously for ways to shape the rules of capitalism and undermine rivals with incompatible capitalist systems. The way for countries to get ahead is the same as that for businesses: be the first to upend the economic apple cart, in this case the prevailing capitalist system. National leaders cannot sustain an advantage by practicing defense. They must go on the offense, disrupt the rival version of capitalism, and force other countries to play catch-up.

Witness how Korea seized the lead in the dynamic random-access memory (DRAM) semiconductor business from Japan in the mid-1990s (after Japan seized it from the United States in the 1980s). Korea incorporated into its capitalist system a series of state-guided efforts to enter the chip industry. Witness how Japan, particularly Toyota, now relentlessly upgrades its manufacturing expertise. Japan, a heavy practitioner of managed capitalism, also encourages the innovative forces of laissez-faire capitalism, to help Toyota achieve success. And witness how Germany has won by reworking its mix of laissez-faire, managed, and social-market capitalism, in particular by reining in an overindulgence in social-market benefits. Witness how China has wrested the solar-panel business from Germany and the United States, as China's leaders specifically targeted national investment to support the building of emerging energy technologies and undermine the advantage of technological leaders, creating a larger domestic market with regulations and using subsidies to throw the advantage toward Chinese firms.

All these countries have been thinking through moves and countermoves among the capitalist systems, not just leaving strategy to their corporations. They have seized the initiative so that they land most of the punches, reducing their rivals to absorbing competitive blows. They have done all this through a methodical strategy to create a superior capitalist system and build superior economic power.

Successful national leaders benchmark and target the best practices in the capitalist systems of their rivals, change the way they think and work, and lead the world to ever-increasing levels of competition based on what they have learned about how capitalist systems compete. As in every other aspect of life today, national leaders must steadily improve their game if they want to stay in the game. They must grasp the imperative of hypercompetition between national capitalist systems, they must overcome fear and exercise imagination, and they must help their nations grow while others languish.

Strategic Capitalism for the United States

In Part 2, I detailed a long list of strategic actions to improve the position of the U.S. capitalist system. Let me highlight 10 of the more counterintuitive or surprising options that U.S. leaders might evaluate and undertake to strengthen the American capitalist system. (I know that many of these will be controversial, but that is precisely my point. It is only by exploring new alternatives and questioning sacred cows that we can hope to regain the initiative that has been lost.)

1. *Embrace economic pragmatism.* Throw out economic ideology and adopt what works. Stop fighting over whether managed, laissez-faire, or social-market capitalism is right. All are potential solutions. Strategists who win make decisions based on facts about how to beat the competition and the effectiveness of the current mixture of generic capitalist strategies.

2. *Rein in overstretch.* Start by balancing ambitions, resources, and threats. Reduce entitlements for healthcare, social services, and retirement in the United States. Narrow the nation's commitments of money and people around the world, principally the military. The United States cannot act as a global security force to fight everyone everywhere all the time. It has to give priority to containing China.

3. *Reduce congressional power over commerce.* Stop Congress from making industrial policy decisions for the nation. Create a nonpartisan autonomous authority (set up in the same way as the Federal Reserve) to craft and execute strategy. This authority, the Federal Industrial Policy Board, could take rational steps to prevent industrial decline. Give the new board power to craft a grand strategy, award funding for R&D, and underwrite emerging and strategic industries. The goals are to create a pipeline of emerging industries that will power long-term economic growth and to manage America's industry portfolio proactively.

4. *Reinvent American capitalism.* End the piecemeal approach to managing the economy and industrial policy making. Recognize that our capitalist system today has become

uncompetitive because of China's strategic capitalism. China is surging because of its forthright economic nationalism and managed capitalism. Western nations, especially the United States, must fashion a blend of capitalisms that increases managed capitalism, modifies laissez-faire capitalism, and reduces social-market capitalism.

5. *Integrate and focus national power.* Integrate all federal policies to advance the United States' grand strategy for economic preeminence. Make every department of government accountable for economic prosperity—from the Department of Commerce to Agriculture to Energy, and from the Department of State to Education to Labor. By using diplomatic and military power more selectively, the United States can strengthen its economy.

6. *Set national economic goals.* Stop assuming that the United States will excel if we simply champion the free market and let the chips fall where they may. We cannot assume that the natural evolution of free markets will yield success. The evolution to date has moved manufacturing overseas. Give Congress and the president quantitative goals, measure their progress, provide salary incentives, and institute term limits for subpar performance. Start by passing a balanced-budget amendment to discipline Congress fiscally.

7. *Create more corporate patriotism.* Stop making shareholder value the prime measure of corporate success. Pass and enforce new tax incentives to invest in America, create jobs in America, and move overseas operations back home. Give corporations the freedom to be patriotic. Reduce the power of shareholders by changing the governance rules, and the power of Wall Street financiers by limiting their pressure on CEOs to focus on short-term quarterly earnings.

8. *Stop going soft at the bargaining table.* Without fanfare or announcement, establish a national strategic intent to recapture the leading position on the global chessboard by rebuilding the American economic sphere of influence.

Acquiescing to China's hardball tactics dooms America to second-class negotiating status. Incrementally erect trade barriers to protect U.S. jobs, and force China to negotiate on opening its domestic markets. Escalate competition slowly by disrupting China's capitalist system.

9. *Throw off the handcuffs.* Re-create the world order by dissolving post–World War II institutions that are spurring a U.S. decline, including the United Nations, the World Trade Organization, the North Atlantic Treaty Organization, and the International Monetary Fund. Replace them with entities that give the United States and other democratic nations an economic advantage.

10. *Restore self-sufficiency.* Insulate the nation from further economic interdependence. Integration through trade with undemocratic nations destabilizes the global economy by risking recession-driven chain reactions of financial and economic panic. Decouple the United States from China and OPEC in multiple ways, and shift trade to less adversarial partners.

Putting It All Together

As this list makes clear, national leaders have to embrace economic realpolitik and dynamic strategic action if they are to succeed. The job is much bigger than many policy makers believe, as it encompasses economics, politics, diplomacy, defense, and other policies. But by thinking big, the United States and other nations can retain and advance the competitive positions of their countries.

Recall the old story about the blind men and the elephant. The first feels the leg and declares the elephant to be a tree. The second feels the ears and declares it to be a manta ray. The third feels the trunk and declares it to be a snake. None of them is able to put it all together. The same goes for many national leaders today. They declare that their nation's problem is one of fiscal management, or failing capitalism, or failing industrial policy, or failing trade and diplomatic policy. None of them sees the big picture. And yet a country today succeeds or fails based on its entire grand strategy for economic prosperity.

In the introduction, I mentioned the damned-if-you-do, damned-if-you-don't complaint by CEOs. Many CEOs have admitted to me that, as American citizens, they don't think it is a good idea to invest in China because it will contribute to the decline of America. But the same people say that, as CEOs with responsibilities to shareholders, they have no choice but to invest in the fastest-growing market in the world. Although they may feel that they have little choice, they are wrong. Worse, this belief in China's inevitable rise has infected too many influential leaders in society. Even consumers think and act the same way: they buy cheap Chinese products, but they close their eyes to their neighbors' job losses and the long-term decline in U.S. wages, job growth, and affluence.

The time has come for us to open our eyes. America's leaders must recognize the inevitability, not of China's hegemony, but of an escalating capitalist cold war. They must see that competition has risen a level. It is no longer only about how one company beats another. Competition is now based on how one country supports and guides its companies relative to another. It involves a host of new actions in which one capitalist system attempts to disrupt and displace another.

National leaders must view their challenge as being more than improving the competitiveness of the existing capitalist system. It is about reinventing the capitalist system to create new competitive advantages. Without this big view, and without corporate, political, and civic leaders who grasp the power of that view, countries will not prevail against rivals who are trying to undermine their capitalist system and change the rules of capitalism.

Leaders who recognize the challenge as one of economic hyper-competition among capitalist systems will replace narrow special and corporate interests with national interests. They will plan a sequence of moves and countermoves to gain and sustain an edge. They will lift their countries to the high ground of geoeconomic and geopolitical superiority. And with their strategic abilities to analyze competition among capitalisms through the four Cs and their abilities to formulate winning capitalist strategies using the four Rs, they will have gained Sun Tzu's mountain of advantage— and they will use the strategy of the ancient Chinese strategist against China. They will, as Sun Tzu said, recognize that "what is of supreme importance . . . is to attack the enemies' strategy."[2]

This is what China has done to Western capitalism. And now, it is our turn.

Endnotes

Introduction

1. Brazil, India, Russia, Japan, South Korea, Australia, and South Africa.
2. Shannon Bond, "US Trade Deficit Reaches Six-Month High," *Financial Times,* February 10, 2012, http://www.ft.com/intl/cms /s/o/5cfbb37c-53fo-11e1-9eac-00144feabdco.html#axzz1mBksGujU.
3. Incomes for many Americans have stagnated for decades. For example, in 2010 dollars, median male income in the United States in 1970 was $33,423. In 2010, it was $32,137. See, for example, data from the 2010 census at http://www.census.gov/hhes/www/income /data/historical/people/2010/P05AR_2010.xls. Household income has increased over the last 40 years, but even here the increase has been paltry, especially in the last 10 years, in which it declined. See "Cutting the Cake," *Economist,* September 14, 2011, http://www .economist.com/blogs/dailychart/2011/09/us-household-income.
4. http://pewresearch.org/pubs/1855/china-poll-americans-want-closer-ties-but-tougher-trade-policy.

Chapter 1

1. A group of companies with interlocking business relationships and shareholdings.

2. Before World War II, each major bank was part of a *zaibatsu* group of companies. As part of a *zaibatsu,* each firm owned parts of other firms in the group, and each acted with the others to compete against other *zaibatsu.* After the war, the occupation government formally broke up the *zaibatsu*, but the big banks still act as central bankers for several companies, often bearing the bank's name.

3. From 1982 to 2000, the Dow Jones Industrial Average measure of stock prices shot from a meager 777 on August 12, 1982, to 11,723 by January 14, 2000. That was more than 1,500 percent.

4. Eamonn Fingleton, "The Myth of Japan's Failure," *New York Times,* January 6, 2012.

5. *Amakudari* is a practice in which top Japanese government officials retire into lucrative posts in industries that they once oversaw. This retiree network gives government a say in company decisions and gives companies a say in government decisions. This facilitates informal communication about, and coordination of, government policy.

6. Sinopec, China's oil giant, announced in December 2010 that it would buy Occidental Petroleum's Argentine assets for $2.45 billion. This followed the October 2010 announcement that Sinopec would buy 40 percent of Repsol's Brazilian assets for $7.1 billion. Between 2000 and 2009, China's imports from Latin America and the Caribbean ballooned from about $5 billion to $44 billion, and 80 percent of this involved commodities. Bolivia, for example, has massive lithium deposits, which China needs to make batteries and other products. Latin America has also become a major export market for China. From 2002 to 2009, the United States' share of exports to Latin American fell almost 50 percent. China's grew about 10 percent. Chinese exports are replacing products made in Brazil, Mexico, and other Central American states. China is also bidding on infrastructure projects, such as roads, bridges, railways, ports, and information technology and telecommunications. The Bank of China is offering attractive financing to help Chinese firms, and the Chinese government is negotiating free-trade agreements with Latin America.

7. One example is the soft loan made in 2004 by the China Export-Import Bank. The loan provided $2 billion to Angola to help build infrastructure. In return, the Angolan government gave China a stake in oil exploration off the coast. China is writing off African national debts to gain influence. And, to attain access to African

resources and markets, China is using its influence with former rebels that were put into power with the help of Chinese support during civil wars and uprisings in earlier decades.

8. "Africa Fears Neo-Colonialism with China's Foray," *Terra Daily*, September 30, 2009, http://www.terradaily.com/reports/Africa _fears_neo-colonialism_with_Chinas_foray_analysts_999.html.

9. "10 Industries Where the U.S. No Longer Leads," *Atlantic Monthly*, February 7, 2011, http://www.theatlantic.com /business/archive/2011/02/10-industries-where-the-us-no-longer -leads/70888/#slide3.

10. Developing Asia, Coggan notes, has gone from 7 percent of world GDP in 1970 to about 28 percent today. This could become as much as 50 percent by 2050. "This is a huge shift and is what 'economics' will be about for the next 30–40 years," says Coggan.

11. Kenneth Lieberthal and Wang Jisi, *Addressing U.S.-China Strategic Mistrust* (Washington, DC: Brookings Institution, John L. Thornton China Center, 2012), http://www.brookings.edu/papers/2012 /0330_us_china_lieberthal.aspx.

Chapter 2

1. I would like to thank Kevin Williams for his research on the capitalist system of Taiwan; Miseon Lee for South Korea; Rodolfo Araujo for Brazil and Indonesia; Sony Mistri, Sasha Vyash, and Subhrajyoti Ghatak for India; and Jerry Shen, Jincheng (JC) Li, and Srivatsan Sivanandan for China.

2. I would like to thank Jens Moebius for his research on the French capitalist system.

3. http://money.cnn.com/magazines/fortune/global500/2010/countries /France.html.

4. I would like to thank Anant Shivraj for his research on the U.K. capitalist system.

5. I would like to thank Dennis Huggins for his research on the Singaporean capitalist system.

6. http://www.doingbusiness.org/rankings.

7. I would like to thank Momoka Osako for her research on the Japanese capitalist system.

8. *World Tariff Profiles 2011: Applied MFN Tariffs*, (Geneva, Switzerland: World Trade Organization, International Trade Commission, and United Nations Conference on Trade and

Development, 2011), http://www.wto.org/english/res_e/booksp_e/tariff_profiles11_e.pdf.

9. I would like to thank Jens Moebius and Lauren Hirsch for their research on the German capitalist system.

10. https://www.cia.gov/library/publications/the-world-factbook/geos/gm.html.

11. *Ideas, Innovation, Prosperity: High-Tech Strategy 2020 for Germany,* (Bonn, Germany: Federal Ministry of Education and Research, 2010), http://www.bmbf.de/pub/hts_2020_en.pdf.

12. http://www.hightech-strategie.de/en/879.php.

13. http://www.hightech-strategie.de/en/432.php.

14. Michael Thöne and Stephan Dobroschke, *WTO Subsidy Notifications: Assessing German Subsidies Under the GSI Notification Template Proposed for the WTO* (Cologne, Germany: FiFo Institute of Public Economics, April 2008), http://www.globalsubsidies.org/files/assets/wto_subsidies_germany.pdf.

15. "2011 Global R&D Funding Forecast," *R&D Magazine*, December 2010, p. 6.

16. "The Third Way Tax Receipt, 2010," http://www.thirdway.org/taxreceipt. Note: The numbers add up to more than 100 percent because gross interest expense excludes interest received on government investments.

17. The 10 elements are business freedom, corruption freedom, financial-sector freedom, government bloat freedom, inflation freedom, investment freedom, labor freedom, property rights freedom, tax freedom, and trade freedom.

18. http://www.heritage.org/Index/PDF/2011/Index2011_Methodology.pdf.

19. Measured using the most common measure of prosperity, GDP per capita. Data from the World Bank, http://data.worldbank.org/indicator/NY.GDP.PCAP.KD.

20. I would like to thank Raj Koganti for collecting the data from public sources, Zongyu (Chuck) Jiang for creating the SAS data sets, and Pen-che Ho for doing the statistical analysis.

Chapter 3

1. Wu Huanshu, "China's First Entrepreneur," China.org.cn, October 8, 2008, http://china.org.cn/china/reform-opening-up/2008-10/10/content_16645148.htm.

2. Chris Hogg, "China's Reluctant First Entrepreneur," *BBC News,* February 20, 2011, http://news.bbc.co.uk/2/hi/8487888.stm.
3. "Capitalist Number One," *Times* (London), February 20, 2011.
4. "Zhang Huamei—China's First Self-Employed Businessman," *CRIENGLISH,* February 20, 2011, http://english.cri.cn/4026 /2008/12/12/146184432173.htm.
5. *China Business News,* May 1, 2011, http://cnbusinessnews.com /chinas-march-fdi-up-32-9-yr-on-yr/.
6. Jason Dean, Andrew Browne, and Shai Oster, "China's 'State Capitalism' Sparks a Global Backlash," *Wall Street Journal,* November 16, 2010, http://online.wsj.com/article/SB100014240527 48703514904575602731006315198.html.
7. Ibid, p. 53.
8. Andrew Szamosszegi and Cole Kyle, *An Analysis of State-Owned Enterprises and State Capitalism in China* (Washington, DC: U.S.-China Economic and Security Review Commission, report prepared by Capital Trade, Incorporated, October 26, 2011), p. 8, Table III-2.
9. Studies of corporate culture by Geert Hofstede since the 1970s confirm that Chinese leaders enjoy this cultural advantage. Hofstede found that China differs sharply from the United States in two telling ways. On a scale that measures individualism, the United States scores a high 91, while China scores a low 20. On a scale that measures long-term orientation, the United States scores a low 29, whereas China scores a high 118, http://geert-hofstede.com /china.html.
10. Szamosszegi and Kyle, *An Analysis of State-Owned Enterprises,* p. 45.
11. Ibid., p. 10.
12. Ibid., pp. 33–34.
13. Ibid., p. 26.
14. Ibid., p. 65.
15. "The Struggle of the Champions," *The Economist,* January 8, 2005, pp. 58–59.
16. Szamosszegi and Kyle, *An Analysis of State-Owned Enterprises,* p. 75.
17. As quoted in Szamosszegi and Kyle, *An Analysis of State-Owned Enterprises,* p. 93.
18. Ibid., p. 3.
19. Ibid., p. 52.
20. Ibid., p. 47.

21. For financial data, see Form 20-F, p. 3, and note 14, p. F-23, http://www.sec.gov/Archives/edgar/data/1191255/000119312511118263/d2of.htm.

22. http://www.ustr.gov/about-us/press-office/press-releases/2011/october/united-states-seeks-detailed-information-china's-i.

23. "2011 Report to Congress on China's WTO Compliance" (Washington, DC: U.S. Trade Representative, December 2011), p. 6, http://www.ustr.gov/webfm_send/3189.

24. Anonymous, personal communication with author, October 2011.

25. Sheo Nandan Pandey, "Labour Unrest in China and Foreboding," Paper no. 4063, September 27, 2010, http://www.southasiaanalysis.org/%5Cpapers41%5Cpaper4063.html.

26. https://chinastrikes.crowdmap.com/main.

27. Jeffrey Wasserstrom, "Strike Out: What the Foreign Media Misses in Covering China's Labor Unrest," *Foreign Policy*, June 18, 2010, http://www.foreignpolicy.com/articles/2010/06/18/strike_out?page=0,0.

28. James Melik, "China Leads World in Green Energy Investment," *BBC News*, September 15, 2011, http://www.bbc.co.uk/news/business-14201939.

29. "Clean Energy Investment Hits Record $260 Billion," Reuters, January 12, 2012, http://www.reuters.com/article/2012/01/12/us-clean-tech-investment-idUSTRE80B1NX20120112.

30. Esther Tanquintic-Misa, "China Leads Global Investments in Renewable Energy," *International Business Times*, December 5, 2011, http://au.ibtimes.com/articles/261083/20111205/china-leads-global-investments-renewable-energy.htm.

31. "An Overview of China's Renewable Energy Market," *China Briefing*, June 16, 2011, http://www.china-briefing.com/news/2011/06/16/an-overview-of-chinas-renewable-energy-market.html.

32. "China," U.S. Department of State, March 22, 2011, http://www.state.gov/r/pa/ei/bgn/18902.htm.

33. "Did Spark Spark a Copycat?" *BusinessWeek*, April 12, 2011, http://www.businessweek.com/magazine/content/05_06/b3919010_mz001.htm.

34. "GM Daewoo Files Suit Against Chery," *China Daily*, U.S. edition, April 12, 2011, http://www.chinadaily.com.cn/english/doc/2005-05/09/content_440334.htm.

35. Guy Dinmore and Geoff Dyer, "Immelt Hits Out at China and Obama," *Financial Times,* July 1, 2010, http://www
.ft.com/intl/cms/s/0/ed654fac-8518-11df-adfa-00144feabdco
.html#axzz1kfZaWDmN.
36. As quoted in James McGregor, "China's Drive for 'Indigenous Innovation': A Web of Industrial Policies," (Global Intellectual Property Center, U.S. Chamber of Commerce, and APCO Worldwide, 2010), p. 4, http://www.uschamber.com/sites/default
/files/reports/100728chinareport_0.pdf.
37. The story has been widely reported. A summary appears in Szamosszegi and Kyle, *An Analysis of State-Owned Enterprises,* pp. 70–71.
38. McGregor, "China's Drive for 'Indigenous Innovation'," p. 5.
39. "China Piracy Cost U.S. Firms $48 Billion in 2009: Report," Reuters, May 22, 2011, http://www.reuters.com/article/2011/05/18
/us-usa-china-piracy-idUSTRE74H6CO20110518.
40. McGregor, "China's Drive for 'Indigenous Innovation,'"
p. 14.
41. Ibid.
42. Robert E. Scott, *Growing U.S. Trade Deficit with China Cost 2.8 Million Jobs Between 2001 and 2010* (Washington, DC: Economic Policy Institute, September 20, 2011), http://www.epi
.org/publication/growing-trade-deficit-china-cost-2-8-million/.
43. "The Most Popular American Companies in China," *24/7 Wall Street,* January 3, 2012, http://247wallst.com/2012/01/03/the-most
-popular-american-companies-in-china/2/.
44. Ibid.
45. http://news.pg.com/blog/bob-mcdonald/pg-makes-new-stride
-innovation-china-ministry-commerce-highly-commends-pg's
-contri.
46. Even Google is looking for a way back into the Chinese market.
47. David Barboza, "Danone Exits China Venture After Years of Legal Dispute," *New York Times,* September 30, 2009, http://www
.nytimes.com/2009/10/01/business/global/01danone.html.

Chapter 4

1. The figures in parentheses represent the percentage of imports plus the percentage of exports as a percentage of the nation's GDP.

2. I would like to thank Raj Koganti for calculating the data in parentheses.

3. In the figures, countries were ranked by looking at the ratio of the country's trade with America (imports plus exports as a percentage of GDP) to the country's trade with China (imports plus exports as a percentage of GDP). A one-to-one ratio indicates equal trade with both superpowers (these nations fall into the black oval in the center of the figure). Countries with ratios greater than 1 fall to the right of the center (the American economic sphere of influence), while those with ratios less than one fall to the left of the center (the Chinese economic sphere).

4. For a summary of China's negotiated settlement in 2001, see http://www.wto.org/english/news_e/pres01_e/pr243_e.htm.

5. http://www.wto.com/what-is-the-wto/.

6. "China and the G20: Taking the Summit by Strategy," *Economist*, April 8, 2009, http://www.economist.com/node/13447015.

7. http://www.iie.com/publications/interstitial.cfm?ResearchID=1982.

8. http://www.swfinstitute.org/research/reformcurrencychina.php.

9. Zhou Xiaochuan, "Reform the International Monetary System," *Bank for International Settlements Review*, 2009, www.bis.org /review/r090402c.pdf.

10. http://professional.wsj.com/article/SB1000142405274870462840457 6264292303686626.html?mg=reno-secaucus-wsj.

11. Ignatius Banda, "To Yuan or Not to Yuan, That Is the Question," allAfrica.com, January 26, 2012, http://allafrica.com/stories /201201261488.html.

12. http://news.xinhuanet.com/english2010/china/2011-09/06/c _131102186.htm.

13. http://professional.wsj.com/article/BT-CO-20110821-706955 .html?mg=reno-secaucus-wsj.

14. "China's Social Welfare Spending," HSBC Global Research, March 6, 2011, http://www.institutionalinvestorchina.com/arfy /uploads/soft/110324/1_0755164271.pdf.

15. "Break India, Says China Think-Tank," *Times of India*, August 12, 2009, http://articles.timesofindia.indiatimes.com/2009-08-12 /india/28195335_1_dai-bingguo-state-councillor-chinese-website.

16. These two figures are modified from graphics prepared by Raj Koganti under the supervision of Richard D'Aveni.

17. John Bussey, "U.S. Attacks China Inc." *Wall Street Journal*, February 3, 2012, http://online.wsj.com/article/SB10001424052970 2046622045771988339249406.html.

18. Andy Grove. "Andy Grove: How America Can Create Jobs," *BusinessWeek*, July 1, 2010, http://www.businessweek.com /magazine/content/10_28/b4186048358596.htm.

Chapter 5

1. Quoted in Charles W. Kegley Jr. and Gregory Raymond, *Multipolar Peace: Great Power Politics in the Twenty-First Century* (New York: St. Martin's Press, 1993).
2. Paul Kennedy, *The Rise and Fall of the Great Powers* (New York: Vintage, 1989), p. 515.
3. Kegley and Raymond, *Multipolar Peace*.
4. As of March 2012. This accounts for the debt held by the public, excluding "intragovernmental debt" held by government agencies in their own accounts, such as in the social security account. Debt held by the public was $10.8 trillion.
5. Carmen M. Reinhart and Kenneth Rogoff, "Debt and Growth Revisited," *VOX*, August 11, 2010, http://www.voxeu.org/index .php?q=node/5395.
6. "The Federal Government's Long-Term Fiscal Outlook: January 2011 Update" (Washington, DC: General Accounting Office, January 2011), p. 1, http://www.gao.gov/new.items/d11451sp.pdf.
7. There is much controversy over what the prudent debt-to-GDP level should be. See, for example, Anis Chowdhury, "Is There an Optimal Debt-to-GDP Ratio?" *VOX* (November 9, 2010), http://www.voxeu.org/index.php?q=node/5764.
8. Carlo Cottarelli, *From Stimulus to Consolidation: Revenue and Expenditure Policies in Advanced and Emerging Economies* (Washington, DC: International Monetary Fund, April 30, 2010), p. 6, fn. 3, http://www.imf.org/external/np/pp/eng/2010/043010a .pdf. Note that there is much controversy among economists about the right ratio. For example, see Chowdhury, "Is There an Optimal Debt-to-GDP Ratio?"
9. A figure suggested by the International Monetary Fund. See Cottarelli, *From Stimulus to Consolidation*.
10. See http://www.tradingeconomics.com/united-states/gdp-growth. This rate is enough to create healthy job growth and steady increases in the standard of living without driving inflation, asset bubbles, or other consequences of excessive exuberance in stock and real estate markets.
11. There is much debate about the natural unemployment rate, but 5 percent is a reasonable target. For a recent discussion, see Justin

Weidner and John C. Williams, "What Is the New Normal Unemployment Rate?" (San Francisco: Federal Reserve Bank of San Francisco, February 14, 2011), http://www.frbsf.org/publications /economics/letter/2011/el2011-05.html.

12. This benchmark is based on the average "charitable commitment" of the 200 largest charities in the United States. See William P. Barrett, "America's Largest 200 Charities," *Forbes.com*, November 17, 2010, http://www.forbes.com/2010/11/16/forbes -charity-200-personal-finance-philanthropy-200-largest-charities -charity-10-intro_2.html.

13. Richard Rahn, "The Optimal Size of Government," *Washington Times*, January 29, 2009, http://www.washingtontimes.com /news/2009/jan/29/the-optimum-government/?page=all.

14. Jim Angle, "Analysis: 'Fair Share' in Taxes? Not by the Numbers," *Foxnews.com*, February 20, 2012, http://www.foxnews.com /politics/2012/02/20/analysis-fair-share-in-taxes-not-by-numbers/.

15. For example, Israel spends 4.43 percent and Sweden 3.78 percent. See http://www.nsf.gov/statistics/seind04/c4/tt04-17.htm.

16. "Life in the Slow Lane," *Economist*, April 28, 2011, http://www .economist.com/node/18620944.

17. This ambitious goal, which would double manufacturing employment in the United States, is suggested by Jeffrey R. Immelt, CEO of GE and a member of the President's Council on Jobs and Competitiveness.

18. Bureau of Economic Analysis, http://research.stlouisfed.org/fred2 /data/PSAVERT.txt.

19. http://epp.eurostat.ec.europa.eu/cache/ITY_OFFPUB/KS-SF-09-029 /EN/KS-SF-09-029-EN.PDF.

20. Dennis Tao Yang, Junsen Zhang, and Shaojie Zhou. "Why Are Saving Rates So High in China?," National Bureau of Economic Research Working Paper 16771, February 2011, http://www.nber .org/papers/w16771.pdf.

21. Jaewoo Lee, Pau Rabanal, and Damiano Sandri, "IMF Staff Position Note: U.S. Consumption after 2008," January 15, 2010, http://www.imf.org/external/pubs/ft/spn/2010/spn1001.pdf.

22. Jahangir Aziz and Li Cui, "IMF Working Paper: Explaining China's Low Consumption: The Neglected Role of Household Income," July 2007, http://www.scribd.com/doc/500177/Chinese -Consumption-Household-Income-IMF-Working-Paper.

23. "The Third Way Tax Receipt, 2010," http://www.thirdway.org /taxreceipt.

24. For the schedule of current rates, which vary by age cohort, see http://mycpf.cpf.gov.sg/Employers/Gen-Info/cpf-Contri/ContriRa .htm.

25. "The Moment of Truth" (Washington, DC: National Commission on Fiscal Responsibility and Reform, December 2010), p. 48.

26. "Third Way's Bipartisan Savings Package for the Joint Select Committee on Deficit Reduction" (Washington, DC: Third Way, September 15, 2011), p. 6, http://content.thirdway.org /publications/442/Third_Way_Letter_-_Deficit_Reduction _Recommendations_to_Super_Committee_.pdf.

27. Ibid., p. 2.

28. Ibid., p. 8.

29. "The Moment of Truth," p. 25.

30. "Third Way's Bipartisan Savings Package," pp. 4–5.

31. "The Moment of Truth," pp. 20–25.

32. Ibid., p. 38.

33. "Doing Business 2011: Making a Difference for Entrepreneurs" (Washington, DC: International Finance Corporation and World Bank, 2010), p. 4.

34. Ibid., p. 202.

Chapter 6

1. I would like to thank MiSeon Lee for her research on the Korean economy.

2. http://www.indexmundi.com/facts/korea/gdp-per-capita.

3. "The Third Way Tax Receipt, 2010," http://www.thirdway.org /taxreceipt.

4. Bill Powell, "Should China and the U.S. Swap Stimulus Packages?" *Time*, March 5, 2009, http://www.time.com/time/business /article/0,8599,1883277,00.html.

5. Numbers vary depending on income and retirement age. The figure cited is for a two-earner couple with one spouse earning an average wage ($43,500 in 2011) and one earning a low wage ($19,500 in 2011). For results using other assumptions, see C. Eugene Steuerle and Stephanie Rennane, "Social Security and Medicare Taxes and Benefits over a Lifetime" (Washington, DC: Urban Institute, June 2011), p. 5, http://www.urban.org/UploadedPDF/social-security -medicare-benefits-over-lifetime.pdf.

6. As it is under the shareholder capitalism we have today, current savers are getting approximately zero percent on their money,

and cheap prices have translated into cheap junk on many store shelves. In addition, numerous stock market bubbles have reduced the pensions of millions of investors. So I don't see what is really improved by being so single-minded about shareholder capitalism.

7. Maxwell Strachan, "Financial Sector Back to Accounting for Nearly One-Third of U.S. Profits," *Huffington Post*, March 30, 2011, http://www.huffingtonpost.com/2011/03/30/financial-profits -percentage_n_841716.html.

8. Kathleen Madigan, "Like the Phoenix, U.S. Finance Profits Soar," *Wall Street Journal*, March 25, 2011, http://blogs.wsj.com /economics/2011/03/25/like-the-phoenix-u-s-finance-profits-soar/.

9. Paul A. Pautler, "The Effects of Mergers and Post-Merger Integration: A Review of Business Consulting Literature" (Washington, DC: Bureau of Economics, Federal Trade Commission, January 21, 2003), p. 6, Table 1, http://www.ftc.gov /be/rt/businesreviewpaper.pdf.

10. Gary P. Pisano and Willy C. Shih, "Restoring American Competitiveness," *Harvard Business Review*, July–August 2009, p. 116.

11. "U.S. Scientific Research and Development 101: Understanding Why These Investments Are Key to Our Future Economic Competitiveness," *Science Progress*, February 16, 2011, p. 2.

12. http://www.uspto.gov/web/offices/ac/ido/oeip/taf/reports.htm.

13. As recommended by the American Energy Innovation Council in 2010. See Martin Grueber and Tim Studt, "2011 Global R&D Funding Forecast." *R&D Magazine*, December 2010, p. 21, http://www.battelle.org/aboutus/rd/2011.pdf.

14. *Federal Support for Research and Development* (Washington, DC: Congressional Budget Office, June 2007), p. 15.

15. Martin Grueber and Tim Studt, "2012 Global R&D Funding Forecast: R&D Spending Growth Continues While Globalization Accelerates," *R&D Magazine,* December 16, 2011, http://www .rdmag.com/Featured-Articles/2011/12/2012-Global-RD-Funding -Forecast-RD-Spending-Growth-Continues-While-Globalization -Accelerates/.

16. Adrian Slywotzky, "Where Have You Gone, Bell Labs?" *BusinessWeek*, August 27, 2009, http://www.businessweek.com /magazine/content/09_36/b4145036681619.htm.

17. Statistical analysis of Department of Education data.

18. National Association for Gifted Children, "State of the Nation in Gifted Education: A Lack of Commitment to Talent Development,"

Washington, DC, November 2011. For an executive summary, see
http://www.nagc.org/uploadedFiles/Information_and
_Resources/2010-11_state_of_states/State%20of%20the%20
Nation%20%20(final).pdf.

19. I wish to thank Jens Moebius for his insightful work in preparing
the U.S. industry portfolio analysis.

20. When used for business strategy purposes, the Boston Consulting
Group (BCG) matrix graphs a company's product divisions using
the growth of the total industry against the market share of the
division. The goal is to display the attractiveness of each product
division in terms of its position or strength within the market
(market share) and the growth of its product industry. Our
analogy replaces market share with profitability, because studies
have shown that market share is often the primary determinant of
profitability.

21. In the case of the United States, the cutoffs between the quadrants
are 7 percent for growth (which ranged from –9 to 23 percent),
and 11 percent for profitability (EBIT), which ranged from 3 to
25 percent. The cutoffs are based on the weighted-average growth
rate and the weighted-average profitability, respectively.

22. I would like to thank Jens Moebius for his research on the German
industry portfolio.

23. Fred Block, "US Industrial Policies, R&D, and the WTO's
Definition of Non-actionable Subsidies," *Intellectual Property
Watch*, December 23, 2010, http://www.ip-watch.org
/weblog/2010/12/23/us-industrial-policies-rd-and-the-wto's
-definition-of-non-actionable-subsidies/.

24. James Manyika et al., *How to Compete and Grow: A Sector Guide
to Policy* (New York: McKinsey Global Institute, 2010), pp. 12–16,
http://www.mckinsey.com/Insights/MGI/Research/Productivity
_Competitiveness_and_Growth/How_to_compete_and_grow.

25. I would like to thank Jens Moebius for his research on the Internet
and capitalisms that fit different stages of an industry life cycle.

Chapter 7

1. https://www.uschina.org/statistics/tradetable.html.

2. The United States cannot "start" a trade war by going on the
offensive. A trade war is already in progress. It has been in
existence for the last decade. There are hundreds of lines of tariffs
in the U.S. tariff schedule. The weighted-average tariff on imported
goods is 1.8 percent. In the European Union, it is 1.2 percent. In

China, it is 4.2 percent. Many individual Chinese tariffs, such as that on cars, run as high as 22 percent. China persists in using subsidies, service market restrictions, import bans, import licensing, complex regulations and standards, intellectual property theft, and corruption-prone customs administration. The question, then, is not whether to fight a trade war, but how intensively, and on what terms, to fight it.

3. B.H. Liddell Hart, *Strategy,* 2nd ed. (New York: Penguin [Meridian], 1991), p. 6.

4. Eric K. Clemons and Jason A. Santamaria, "Maneuver Warfare: Can Modern Military Strategy Lead You to Victory?" *Harvard Business Review*, April 2002.

5. David B. Yoffie and Michael A. Cusumano, "Judo Strategy: The Competitive Dynamics of Internet Time," *Harvard Business Review*, January–February 1999.

6. http://www.upi.com/Business_News/Energy-Resources/2012/01/18 /Ethiopia-Thousands-driven-out-in-land-grab/UPI -60071326912191/.

7. Benjamin Lin, "China May Cut Spending on Strategic Industries," Reuters, July 7, 2011, http://www.reuters.com/article/2011/07/07 /us-china-industries-idUSTRE7660XO20110707.

8. Richard D'Aveni, *Hypercompetition: Managing the Dynamics of Strategic Maneuvering* (New York: Free Press, 1994), p. 87.

9. As quoted in James McGregor, "China's Drive for 'Indigenous Innovation': A Web of Industrial Policies" (Global Intellectual Property Center, U.S. Chamber of Commerce, and APCO Worldwide, 2010), p. 4, http://www.uschamber.com/sites/default /files/reports/100728chinareport_0.pdf.

10. Ibid, p. 5.

11. http://www.nsf.gov/statistics/infbrief/nsf12303/.

12. http://siteresources.worldbank.org/INTINTERNATIONAL /Resources/1572846-1253029981787/6437326-1253030199852 /Piacentini_Gaule.pdf and http://www.nsf.gov/statistics/seind10/c2 /c2h.htm.

13. Michael G. Finn, "Stay Rates of Foreign Doctorate Recipients from U.S. Universities, 2005," Oak Ridge Institute for Science and Education, 2007, p. 1, http://orise.orau.gov/files/sep/stay-rates -foreign-doctorate-recipients-2005.pdf.

14. Joseph Casey and Katherine Koleski, *Backgrounder: China's 12th Five-Year Plan* (Washington, DC: U.S.-China Economic and

Security Review Commission, June 24, 2011), p. 9, http://www
.uscc.gov/researchpapers/2011/12th-FiveYearPlan_062811.pdf.

15. Carl von Clausewitz, *On War* (Princeton, NJ: Princeton University
Press, 1989).

16. George Stalk, Jr., and Rob Lachenauer, "Hardball: Five Killer
Strategies for Trouncing the Competition," *Harvard Business
Review*, April 2004.

17. http://www.futureofuschinatrade.com/article/issues-in-depth-china
-is-rising.

18. "EU Prepares to Challenge China Export-Credit Sources," Reuters
Africa, January 13, 2011, http://af.reuters.com/article
/energyOilNews/idAFLDE70C2G220110113?pageNumber=2&
virtualBrandChannel=0&sp=true.

19. Einar Tangen, "Dispatches from China: China's Infrastructure
Investments Will Be Huge," *BizTimes.com*, April 29, 2011,
http://www.biztimes.com/news/2011/4/29/dispatches-from-china
-chinas-infrastructure-investments-will-be-huge.

20. Brina Milkowsky, "Transportation Infrastructure Report 2011:
Building America's Future, Falling Apart and Falling Behind"
(Washington, DC: Building America's Future Educational Fund,
2011), pp. 11, 25, http://www.bafuture.com/sites/default/files
/Report_0.pdf.

21. Ibid., p. 31.

22. Ibid., p. 33.

23. Klaus Schwab, "The Global Competitiveness Report" (Geneva,
Switzerland: World Economic Forum, 2011), p. 362, http://reports
.weforum.org/global-competitiveness-2011-2012/.

24. Ibid., pp. 413–416.

25. Danielle Kurtzleben, "Are Infrastructure Projects the Answer to
America's Jobs Problem?," *U.S. News & World Report*, August 22,
2011, http://www.usnews.com/news/articles/2011/08/22/are
-infrastructure-projects-the-answer-to-americas-jobs-problem.

26. http://foreignaffairs.house.gov/112/bro030911.pdf.

27. Peter Brookes, "Legions of Amateurs: How China Spies," Heritage
Foundation, May 31, 2005, http://www.heritage.org/research
/commentary/2005/05/legion-of-amateurs-how-china-spies.

28. http://www.chinadaily.com.cn/business/2010-03/30/content
_9661921.htm.

29. "Foreign Direct Investment in China in 2010 Rises to Record
$105.7 Billion," *Bloomberg News*, January 17, 2011, http://www

.bloomberg.com/news/2011-01-18/foreign-direct-investment-in
-china-in-2010-rises-to-record-105-7-billion.html.

30. Kevin Brady, "Hearing on the U.S.-China Economic Relationship,"
Trade Subcommittee of the U.S. House Ways and Means
Committee, October 25, 2011, http://waysandmeans.house.gov
/UploadedFiles/Brady_China_Hrg_Statement.pdf.

Chapter 8

1. Ken Sofer, "China and the Collapse of Its Noninterventionist
Foreign Policy: Past Diplomatic Practices Collide with Rising
Economic and Political Realities," Center for American Progress,
March 8, 2012, http://www.scribd.com/doc/84498902/China-and
-the-Collapse-of-Its-Noninterventionist-Foreign-Policy.

2. I would like to thank Colin Carrihill and Georgios Savvidis for
their ideas concerning the geoindustry and geoproduct chessboards
shown in Figures 8-1 to 8-4. The grids in the figures are modified
versions of the grids submitted to me, and the strategic intents listed
in the boxes have been changed to reflect my research. But the basic
idea was theirs.

3. "Cosco Signs Deal with Greek Port," *China Daily*, November 27,
2008, http://www.chinadaily.com.cn/china/2008-11/27
/content_7244698.htm.

4. Andrés Cala, "Spain Welcomes Chinese Investment Even with
Strings Attached," *Christian Science Monitor*, January 6, 2011,
http://www.csmonitor.com/World/Europe/2011/0106/Spain
-welcomes-Chinese-investment-even-with-strings-attached.

5. Fu Jing, "Ambassador Calls for More Hungary-China Trade,"
China Daily, June 25, 2011, http://www.chinadaily.com.cn
/cndy/2011-06/25/content_12773880.htm.

6. Thom Shanker, "Defense Secretary Warns NATO of 'Dim' Future,"
New York Times, June 10, 2011, http://www.nytimes
.com/2011/06/11/world/europe/11gates.html.

7. Vivian Ni, "China's Demand for Resources Brings Brazil Closer,"
China Briefing, June 3, 2011, http://www.china-briefing.com
/news/2011/06/03/chinas-demand-for-resources-brings-brazil-closer
.html.

8. Tom Phillips, "Brazil's Huge New Port Highlights China's Drive
into South America," *Guardian* (Manchester, U.K.), September 15,
2010, http://www.guardian.co.uk/world/2010/sep/15/brazil-port
-china-drive.

9. Address to the Senate on January 22, 1917. For the full text of Wilson's speech, see http://www.mtholyoke.edu/acad/intrel/ww15 .htm.

10. New agreements between Russia and China in October 2011 are reported to promise $100 billion in bilateral trade by 2015, http://news.xinhuanet.com/english2010/china/2011-10/12/c _131187753.htm.

11. Harley Balzer and Maria Repnikova, "Migration Between China and Russia," *Post-Soviet Affairs* 26 (2010).

12. Richard Weitz, "China-Russia Security Relations: Strategic Parallelism Without Partnership or Passion?" (Carlisle, PA: Strategic Studies Institute, August 2008).

13. "America's Image Remains Strong: India Sees Threat from Pakistan, Extremist Groups," Pew Research Center, October 20, 2010, http://www.pewglobal.org/2010/10/20/indians-see-threat-from -pakistan-extremist-groups/.

14. http://www.forbes.com/forbes/2012/0312/thoughts-opinions -proverbs-chess.html.

Conclusion

1. Quotations from *The Art of War* come from many different translations. For this translation, see http://sun-tzu-aow.blogspot .com/2009/05/chapter-5-strategic-military-power.html.

2. Sun Tzu, *The Art of War* (Ware, Hertfordshire, UK: Wordsworth Editions, 1998), p. 26.

Acknowledgments

I would like to thank the many individuals who contributed to the development of this project. My heartfelt thanks go to Bill Birchard, whose logic, research, editorial, and writing skills helped me pull all of my ideas together into the book you see today. In addition, I thank Stuart Crainer and Des Dearlove for their editorial help in condensing earlier drafts and making the book readable. They clarified my arguments beautifully. I also greatly appreciate Bill, Stuart, and Des's willingness to share ideas. They made invaluable contributions, not just to the book's writing, but to its content. Thanks also to Des and Stuart for helping with the original framing of the book. While the book has evolved from the original concept, the original theme remains, and the hardest step is always the first.

My thanks go out to Knox Huston at McGraw-Hill for publishing the book, for his patience and faith in me when I missed deadlines, and for his valuable comments that improved the book immensely. And thanks also go to John Landry, who, as a subject-matter expert, critiqued the book's contents, saving me from many errors and sharpening my point of view considerably. I also appreciate the help of Kim Keating, Kent Holland, and Jill Totenberg. They contributed greatly to the positioning of the book and to my understanding of the book's audience and message.

Several CEOs made important contributions to the book. I cannot tell them how much I appreciate their time and effort. All were very thoughtful and diligent about their commentaries, writing them personally and responding to my many questions about how to fix America. So I greatly thank Bill Achtmeyer, founder and managing director, The Parthenon Group; Fernando Aguirre, chairman and CEO, Chiquita Brands International; Steve Angel, chairman, president, and CEO, Praxair, Inc.; George S. Barrett, chairman and CEO, Cardinal Health, Inc.; David M. Cote, chairman and CEO, Honeywell Corporation; Michael T. Dan, recently retired chairman, president and CEO, The Brink's Company; Daniel R. DiMicco, chairman and CEO, Nucor Corporation; Salvatore D. Fazzolari, former chairman, president, and CEO, Harsco Corporation; J. Erik Fyrwald, president, Ecolab, and former president and CEO, Nalco Company; Jim Goodnight, CEO, SAS Institute, Inc.; John H. Hammergren, chairman, president, and CEO, McKesson Corporation; Christopher J. Kearney, chairman, president, and CEO, SPX Corporation; Gregory T. Lucier, chairman and CEO, Life Technologies, Inc.; Michael G. Morris, chairman and former CEO, American Electric Power; Peter M. Nicholas, cofounder and chairman of the board, Boston Scientific Corporation; Bill Nuti, chairman and CEO, NCR Corporation; Dinesh C. Paliwal, chairman, president, and CEO, Harman International Industries, Inc.; Patrick M. Prevost, president and CEO, Cabot Corporation; and John M. Stropki, chairman, president, and CEO, Lincoln Electric Holdings, Inc.

My research assistants have made significant contributions to the book. As for the empirical analysis, I wish to thank Pen-che Ho for his computer programming and statistical analysis, Zongyu (Chuck) Jiang for his help with database creation, and Raj Koganti for his data collection efforts and preparation of some figures. I also wish to acknowledge the contributions of numerous research assistants footnoted throughout the book. I am grateful for the diligent and thoughtful help of Rodolfo Araujo, Subhrajyoti Ghatak, Lauren S. Hirsch, Dennis L. Huggins, Raj Koganti, MiSeon Lee, Jincheng (JC) Li, Xiaojun (Patrick) Li, Jens M. Moebius, Soni J. Mistry, Momoka Osako, Yizhou (Jerry) Shen, Anant Shivraj, Srivatsan Sivanandan, Sasha Vyash, Kevin G. Williams, and three Chinese nationals who wish to remain anonymous. I also wish to thank two students who suggested ideas within the context of my courses at the Tuck School of Business: Colin Carrihill and Georgios Savvidis. I want to give special thanks to Jens M. Moebius, who completed complex tasks even when he had serious family matters to attend to.

My research assistants and students provided me with facts, figures, and frameworks; however, the words in this book are my responsibility only. I used my own judgments and have come to my own conclusions based on their analyses. No one and no government should hold my research assistants or my students responsible for the conclusions or recommendations in this book. I carry sole responsibility for these conclusions and recommendations.

On my research visits to China, I met with a large number of people. Many of them were former students of mine from many different MBA and executive programs around the world. Approximately half were Chinese nationals, and half were foreigners doing business in China. I wish to thank all of them for their insights and the examples they gave me about China. They were insightful, instructive, and positive. I could not have done this book without their thoughts, factory tours, government contacts, and meetings within their companies or universities. Since they live and work in China, I will leave their names out of the book. But I thank them nevertheless.

The Tuck School of Business has provided a great deal of support for this project. First, I would like to thank Dean Paul Danos and Senior Associate Dean Robert G. Hansen for the research funding they provided for this book. Without their support for academic freedom and their long-term investment in this book, it would never have been done. I would also like to thank Zdenek Bakala for funding my chair and for his encouragement of and excitement about my work on the topic of capitalism. He grew up under Communist rule, was a former student at Tuck, and is now one of the world's most important capitalists in Europe. He is listed on the Forbes Global 1000. I honor his achievement and his generosity to the Tuck School.

Tuck's support structure has played a very important role in getting this book done. First, Kimberly A. Hayward, my academic coordinator at Tuck, has been great. She worked on scheduling meetings with my research assistants, no easy task given how many there were. Kim also helped with my travel arrangements, visas, and scheduling while I was in China, again no easy task given how many appointments she had to juggle. Her support and hard work was pure dedication. Many thanks go to her.

Second, the Dartmouth Library System has been a great resource during this project. Feldberg librarians have provided so much support that I cannot even describe it. I would like to thank the head librarian, James (Jim) Fries, as well as reference librarians Anne Esler, Richard Felver, and Karen Sluzenski for all their help. I would also like to give a special thanks to Sarah Buckingham, who recently passed away from cancer. We shall miss her.

There are two more groups I would like to thank. The first are the people whose ideas inspired or shaped this book. The works of Zbigniew K. Brzezinski have helped frame my thinking, including *The Grand Chessboard: American Primacy and Its Geostrategic Imperatives* and *Strategic Vision: America and the Crisis of Global Power*. So have the works of Clyde V. Prestowitz, including *The Betrayal of American Prosperity* and *Three Billion New Capitalists: The Great Shift of Wealth and Power to the East*. Martin Jacques's book, *When China Rules the World*, stimulated my ideas as well. Henry Kissinger's book *On China* was also a key inspiration for the book. Ian Bremmer's books *Every Nation for Itself: Winners and Losers in a G-Zero World*, *The End of the Free Market: Who Wins the War Between States and Corporations?*, and *The J Curve: A New Way to Understand Why Nations Rise and Fall*, were also critical to my analysis.

And, of course, my long-term love affair with the strategic works of Sun Tzu, Carl von Clausewitz, Gary Hamel, Tom Peters, Michael Porter, Adrian Slywotsky, and George Stalk played a big part in formulating my view of what a "good strategy" is.

The last, but certainly not least, group that I would like to thank is my family. I draw inspiration and the reason to write from the love and support of my parents, Anthony R. and Marion E. D'Aveni, as well as my children, Ross and Gina D'Aveni; my stepdaughter, Tanya Tudan; and her husband, Chris Jones. I love them all.

Index

About the Author

Richard A. D'Aveni is among the top 50 business thinkers in the world for the past 6 years running, according to CNN, *Forbes*, the *Times* (London), and the *Times of India*. Best known for his work on hypercompetition, D'Aveni is the Bakala Professor of Strategy at the Tuck School of Business at Dartmouth College and a winner of the prestigious A. T. Kearney Award for his research. He has been a World Economic Forum Fellow.

He holds a PhD from Columbia University, a JD from Suffolk University, an MBA from Boston University, and an AB in government from Cornell University. He is also a CPA (expired) and a member of the bar (inactive) in Massachusetts.

Professor D'Aveni is one of the top three experts on competitive strategy in the world. His field looks for the principles of power and success in competition between individuals, teams, corporations, militaries, or nations.

D'Aveni is the author of several highly influential articles in the *Harvard Business Review*, *MIT Sloan Management Review*, the *Wall Street Journal*, and the *Financial Times*, as well as the bestselling book *Hypercompetition*, which is available in 12 languages. His follow-up book, *Strategic Supremacy*, is available in four languages. His last book, *Beating the Commodity Trap*, was published in 2010 and is available in five languages.

D'Aveni's writings are credited with creating a new paradigm in the field of strategy based on temporary advantages—using rapid maneuvering rather than defensive barriers. He is also credited with building new paradigms of business strategy using the principles of military science and international relations.

For more information about Richard D'Aveni and his books, go to his website: www.radstrat.com